Natural Medicine 101

How to Win the Medical Information War, and Take Control of Your Health

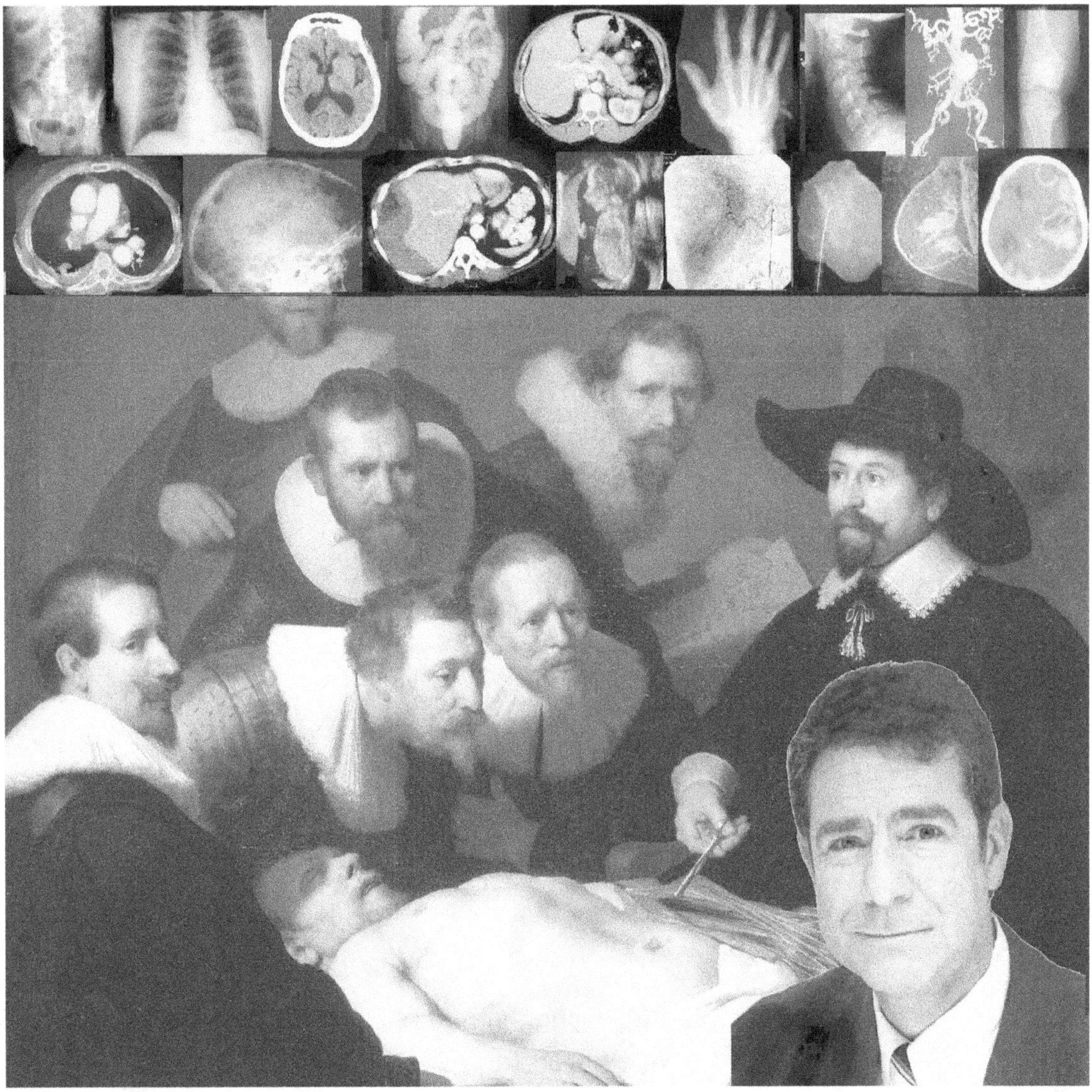

By Jeffrey Dach MD

ISBN: 1-4392-1122-1
ISBN-13: 9781439211229

Visit www.booksurge.com to order additional copies.

Table of Contents

Introduction by William Davis MD

With *Natural Medicine 101*, Dr. Jeffrey Dach has drawn a line in the sand. On one side is the prescription drug industry, international, well-funded, and deep into the pockets of government. And on the other side is what Dr. Dach calls the forces of "Natural Medicine," smaller and without a concerted voice, but with a message that is beginning to resonate with the public, increasingly skeptical of the heavy-handed marketing tactics of the drug industry, not to mention repeated instances of overstated benefits, understated adverse effects, and over-the-top profits.

In *Natural Medicine 101*, Dr. Dach establishes himself as a champion of the Natural Medicine movement, a crusader for natural treatments that encompasses nutritional supplements, vitamins, bio-identical hormones, and other non-patentable substances. This struggle pits the proponents of Natural Medicine squarely against the drug industry, with its paradigm of patent-protectable, and highly profitable synthetic substances.

Dr. Dach predicts that the age of the pre-eminence of drugs will draw to a close. While the financial war chest amassed by the drug industry will ensure their power and position for years to come, Dr. Dach predicts that it will soon begin to erode. And it will erode due to the public's growing recognition of the power of natural substances, and methods that are, by definition, closer to real human substances and thereby promising fewer side-effects while providing greater benefits.

While TV airwaves are filled with billions of dollars of direct-to-consumer advertising for prescription drugs, the Information Age has permitted the much less-powerful Natural Medicine movement to broadcast its message. Information access has never been faster, with the playing field leveled by the World Wide Web and voices like Dr. Dach.

Dr. Dach accurately depicts it as a battle, a battle fought by the drug industry struggling to maintain its dominance, while the Natural Medicine movement gains traction with the public through education and an appeal to reason, such as that provided through Dr. Dach's *Natural Medicine 101*.

The present battle between natural, "bio-identical," hormones versus synthetic hormones (e.g., Premarin®) is serving as a testing ground for this emerging confrontation. Dr. Dach has been a vocal critic of the medical community's non-sensical preference for synthetic pharmaceutical versions of male and female hormones, when the natural substances are readily available–at much reduced cost. (Pharmaceutical giant Wyeth Pharmaceuticals' recent bid to compel the FDA to prohibit physician prescription and compounding pharmacy-dispensing of natural human hormones shows that the battle is well underway.) It's time to declare which side of the battle you stand, and Dr. Dach stands firmly on the side of Natural Medicine, carrying the flag to make sure the public continues to have access to natural alternatives.

It is Dr. Dach's philosophy of heart health that brought his work to my attention, since his approach has proven perfectly compatible with my program, Track Your Plaque. While my cardiology colleagues have been slow to embrace this unique approach to coronary plaque detection, control, and reversal that maximizes reliance on natural strategies while minimizing drugs, Dr. Dach grasped the concepts immediately and has added his own unique insights.

Natural Medicine 101 serves as a "how-to" and "why" guidebook for anyone starting out on this philosophical and health conversion, as well as an in-depth reference for anyone already underway in their quest for better Natural Health.

Dr. William Davis *is a vocal advocate for early heart disease detection and prevention. He is one of the nation's leading authorities on CT heart scans and how they can be used to powerfully impact on heart disease risk. He is author of Track Your Plaque: The only heart disease prevention program that shows how to use the new CT heart scans to detect, track, and control coronary plaque.*

The Track Your Plaque program has provided control—and reversal—of coronary heart disease to a growing number of people using nutrition, nutritional supplements, and other novel techniques. His innovative ideas are also actively promoted to the public, employers, and wellness organizations through his web-based educational site, www.trackyourplaque.com, as well as his Heart Scan Blog at http://heartscanblog.blogspot.com.

Dr. Davis speaks on how heart disease detection and prevention has entered a new age of self-empowerment. He has been quoted and interviewed nationwide, including in the Ladies' Home Journal, CBS News, and NPR. He is a frequent expert contributor to Life Extension Magazine and a member of the Life Extension Medical Advisory Board. He also writes for the HealthCentral.com and Wellness.com websites, among others.

Dr. Davis is a graduate of the St. Louis University School of Medicine and obtained his postgraduate training in internal medicine and cardiology at the Ohio State University Hospitals, with additional postgraduate training at the Case-Western Reserve University hospital system. He helped start Wisconsin's first heart scan device. He practices cardiology and lives in suburban Milwaukee with his wife, three children, and two Boston terriers.

Introduction by Russell Jaffe MD

Jeffrey Dach's approach to medical practice is a breath of fresh air. Evidence based and competent, he is equally caring and open-minded. This means he looks deeply and broadly for useful, safer, more effective therapies. Next, he applies them in his practice and educates his clients and the world at large through his informational website and blog.

His writing style in *Natural Medicine 101* is lucid and accessible, and the book has useful information about applying both natural medicine and conventional medicine for better outcomes. This includes using technology in a functional and integrative way. This means that Dr. Dach's mode of thinking has evolved beyond the reductionist bind, beyond the Descartean error, and beyond the mechanistic limitations.

Reductionism treats the human body like a machine, however elegant, that inevitably wears out and breaks down. Rather, we are more than machines. We are self-renewing, self-sustaining biological entities, aptly described by John Berry as 'a communion of souls, not a collection of objects'.

Rene Descartes, the brilliant 18th century philosopher and scientist, considered the human body analogous to a complex mechanical watch. Subsequently, a century and a half later, we have learned that biological systems are more than mechanical watches. We cannot be reduced to mechanistic elements or rebuilt from them. For example, Albert Einstein commented that 'there is awareness or consciousness in the experience of every cell'. Albert Szent Gyorgy considered the 'unsaturated electron shell' as the key to understanding the phenomenon of life. Biology is quite different and more complex than engineering mechanics.

Using the breakthroughs of Kepler, Newton, Galileo and Copernicus, early scientists applied the laws of Newtonian mechanics to the movement of planets and stars as observed through the telescope. With the invention of the microscope, and the smaller scale of Nano particles, we are in a quite different realm of quantum physics and electrodynamics. While modern physics has made this transition, biomedical research and medical practice remains firmly rooted in 19th century principles and practices of Mechanics. We have surely polished and perfected them. And yet, we have yet to see the full fruits of this transition of medicine into the 21st Century. A new renaissance in medicine, created by the Internet and the Human Genome Project, unfolds as you read this.

In acute illness, the 19th century mechanical approach has proven greatly successful. However, it has been a failure for chronic illness. The application of mechanical or chemical treatment for chronic disease has produced a diminishing return on our investment dollar, as well as intolerable levels of adverse events. In America in 2008,

40% of annual healthcare expenditure (one trillion dollars) will be spent on ineffective or unnecessary treatments leading to unacceptable morbidity and mortality.

The Dartmouth Heath Atlas concludes that America has become dependent upon high tech, high cost, high morbidity and high mortality solutions. This is largely due to a lack of transparency in decision making, as well as a lack of quality measures. For example, you could be cared for in Green Bay, Wisconsin and pay ten per cent as much compared to Newark, New Jersey, and achieve better net outcomes to boot. As John Wennburg and David Eddy have pointed out, beyond a thresshold level for national healthcare expenditure, the complication rate outstrips any benefits achieved in the healthcare system.

Jeffrey Dach is an integrative physician, investigating and researching what is best for each patient seeking his care, and bringing together an appropriate mix of therapies, insights, and follow-up designed to evoke the healing response of each individual. He walks his talk and practices what he preaches. From my personal and professional contact with Jeffrey Dach, I would say that his community is fortunate to have him. His book, *Natural Medicine 101,* will help speed the transition in medicine from sickness care to healthful caring, the transition from high tech medical care to low tech preventive care.

This book, *Natural Medicine 101,* covers broad topics from bio-identical hormones, the low thyroid condition, heart disease prevention, vitamin deficiency, to disease mongering by the drug companies; from living healthfully in a toxic world, to how to bust stress. If you want to live well and happy, and avoid the pitfalls of our medical system, read this book. There is a medical information war going on in the media, and this book will show you how to win it. This book of essays will inspire you and enlighten you. In the writing style of a renaissance artist–physician, Dr. Dach's book, *Natural Medicine 101,* is the opening prelude to the symphony of a 21st century medical renaissance.

RUSSELL M. JAFFE, MD, PH.D.

Dr. Russell M. Jaffe is Lab Director of ELISA/ACT Biotechnologies LLC, Director of PERQUE LLC, and Fellow of the Health Studies Collegium. Through his expertise in non-invasive studies of cells, he developed novel tests for blood platelet survival, fibrinogen survival, platelet aggregation, and lymphocyte response (LRA by ELISA/ACT®). Dr. Jaffe received his BS, Ph.D., and MD from the Boston University School of Medicine in 1972. He completed residency training in clinical chemistry at the National Institutes of Health (1973 - 1979) where he was on the permanent staff as a practicing molecular biologist and molecular pathologist, and is board certified in both Clinical Pathology and in Chemical Pathology. Dr. Jaffe is the recipient of the Merck, Sharp & Dohm Excellence in Research Award, the J.D. Lane Award, and the U.S.P.H.S. Meritorious Service Award. He was also named an

International Scientist of the Year (2003) by the International Biographical Commission, and was the founding chairman of the Scientific Committee of the American Holistic Medical Association.

Russell Jaffe MD PHD, Nutrition for Optimal Health Association
P.O. Box 380 Winnetka, IL 60093 http://www.nutrition4health.org/
Phone: 847-60HEALTH (847-604-3258)

Introduction by Joel Kauffman PhD

It is difficult to find an active medical practitioner such as Jeffrey Dach, MD, who advocates the use of dietary modification and nutritional supplements rather than drugs to treat common medical conditions. His highly readable new book, *Natural Medicine 101*, leads the reader on a remarkable journey through both mainstream and natural medicine. This is indeed a rare find among self-help medical books, fully documented with copious references to back up all claims. There are hot links to many of the citations that lead the reader to the abstracts of papers in medical journals. These hotlinks can be found on the his web sites www.jeffreydach.com and www.naturalmedicine101.com . Even if you don't have time to use the hyperlinks to look up the original articles yourself, your own doctor or other health professionals may use the opportunity to learn about unfamiliar treatments mentioned in the book.

One of the major themes in *Natural Medicine 101* is that bio-identical hormones are better than synthetic hormones with altered chemical structures. It is better to use the same exact substance that your body has stopped making. Doing so is more likely to benefit and entail less risk than a chemically altered prescription drug with adverse side effects. Examples of bio-identical hormones listed in the book are thyroid hormone, progesterone, estradiol, cortisol, testosterone and insulin.

Another theme in the book is a concept originating in orthomolecular medicine. This recognizes the role of vitamin cofactors which assist enzymes in biochemical reactions at the cellular level. Genetic variations cause differing levels of enzyme efficiency leading to disease states which can be treated with the intake of vitamin cofactors which increase enzyme affinity driving cellular biochemistry and restoring health.

When it comes to health benefits, the optimal dose of a vitamin may actual exceed the RDA by a large margin. For example, a minimal amount of Vitamin C may prevent the deficiency disease, scurvy. However, this minimal dose is unlikely to result in maximal health benefit. For another example is Vitamin D which prevents rickets. Observational trials now show greater health benefits with Vitamin D intake exceeding the government RDA (recommended daily allowance) designed to prevent rickets.

In his book, Dr. Dach examines the medical literature and gives examples of biased medical studies and drug trials. Techniques and gimmicks to make the outcome of drug tials favor the drug include biased design, early termination to avoid poor outcome, and a mathematical gimmick called relative risk (instead of absolute risk). The use of relative risk in the medical publication leads to inflated relative risk numbers in the advertising materials. In my book, *Malignant Medical Myths*, 2006, p8, I listed 15 different methods used to pervert a clinical trial, or its report. *Natural Medicine 101* adds a few more such as: placebo washout, in which subjects are pre-tested and those who react favorably to the placebo are eliminated from participation in the drug trial!!

Another theme, disease mongering is covered, and *Natural Medicine 101* exposes Restless Leg Syndrome in which a simple supplement is shown to solve the problem at low cost. Statin drugs to lower cholesterol are examined, revealing cholesterol to be an innocent and essential substance in the body. Very few people taking statin drugs actually benefit from them.

The book examines medical testing such as screening mammograms, shown not to prevent breast cancer or increase lifespan. Many medical conditions are misdiagnosed or ignored. For example, many of us have unrecognized under-active thyroid glands. These are easily treated with natural thyroid hormone and iodine supplements. The book goes into great detail about drug trials that showed real harm from the synthetic chemically altered hormones, and explains that natural testosterone does not cause prostate cancer. Bone healing, infertility, chronic fatigue syndrome, heart disease, depression, diabetes, blood pressure and many other conditions are shown to be treatable with supplements and/or diet. Drugs are sparingly advocated when nothing else is available.

There is a biographical quality to some of the passages in the book, documenting a personal journey into natural medicine, and Dr. Dach has included some of his life experiences as a surgeon and radiologist. He also reviews at length a number of other medical self-help books on specific topics for those who want to educate themselves or their physicians. The amount of work and the courage to put together and publish such a work can hardly be imagined by those who have not actually done it. So get set for a brave and accurate expose of medical mayhem and a myriad of useful treatments.

Joel M. Kauffman, Berwyn, PA, 16 Jul 08

Joel M. Kauffman PhD, is the author of the book, Malignant Medical Myths, 2006, which exposes fraud in medicine. Dr. Kauffman obtained a BS in Chemistry from the Philadelphia College of Pharmacy and Science, now called University of the Sciences in Philadelphia (USP), and a PhD in Organic Chemistry from the Massachusetts Institute of Technology. After 11 years of experience in the chemical industry, Dr. Kauffman joined USP in 1979, rising to Professor of Chemistry in 1990, spending 10 years in exploratory drug development. His grants and contracts include the National Institutes of Health, the Department of Energy, the Office of Naval Research and the Army Research Office and several manufacturing companies. Dr Kauffman holds 11 patents and is the author of 80 publications.

Introduction by Larry J. Frieders, RPh

Certain people in the community possess talents used to help others. Dr. Dach is one of those people, and he is truly a man of medicine, blending both the art and science. While having an extensive knowledge of the science of medicine, Dr. Dach vigorously retains a solid grip on the art of medical practice.

I recall one dialogue we had about thyroid, during which I lamented that many people who visit our pharmacy complain of symptoms that clearly reflect a low thyroid condition, yet go untreated. The standard practice of doing a TSH test (thyroid stimulating hormone) may be notoriously inaccurate, as the standards for "normal" have changed over the years. People with normal TSH levels can in fact be low thyroid. Many of these people improve when offered even tiny supplemental doses of thyroid medication. Unfortunately, for such a patient the vast majority of doctors would tell them their TSH levels are fine, they don't require treatment, and they should probably learn to live with the symptoms. However, Dr. Dach knows symptoms don't always match lab values, and a trial of thyroid treatment is not refused. People benefit from the care of this kind of doctor.

There is an ongoing battle about hormone replacement, particularly as it applies to menopause. The standard of care in conventional medicine insists on chemically altered hormones that are not found in the human body. The reason for this is chemically altered substances can be patented, providing protection from competition and financial muscle for marketing. It just so happens that scientists discovered how to make hormones that are structurally identical to the hormones we all make ourselves. These are referred to as bio-identical hormones. Again, where the medical majority act in lockstep with Drug Company marketing, Dr. Dach takes a different and more logical approach, offering bio-identical hormones instead of chemically altered ones. He clearly recognizes that REAL hormones are better than synthetic chemically altered versions.

Doctors like Jeffrey Dach have become a very rare commodity, and we should be thankful that this man is making the effort to put his approach to health and medicine into writing. I surely recommend Dr. Dach's book, *Natural Medicine 101*. It offers useful ideas and practical ways to achieve and maintain health, our most precious commodity.

Larry Frieders obtained a B.S. in pharmacy from the University of Illinois College of Pharmacy in 1971, and masters in Management from Northwestern University in 1975. He has a masters degree in Philosophy, and Medical Ethics from Loyola University in 1998. Larry worked as a staff pharmacist at Cook County Hospital from 1969 - 1975, and at Jackson Park Hospital 1975 – 1982. Larry founded his own pharmacy in 1983, presently known as The Compounder, Inc., in Aurora, specializing in Compounding, and hormone replacement. Larry is a Certified Menopause Educator and frequent speaker at medical meetings. He is a consultant to the Ethics Committee and member of the Institutional Review Board at Provena Mercy Medical Center, Aurora, IL.

Larry J. Frieders, RPh
http://www.thecompounder.com/
340 Marshall, Unit 100
Aurora, IL 60506
Telephone 630-859-0333

Introduction by Jeffrey Dach MD

A Note on the References:

Please be advised that all references are hyperlinked and can be found at www.jeffreydach.com and www.naturalmedicine101.com, where you can easily read the original references articles with a simple mouse click on the hyperlinked reference.

Why Write a Book About Natural Medicine?

You might ask, why even write a book about Natural Medicine? Firstly, this book serves as an educational tool for new patients explaining testing and treatment programs, and what to expect during the first office visit. Secondly, the book serves as an educational tool for the general public, presenting the ideas of natural medicine. There is a medical information war going on in the media between the views of the drug industry and natural medicine. These drug industry views are supported by huge amounts of advertising dollars, while the small voice of natural medicine is often ignored. This book will present the natural medicine side of the debate, and attempt to dispel the myths and falsehoods promotes by drug advertising in this media information war. Thirdly, other health care professionals may find the book useful, since natural medicine is the next medical paradigm.

Lastly, this book represents about one year's work writing each chapter which was sent out in the form of e-mail newsletters and then posted on my blog at www.jeffreydach.com from May 2007 to July 2008. Unlike the old days when books appeared in print first, and later to be posted on the internet (without the hyperlinks), this book was written first on my blog on the internet with references hyperlinked to the original sources. The advantage of the internet is the hyperlinked references which allow the reader to jump to the original article with a mouse click. Therefore, you may find it helpful to refer to the references at my blog www.jeffreydach.com for the convenience of the hyperlinked references, and also for the larger number of illustrations scattered throughout the text.

Training in Conventional Methods

My background and training is that of hospital based, mainstream physician. After working in the hospital for 25 years, my approach to diagnosis and treatment is much the same as any other conventional trained physician which includes a detailed medical history, physical examination, laboratory evaluation and careful follow up. You will find a similar approach at most conventional medical offices.

Lab Testing: Combined Conventional and Non-Conventional

Our office departs from strict conventional medicine regarding lab testing. Most of our lab tests are standard Quest and LabCorp tests which, by definition, are in mainstream medicine. However, some of our lab tests are outside of mainstream medicine, such as the salivary cortisol test which is quite useful, and in many ways superior to the cortisol blood test. Salivary cortisol testing has been accepted and widely used in medical research for 30 years. For example, NASA uses salivary cortisol testing on the astronauts on the space shuttle. Amazingly it is not accepted by mainstream medicine, and your doctor may not even be aware of it. For Celiac testing, we have found that it is necessary to use outside labs such as Enterolabs.

Treatment Protocols

Our treatment protocols are mostly outside of mainstream medicine because we prefer to use natural treatments such as bio-identical hormones, natural desiccated thyroid, vitamins and minerals for deficiency states. There is no question in my mind that natural treatments are by and large more effective and superior to chemically altered drugs. For example, in the patients who have made the transition from synthroid to natural thyroid medication, we have seen superior clinical results.

The Great Achievements of Modern Medicine

No doubt, modern medicine has had some great achievements, and perhaps the greatest achievement of modern medicine has been the conquest of infectious disease with antibiotics and vaccines. Perhaps these great achievements would not have been possible without the drug patent system which provides financial incentives to bring new drugs to market. Unfortunately this financial clout has produced a mainstream medical system controlled and dominated by the pharmaceutical industry. This domination is achieved by infusions of cash for research funding, advertising, marketing, educational meetings, and of course a massive network of sales representatives who make face to face visits with the doctors to present "educational" literature.

The Patented Drug Paradigm

Patented drugs are chemically altered versions of natural substances which are not found in nature or in the human body. They are foreign to the human body. For centuries, medicinal substances came from the natural world. It was is only recently in the 19th and 20th centuries that this paradigm changed because of a quirk in our legal system which allows patent protection for new chemical structures not found in nature. While the legal system allows patent protection for a synthetic, chemically altered drug, the legal system also says that all natural substances reside in the public domain and therefore cannot be patented. For example, both Vitamin C and bio-identical hormones reside in nature and cannot be patented. However there is a small loophole which can be used to patent a natural substance. A patent can be obtained for the manufacturing process to make a natural substance (such as human insulin or human growth hormone), but not on the chemical structure. I think we will see more manufacturing patents for natural substances in the future.

Patent protection restricts competition and allows huge profits from drug sales. This has created the most profitable industry in the history of the world, the US pharmaceutical industry. Like any other self-interested corporation, the drug industry uses standard business practices to increase profit margins. As patents on old drugs expire, the profitability of the industry relies on a steady stream of new drugs in the pipeline. In order to bring these new drugs to market, medical studies must be submitted for FDA approval showing benefit greater than placebo. Once approved, the next step is a massive advertising campaign to convince both the public and the medical professionals they need the drug.

Somewhere along the line things went wrong, and we find the medical studies are manipulated to show benefit for drugs which are marginal, ineffective or actually harmful. We find the drug marketing advertising to be deceitful and misleading. We also find that drug companies behave like any other self interested corporation. They lobby the government and peddle influence to gain favor for their products, while using their clout with the government to suppress competitors in natural medicine.

Two examples: the GAG Rule, and Request to Ban Bio-Identical Hormones
An FDA "gag rule" makes it unlawful for vitamin companies to give information to the public about their products. Because of this FDA rule, it is illegal for manufacturers to inform the public about the usefulness of vitamins, supplements and natural medicines. Some say this rule is an unconstitutional infringement on the right of free speech. This "gag rule" is one example of the power of the drug lobby to influence government to suppress its competition and increase profits at the expense of the constitutional right of free speech.

Another example is the "Citizens' Complaint" filed by Wyeth with the FDA, asking the FDA to ban bio-identical hormones. Following the 2002 Women's Health Initiative study, halted early because the synthetic chemically altered hormone pills caused cancer and heart disease, millions of women abandoned the synthetic hormones and switched to the safer bio-identical (natural) human hormones. The massive switch away from their synthetic product resulted in 4 billion dollar loss for Wyeth, as discussed in the chapter entitled, the FDA Declares War on BioIdentical Hormones.

The FDA Cannot Protect the American Public
The FDA, the government agency designed to be a drug watchdog and protect the American Public, is sadly under the thumb of the pharmaceutical industry. According to the Director of Drug Safety at the FDA, David Graham, the FDA cannot protect the American Public from bad drugs. One example is the case of chemically altered synthetic hormones. These monstrosities clearly should never have been approved nor marketed to the American people. Since their discovery and routine use over 70 years ago, natural bio-identical hormones have always been found to be superior to synthetic chemically altered versions of hormones, which are the ones offered by the mainstream medical system. As this book is written, deceptive television advertising touting the benefits of synthetic hormones can be viewed daily. These monsters should be banned immediately.

Natural Medicine, the Next Paradigm

Substances found in medicinal plants form the basis for many of our drugs used in conventional medicine. For example, aspirin comes from the willow tree, digitalis comes from foxglove plant, morphine from the poppy plant, quinine from the cinchona plant, Taxol comes from the Yew tree native to the Pacific Northwest, and the diabetes drug Metformin from the French Lilac plant. In general, a natural substance is more effective than the synthetic drug made from it. For example, all man made antibiotics eventually cause antibiotic resistant bacteria such as the MERSA organism (methicillin resistant staph aureus). However, anti-microbial essential oils from plants, such as carvacrol and thymol in oregano, are superior antibiotics because they do not create antibiotic resistant bacteria.

As we have seen in the case of natural hormones, whenever the market-place recognizes the natural version of a drug to be safer and more effective than the drug, this spells financial disaster for the drug. On an open playing field, the natural version always wins. This creates an economic rivalry between the drug industry and natural medicine which can be won only at the expense of the truth, by waging a medical information war. This book will show you how to win this medical information war and take control of your health.

The Information War between Drug Medicine and Natural Medicine

The drug industry is waging a medical information war in the media to win the hearts and minds of the public. One obvious theme is the rejection of vitamins. For example, the chapter entitled, "My Vitamins Are Killing Me", reveals how a flawed medical study published in JAMA concludes that vitamins are killing people. This ridiculous conclusion was then picked up and amplified by the media.

We are bombarded with print and television misinformation blaring out the continuous messages, telling us that drugs are beneficial, and natural substances are bad for us. In reality, these medical myths created by the media. This book is intended to dispel those myths, thereby winning the medical information war.

Television and Print Advertising

The drug industry, like any corporate entity, utilizes sophisticated Madison Avenue television advertising techniques (also known as disease mongering) to sell more product to the public. With the exception of New Zealand, the US is the only country that allows Direct to Consumer Television drug advertising which has been banned elsewhere because it is deceptive, misleading and harmful to the public interest. Read more about disease mongering by the drug industry in the chapter on Restless Leg Syndrome, Requip and Disease Mongering.

Prior to the Internet Revolution which has created a Renaissance in free information, the medical information war was very one sided. Despite false and deceptive messages in print and television, the drug industry ran its advertising without watchdog criticism. However, this has changed with the Internet Revolution providing alternative media which reveals these myths and deceptive untruths, breaking the stranglehold of the drug industry on the media, and creating a renaissance in medical information at the grassroots level.

The open information on the internet has changed the rules of the game, with greater public scrutiny of the media. Disease mongering advertising for marginal or ineffective drugs is now effectively opposed by information on the Internet which ridicules and satirizes the drug ads. The eyes of the public have been opened by the Internet Medical Information Revolution to all the tricks of media manipulation, false advertising and deceitful conduct of the pharmaceutical industry, and it is not a pretty picture. All this is quite obvious to the millions of internet savvy e-patients who are drawn towards natural medicine, away from the chemically-altered synthetic drug paradigm. The e-patient has learned the obvious truth that natural medicine is more effective and yields better results than the synthetic counterparts.

The Demise of the Patented Drug Paradigm

As discussed in the Chapter on the Future of Medicine, rapid advances in science will make the chemically altered drug paradigm obsolete. These advances are in the fields of biotechnology, personalized medicine, genomic medicine and orthomolecular medicine, and they involve DNA expression and protein synthesis. Advancing technology is driving change in medicine towards the natural medicine paradigm involving human gene expression of proteins, hormones, and vitamin co-factors.

To survive, mainstream medicine must transform itself and embrace the renaissance in natural medicine. This transformation is not as difficult as you might think. There are many examples of natural medicine in mainstream medicine such as: Blood transfusions, Intravenous fluids, hormones such as human insulin, and growth hormone made with recombinant technology, Slo-Niacin (B3), L-arginine and Omega 3 oils for reversal of heart disease, Lithium for depression, IV magnesium for eclampsia, silver for wound healing, electric stimulation for bone fracture union, etc. As mentioned above, most synthetic drugs are based on original versions found in nature.

Modern Surgery and Natural Medicine Similarities

I have observed over the years that the specialty of internal medicine has always been under the influence of the drug industry, the surgical specialties have always been somewhat independent of drug company influence. In this way, perhaps the specialty of surgery may have something in common with natural medicine, as they are both independence of drug company influence. Surgical techniques cannot be patented or even submitted for FDA approval, as they change and evolve rapidly based on effectiveness. Over the past few decades, new surgical procedures have replaced old ones. Some procedures were shown to be sham, such as arthroscopy for Osteoarthritis. Some procedures were victims of advancing technology, as in the replacement of many open surgery procedures with laparoscopic techniques.

One thing I have learned over the years is:

Never underestimate the ability of medicine to change.

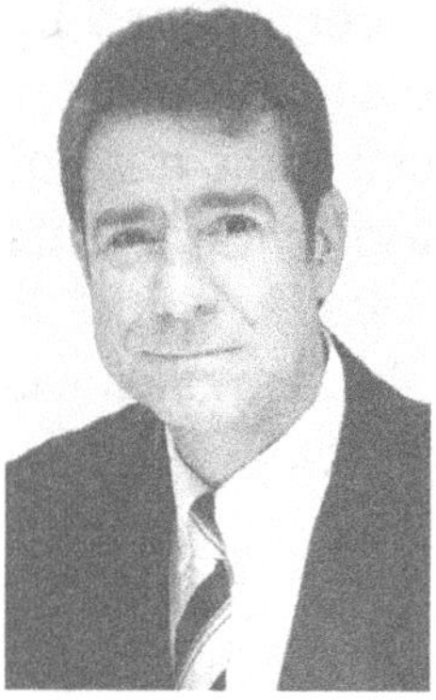

Jeffrey Dach MD

Jeffrey Dach MD obtained his MD degree from the University of Illinois. His training includes a medical/surgical internship and radiology residency at Rush Presbyterian Hospital in Chicago, a fellowship in CAT Scan, Ultrasound and Interventional Rdiology at the University of Miami Jackson Memorial in 1981. Dr Dach served on the hospital staff as an Inteventional Radiologist for 25 years in the Memorial Hospital System in Hollywood Florida. After retiring from radiology in in 2005, Dr. Dach founded TrueMedMD, a clinic specializing in natural medicine, and bioidentical hormone therapy. References for this book can be found at his web sites:www.jeffreydach.com and www.naturalmedicine101.com

Acknowledgements:

First of all, I wish to thank my wife Judith who is the light of my life, and without her help this book would not have been possible. This book is dedicated to my children Ari, Benjamin and Karina who are in the process of picking up the gauntlet for the next generation.

I wish to thank all the people who have influenced this book, my friends, colleagues, and mentors: Russell Jaffe, Joel Kauffman, David Brownstein, George Flechas, Erika Schwartz, Larry Frieders, Sangeeta Pati, Harvy Bialy, Jonathan Wright, Julian Whitaker, CW Randolph, Mark Starr, Dan Clark, William Davis, James Roberts, Joseph McWherter, Uzzi Reiss, Eugene Shipman, Ron Rothenberg, Jacob Teitelbaum, Kent Holtorf, Sheri Lieberman, and Abram Hoffer. Also thanks to John R Lee, Broda Barnes, William Mc Jefferies, and Linus Pauling.

Also thanks goes to Richard Beckman, the marketing and advertising guru responsible for keeping my cardiovascular system in order by forcing me to chase after a yellow tennis ball. And thanks to my close friends, Ellis Sinyor, Ben Fireman, Alan Wolf, and Howie Wolkowitz, whose input has also influenced this book.

Also thanks and acknowledgement goes to Jenny Ruhl, Merrill Goozner, Aubrey Blumsohn, Sally Pacholok, Eddie Vos, Bob Fiddaman, Ed Silverman, and the many people on the internet blogs and message boards who have interacted, communicated, shared knowledge and influenced this book. Medical education continues after medical school as an ongoing process without end. My second medical education began with installation of high speed internet, the required gateway to our current medical information explosion. Health professionals who ignore this necessary internet interface will be marginalized to the sideroads while the rest of us cruise the medical information superhighway.

Finally I must acknowledge that this book will never be finished, as the history of medicine will march into the future and will continue to evolve. However, we have made our best effort for a beginning. As Winston Churchhill said, "Now this is not the end. It is not even the beginning of the end. But it is, perhaps, the end of the beginning."

Front Cover Image: The Anatomy Lesson of Dr. Nicolaes Tulp, 1632, by Rembrandt courtesy of the Mauritshuis museum in The Hague, the Netherlands.

Disclaimer:

This book is not intended as medical advice nor should it be regarded as such. It is important to discuss any treatment plan with your personal physician. Do not start or stop a treatment, drug, supplement or lifestyle change based on information from this book. Even if a drug is on a ligation, recall or black box list, any decision to start or stop a drug should be made in consultation with your own doctor, who should help you weigh the comparative risks and benefits to arrive at an informed decision.

The information contained in this book is NOT intended to diagnose or treat any existing disease or ailment, or to replace in any way the patient /physican relationship with your own personal physician.

Regarding the nutritional supplements which may be mentioned: These have not been evaluated by the FDA and are not intended to treat disease. Any comments made about nutritional supplements are of a general nature and not intended to provide personal advice. The reader should seek the advice of a trusted health care professional regarding the use, risks, benefits, indications, and contra-indications of the various nutritional supplements which may be mentioned.

Regarding FDA approved pharmaceutical drugs mentioned: Any comments made about drugs are of a general nature and not intended to provide personal advice. The reader should seek the advice of a trusted health care professional regarding the use, risks, benefits, indications, and contra-indications of drugs.

The reader is advised to discuss the comments on these pages with his/her personal physicians and to only act upon the advice of his/her personal physician

Some treatment options do not require a prescription and can be obtained over the counter. Even so, it is recommended that one should always work closely with a knowledgeable physician, found by consulting one of the following organizations:

Find A Physician in Your Area

http://www.worldhealth.net/
American Academy of Anti-Aging Medicine
(Chicago Office)
1510 W. Montana Street
Chicago, IL 60614 USA
Directory of members, to find a doctor:
Telephone is 800-558-1267

http://www.acamnet.org/
ACAM - Americal College for the Advancement of Medicine
24411 Ridge Route Ste 115
Laguna Hills, CA 92653
ACAM doctor's directory to find a physician:
Toll free telephone: 800-532-3688

http://icimed.com/
International College of Integrative Medicine
122 Thurman St. Box 271, Bluffton, OH 45817
Telephone: (866) 464-5226,
(419) 358-0273, ICIM doctor's directory

http://www.holisticmedicine.org/
American Holistic Medical Association
One Eagle Valley Court, Suite 201
Broadview Heights, Ohio 44147
Phone: (440) 838-1010

Chapter One

My Vitamins are Killing Me

Vitamins Courtesy of Wikimedia Commons

Rather than making you healthier, you might be surprised to know that the vitamins you take every day are actually killing you. This news story has been running in the media based on a meta-analysis published in 2007 JAMA by Bjelakovic. *(1A)(10)(12)(13)(1).*

The problem is that this JAMA article was a flawed hatchet job not worth the paper it was written on. Out of 748 vitamin studies, the researchers selected only 67 focusing on high dose synthetic vitamins, and excluded all the others showing benefit. This is called selective sampling. *(1B)(1C)(1D)(11)*

Selective Sampling: How to Prove There is No Water in the Ocean

Using this same research technique, you can prove there is no water in the ocean. Merely go down to the beach front, wade into the water up to your ankles and collect a sample for analysis. Reach under the surface, pick up a few pebbles from the ocean floor, and take them back to your laboratory for sophisticated chemical analysis with nuclear magnetic resonance. Amazingly, the print out shows no water! You have thereby proven there is no water in the ocean, and can publish your report in a prestigious journal. Sadly, this is the current state of our medical journals, and now you can understand how the public is easily deceived.

Proven Health Benefits of Vitamins

Negative vitamin stories are frequently run in the mass media. These are usually studies which are funded by drug companies, and the researchers are paid to come

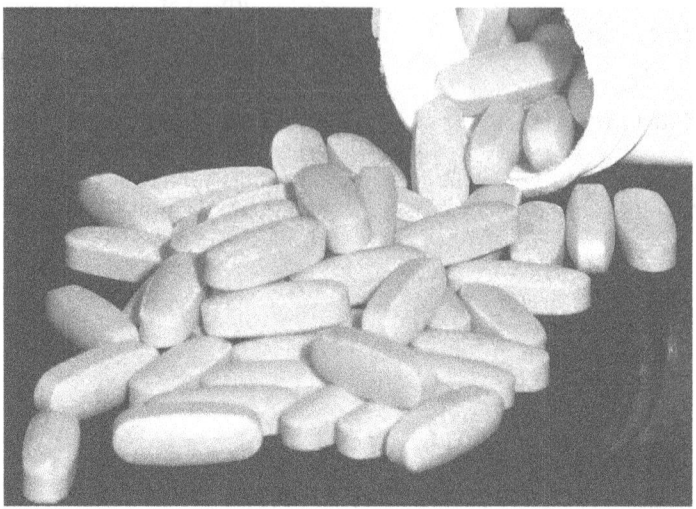

up with negative findings in order to discredit vitamins so people will take more drugs. It is a simple matter of "follow the money trail".

When the medical studies are done by a neutral party, such as the Chinese government, the results are closer to reality. A study from Linxian province in China showed a 9 per cent reduction in mortality from only three vitamins: A, E and Selenium. They also showed a 13% reduction in cancer mortality, and a 21% reduction in gastric cancer mortality.*(2)* Another study showed selenium supplementation prevented esophageal cancer, heart disease, stroke, and total death.*(3)*

Folate supplementation in pregnant mothers prevents Neural Tube birth defects in the developing fetus.*(4)(5)* Vitamin C prevents coronary artery disease and a variety of other chronic diseases.*(6)(7)* Vitamin B-12 supplementation is recommended by the USDA for everyone over the age of 50. (US dept of Agriculture 2005 Food Guidelines)*(14)(8)* In fact there are volumes of research data showing benefits of vitamin supplementation.*(9)*

The Bottom Line, Be Skeptical of News Media

Bottom line is that you can't believe the newspapers or media when it comes to vitamin, mineral or nutritional supplements. The media depends on advertising revenue from the drug companies, and will therefore tend to run stories negative about vitamins and supplements, making drugs look good. The reality is that by and large, vitamins are safe, and drugs are dangerous. Adverse effects from drugs cause 140,000 deaths and 76 billion dollars a year in health care costs.*(15)(16)*

Be skeptical of news media stories which have a hidden agenda. Direct-to-Consumer drug advertising is largely deceptive and misleading, and should be banned here in the US, as it has been banned in all other countries (with the exception of New Zealand).

Which Vitamins Require Caution?

The water soluble vitamins (C and B complex) are readily excreted in the urine and therefore can be taken at high doses with no ill effects. The fat soluble vitamins A and D, however, can accumulate and cause toxicity at high doses over prolonged periods, so these must be monitored. We routinely measure vitamin D blood levels, and supplement Vitamin D with serial monitoring of blood levels. Also, Vitamin E and fish oils have a blood thinning effect, which can cause bleeding tendencies. Most anesthesiologists recommend avoiding Vitamin E and fish oils prior to elective surgery.

All references are hyperlinked at www.jeffreydach.com and www.naturalmedicine101.com.

References for Chapter One:

(1) http://news.bbc.co.uk/1/hi/health/6399773.stm
Vitamins 'could shorten lifespan' Research has produced mixed results, Taking certain vitamin supplements may adversely affect people's lifespan, researchers have suggested. BBC News 28 February 2007

(1A) http://jama.ama-assn.org/cgi/content/abstract/297/8/842
Mortality in Randomized Trials of Antioxidant Supplements for Primary and Secondary Prevention. Systematic Review and Meta-analysis, by Goran Bjelakovic, MD, et al. JAMA 2007;297:842-857.

(1B) http://oregonstate.edu/dept/ncs/newsarch/2007/Feb07/vitaminstudy.html
02-27-07 Media Release Linus Pauling Institute: Study Citing Antioxidant Vitamin Risks Based on Flawed Methodology

(1C) http://www.organicconsumers.org/articles/article_4399.cfm
Alliance for Natural Health Critiques JAMA Study Claiming Synthetic Vitamins Can Kill You JAMA - 'vitamins kill' - no they don't! Alliance for Natural Health (UK), Mar 5, 2007 Straight to the Source

(1D) http://www.alliance-natural-health.org/_docs/ANHwebsiteDoc_270.pdf
Poor methodology in meta-analysis of vitamins. Dr Steve Hickey, Dr Len Noriega and Dr Hilary Roberts Faculty of Computing, Engineering and Technology, Staffordshire University; School of Biology, Chemistry and Health Science, Manchester Metropolitan University.

(2) http://www.ncbi.nlm.nih.gov/pubmed/8360931
J Natl Cancer Inst. 1993 Sep 15;85(18):1483-92. Nutrition intervention trials in Linxian, China: supplementation with specific vitamin/mineral combinations, cancer incidence, and disease-specific mortality in the general population. Blot WJ etal.

(3) http://www.ajcn.org/cgi/content/full/79/1/80
ORIGINAL RESEARCH COMMUNICATIONS Prospective study of serum selenium concentrations and esophageal and gastric cardia cancer, heart disease, stroke, and total death. Wen-Qiang Wei et al. We found significant inverse associations between baseline serum selenium and death from ESCC (RR: 0.83; 95% CI: 0.71, 0.98) and GCC (0.75; 0.59, 0.95)

(4) http://www.fda.gov/Fdac/features/796_fol.html
FDA web site: How Folate Can Help Prevent Birth Defects by Paula Kurtzweil

(5) http://www.ebmonline.org/cgi/content/full/226/4/243
Experimental Biology and Medicine 226:243-270 (2001) Folate, Homocysteine and Neural Tube Defects: An Overview Nathalie M.J. van der Put1,Henny W.M. van Straaten, Frans J.M. Trijbels

(6) *http://www.internetwks.com/owen/Synopsis.pdf*
Linus Pauling Protocol for Reversing Heart Disease by Owen Fonorow 2005

(7) *http://lpi.oregonstate.edu/infocenter/vitamins/vitaminC/*
Vitamin C Information Linus Pauling Institute Oregon State University

(8) *http://www.drinkyourvitamins.com/rk_articles/art09-b12underapr.htm*
Vitamin B12 by Richard A. Kunin, M.D. 2000

(9) *http://www4.dr-rath-foundation.org/NHC/researcharchive.html*
List of Clinical Studies that document the importance of micronutrients and nutrition in maintaining optimum health. Dr Rath Foundation.

(10) *http://www.aidstruth.org/Mortality-with-antioxidants.pdf*
Full pdf of JAMA article, Mortality with antioxidants

(11) *http://en.epochtimes.com/news/8-4-22/69603.html*
Dr. John Briffa is a London-based doctor and author with an interest in nutrition and natural medicine.

(12) *http://news.yahoo.com/s/nm/20080416/lf_nm_life/britain_vitamins_dc_1*
Vitamin pills can "increase rate of mortality" Reuters. Scientists reviewed 67 studies on 230,000 people to see whether so-called antioxidant vitamins prolonged life expectancy.

(13) *http://www.foxnews.com/story/0,2933,351443,00.html*
FOXNEWS. Mom, This Study Says I Don't Have to Take My Vitamins! April 16, 2008. The Health Food Manufacturers' Association told Sky News online that the study was "in essence, systematically flawed." "The analysis focused on one broad category of study, then evaluated just 67 of the 748 studies that could be included in the review," according to the Association.

(14) *http://www.health.gov/dietaryguidelines/dga2005/document/html/executivesummary.htm*
Dietary Guidelines for Americans 2005, USDA. Key Recommendations for Specific Population Groups. People over age 50. Consume vitamin B12 in its crystalline form (i.e., fortified foods or supplements).

(15) *http://archinte.ama-assn.org/cgi/content/abstract/155/18/1949*
Drug-related morbidity and mortality. A cost-of-illness model. Arch Int Med Vol. 155 No. 18, October 9, 1995. J. A. Johnson and J. L. Bootman Center for Pharmaceutical Economics, College of Pharmacy, University of Arizona, Tucson, USA. Drug-related morbidity and mortality was estimated to cost **$76.6 billion** in the ambulatory setting in the United States.

(16) *http://www.healthsentinel.com/briefs.php?id=010&title=Adverse+Drug+Events+a nd+Hospital+Acquired+Infections&event=briefs_print_list_item*
Adverse Drug Events in Hospitalized Patients: Excess Length of Stay, Extra Costs, and Attributable Mortality", Classen, David C. et al.. JAMA, Jan 22, 1997, V277, N0, p301-306

Chapter Two

Vitamin C and Stroke Prevention

One of my friends was hospitalized recently after a sudden paralysis of his right arm and leg which was found to be a stroke on his CAT scan. He is about my age and was previously healthy with none of the usual risk factors of high blood pressure, smoking or obesity. Thankfully, he recovered quickly, and was soon back to normal at home.

What is a Stroke?

Why did my friend get a stroke? What is a stroke and how can it be prevented? There are two kinds of stroke, the first kind is the ischemic stroke, in which blood flow is blocked off by a clot or small plug, and the second kind is the hemorrhagic stroke, in which a small crack in the artery leaks blood into the surrounding brain. Stroke is quite common with about 700,000 strokes annually in the United States. Both heart attacks and strokes are caused by atherosclerotic vascular disease.

Stroke Prevention

Stroke prevention by the medical system usually consists of blood thinners such as coumadin and aspirin, usually started after the first stroke in hopes of preventing a second stroke. An often ignored, yet more important preventive measure is Vitamin C which is cheap and plentiful, so there is no financial incentive to anyone to recommend it.

Vitamin C Beneficial for Stroke Prevention

Here are two of many recent studies published in the medical literature showing Vitamin C to be beneficial in reducing the risk of stroke. This first study was carried out in rural Japan, and the highest blood levels of Vitamin C had 70 per cent fewer strokes.*(1)* A second study done in Finland in 2002 showed the same findings *(2)*. Those people with the lowest vitamin C blood levels had 2.4 times greater risk of stroke. If high blood pressure and obesity were added factors, there was even higher risk for stroke.

How Does Vitamin C Work? - Collagen Synthesis

How does Vitamin C work to make our arteries stronger? The arteries are made of a connective tissue substance called Collagen, and vitamin C is the key nutrient for collagen synthesis. In addition, Vitamin C is a major player as an anti-oxidant, important for quenching free radicals from oxidative metabolism.

Vitamin C Deficiency

Now that you are convinced that Vitamin C is beneficial in preventing stroke, perhaps you might think that we all get enough vitamin C in our diets. A new study of 15,769 people aged 12 to 74 years in the American Journal of Public Health says otherwise. This study found a distressing 10 percent of women and 14 percent of men to be deficient in Vitamin C.*(3)*

Is the Recommended Dietary Allowance for Vitamin C Too Low? How much Vitamin C is enough? Recommendations differ depending on the source:

Daily Vitamin C	Source of Recommendation
60-95 mg	U.S. Government RDA *(15)*
200 mg	Levin/NIH *(16)*
400 mg	Linus Pauling Institute *(7)*
2500 mg	Hickey/Roberts *(12)*
4000 mg	Robert Cathcart MD III *(4)*
6-12 grams	Thomas E Levy, MD, PHD *(6)*

Except Primates, All Animals Can Make Vitamin C from Glucose

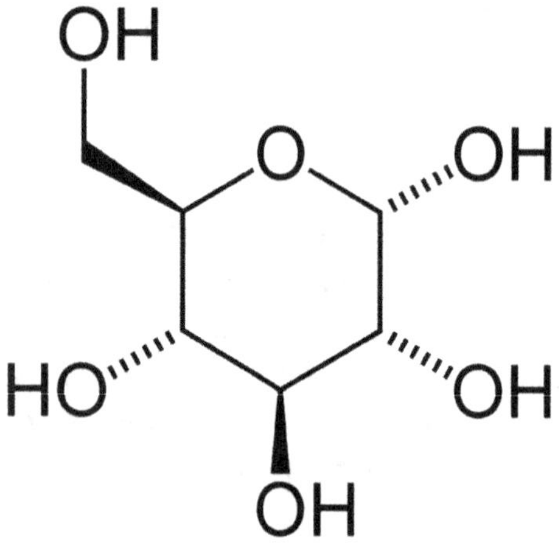

Left Image Glucose

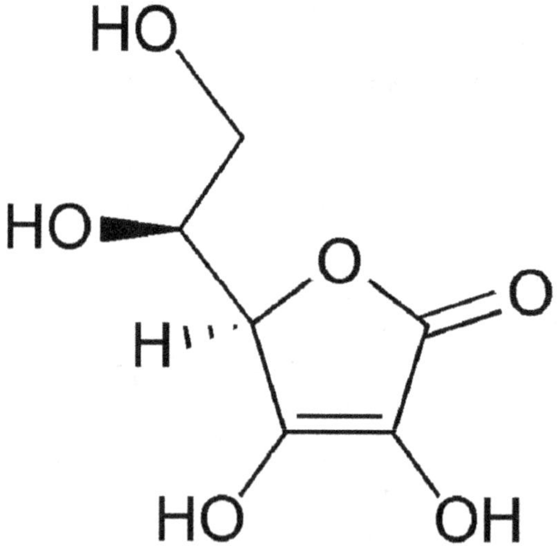

Right Image Vitamin C - Ascorbate

All animals are able to convert glucose into ascorbate vitamin C with the use of three enzymes located in their liver. Primates including us humans had a mutation about 40 million years ago, and we lack the final enzyme step needed to make our own Vitamin C. This last enzyme is called GLO (gulano lactone oxidase).*(13)(14)* You might ask the question: how much vitamin C would we make every day if the GLO enzyme was present and doing its job to convert glucose into vitamin C? Perhaps the best answer comes from studying how much vitamin C animals produce. Based on animal vitamin C data, estimates are that healthy adult humans would produce about 2 to 4 grams (2,000 to 4,000 milligrams) of vitamin C daily. Other primates (gorillas, orangutans, chimpanzees) cannot make their own vitamin C, and they typically consume 3 to 4 grams of vitamin C daily (calculated on a "human-weight basis").*(6)*

Vitamin C Bowel Tolerance Test

Determining how much supplemental vitamin C will meet your individual requirements is fairly easy using a tolerance-test technique developed by Dr. Cathcart.*(4)* The tolerance test starts with a dose of 2 grams of vitamin C per day. Then, slowly increase your Vitamin C dose each day until you start experiencing excess gas or loose bowels. At that point, your body isn't absorbing or able to use that much vitamin C, so you should scale back to the largest amount that doesn't produce these symptoms.

Vitamin C comes from citrus fruits such as oranges, lemons and limes, etc. To take supplemental Vitamin C, a buffered, 100% pure (L) isomer of Vitamin C (ascorbate) is recommended. In terms of medical prevention bang for the buck, you can't beat it.

All references are hyperlinked at www.jeffreydach.com and www.naturalmedicine101.com.

References For Chapter 2

(1) http://stroke.ahajournals.org/cgi/content/full/31/10/2287
Stroke. 2000;31:2287. Serum Vitamin C Concentration Was Inversely Associated With Subsequent 20-Year Incidence of Stroke in a Japanese Rural Community The Shibata Study Full text

(2) http://stroke.ahajournals.org/cgi/reprint/33/6/1568.pdf
Plasma Vitamin C Modifies the Association Between Hypertension and Risk of Stroke. Stroke, 2002;33:1568-1573 S. Kurl, MD; T.P. Tuomainen, MD; J.A. Laukkanen, MD; K. Nyyssönen, PhD;

(3) http://www.ajph.org/cgi/content/full/94/5/870
Hampl JS, Taylor CA, Johnston CS. "Vitamin C deficiency and depletion in the United States: the Third National Health and Nutrition Examination Survey, 1988 to 1994." Am J Public Health 2004; 94(5): 870-875

(4) http://www.orthomed.com/titrate.htm
Cathcart RF. Vitamin C, Titrating To Bowel Tolerance, Anascorbemia, and Acute Induced Scurvy. Medical Hypotheses 1981; 7: 1,359-1,376

(5) http://en.wikipedia.org/wiki/Vitamin_C#_note-UKFSA_Risk
Vitamin C, the L and R isomers: Wikipedia

(6) http://tomlevymd.com/vcone.htm
Thomas Levy MD on Vitamin C

(7) http://lpi.oregonstate.edu/infocenter/vitamins/vitaminC/crefs.html
Linus Pauling Institute References for Vitamin C

(8) http://www.ajcn.org/cgi/content/abstract/80/6/1508
Knekt P, et al. "Antioxidant vitamins and coronary heart disease risk: a pooled analysis of 9 cohorts." Am J Clin Nutr 2004; 80(6): 1,508-1,520.

(9) http://www.seanet.com/~alexs/ascorbate/194x/klenner-fr-southern_med_surg-1949-v111-n7-p209.htm
Klenner FR. "The Treatment of Poliomyelitis and Other Virus Diseases with Vitamin C." Southern Medicine & Surgery 1949: 209

(10) http://faculty.washington.edu/ely/JOM4.html
Ascorbic Acid and Some Other Modern Analogs of the Germ Theory. Journal of Orthomolecular Medicine, 1999; Vol 14 (3): 143-56. John T. A. Ely, Ph.D.Radiation Studies, Box 351310 University of WashingtonSeattle, WA 98195

(11) http://www.orthomed.com/publications1.html
Publications by Robert F. Cathcart MD

(12) http://www.lewrockwell.com/sardi/sardi29.html
Is the Recommended Dietary Allowance for Vitamin C Too Low? by Bill Sardi
Dr. Hickey and Roberts Vitamin C recommendations

(13) http://jn.nutrition.org/cgi/content/full/137/10/2171
American Society for Nutrition J. Nutr. 137:2171-2184, October 2007
Critical Review New Developments and Novel Therapeutic Perspectives for Vitamin C. Yi Li and Herb E. Schellhorn.

(14) http://www.jbc.org/cgi/content/abstract/269/18/13685
J. Biol. Chem., Vol. 269, Issue 18, 13685-13688, 05, 1994

(15) http://www.pubmedcentral.nih.gov/articlerender.fcgi?artid=55540
Proatl Acad Sci U S A. 2001 August 14; 98(17): 9842–9846. A new recommended dietary allowance of vitamin C for healthy young women-90 mg Mark Levine, Yaohui Wang, Sebastian J. Padayatty, and Jason Morrow

(16) http://www.nih.gov/news/pr/apr99/niddk-20.html
NIH Research Shows 100 to 200 Mg of Vitamin C Daily May Benefit Healthy Adults.

Chapter Three Vitamin D

Vitamin D Deficiency, the Ignored Epidemic of the Developed World

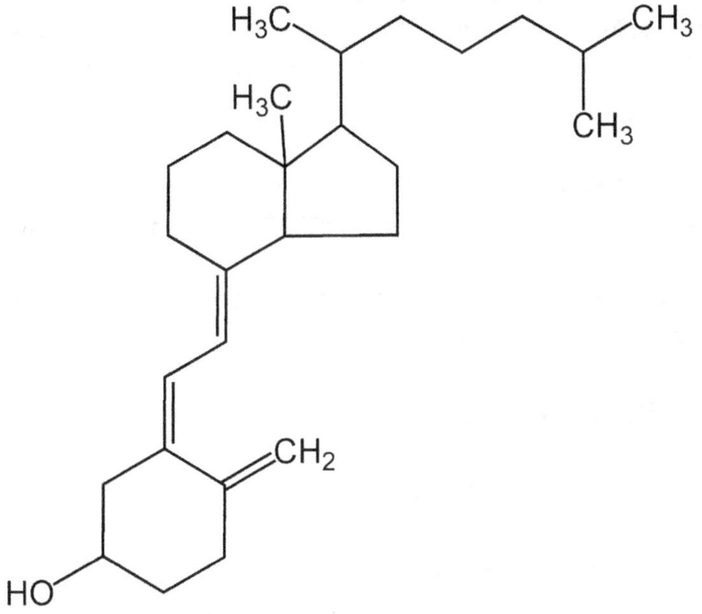

Vitamin D Chemical Structure

Is it a New Bio-Tech Drug, or is it Vitamin D?

What if I told you I discovered a Bio-Tech company with a new drug that could reduce the number of cancer deaths in the US by 43,000 annually, reduce colon cancer by 50%, and breast and ovarian cancer by 30%. Would you be impressed? What if I then told you this same drug could safely prevent or alleviate the following medical conditions: Osteoporosis, Hypertension, Cardiovascular disease, Cancer, Depression, Epilepsy, Type One Diabetes, Insulin resistance, Autoimmune Diseases, Migraine Headache, Polycystic Ovary Disease (PCOS), Musculoskeletal and bone pain, Psoriasis, and Rheumatoid Arthritis, Inflammatory Bowel Disease (Cohn's), chronic lymphocytic leukemia (CLL)*(15)*, as well as improve calcium absorption and reduce hip fractures.*(5A)*

Would you then be even more impressed, and rush out to buy the company stock and get rich quick? Of course you would, but we don't need a new Bio-Tech drug to do this, because, all of the above benefits can be obtained with Vitamin D, an inexpensive vitamin which is free with sun exposure.

Vitamin D Deficiency in Florida, Surely You must Be Joking:

We all know it's a fact: Everyone in Florida gets plenty of Vitamin D from the Florida Sun. This would have been true except for the fact that as Floridians, we are all told to avoid the sun to prevent solar skin damage (brown wrinkling) and to avoid skin cancer.

So the question remains, do we get enough Vitamin D from sun exposure? To answer this question, we actually measured blood Vitamin D levels, and we were surprised to discover that the **majority** showed Vitamin D deficiency (less than 20 ng/ml), or insufficiency (less than 40 ng/ml).

What if you are not fortunate to live in sunny Florida and you live up north above the Mason Dixon Line, in Boston, New York, Chicago, Canada or Scandinavia? Northern latitudes have an even more serious vitamin D deficiency because of the lack of UV sunlight during the winter months. The angle of the sun through the atmosphere closes off the UltraViolet Light from reaching the earth.

An Epidemic of Vitamin D Deficiency

Vitamin D deficiency has been reported in 57% of 290 medical inpatients in Massachusetts, 93% of 150 patients with overt musculoskeletal pain in Minnesota, 48% of patients with Multiple Sclerosis, 50% of patients with lupus and fibromyalgia, 42% of healthy adolescents, 40% of African American Women, and 62 % of the morbidly obese, 83% of 360 patients with low back pain in Saudi Arabia, 73% of Austrian patients with Ankylosing Spondylitis, 58% of Japanese girls with Graves's Disease, 40% of Chinese adolescent girls, 40-70% of all Finnish medical patients. *(5A)*

Vitamin D Toxicity

Vitamin D excess and toxicity requires daily dosage in excess of 40,000 units over a period of months, so 5,000 units a day is safe and far below the level needed to develop vitamin D toxicity. Remember Vitamin D is a fat soluble vitamin, so toxicity is possible with massive doses over long periods of time. Vitamin D toxicity causes elevated calcium levels. That's why Vitamin D supplementation should be done only under your physician's supervision with monitoring of serum 25-Hydroxy Vitamin D levels.

Space Satellite Maps

If you take NASA space satellite photos of North America and color code the UV sunlight exposure as Dr. Grant has done on his *web site, Sunarc.org (3)*, you will see a pattern remarkably similar to the incidence of cancer and multiple sclerosis. This is thought to be due to differences in Vitamin D levels. The farther north with less sun exposure and lower Vitamin D levels, there is an increased incidence of cancer and multiple sclerosis.

Diseases Caused By, or Associated With Vitamin D Deficiency:

Again here is the list: Osteoporosis, Hypertension, Cardiovascular disease, Cancer, Depression, Epilepsy, Type One Diabetes, Insulin resistance, Autoimmune Diseases, Migraine Headache, PolyCystic Ovary Disease (PCOS), Musculoskeletal and bone pain, Psoriasis, and chronic lymphocytic leukemia (CLL)*(15)*.

The current recommendation for Vitamin D deficiency in those people who must avoid the sun is 5,000 IU of Vitamin D per day which costs 5 cents a day.

Vitamin D is not really a Vitamin, it is a Hormone.

Like all other steroidal hormones, vitamin D is made from a cholesterol precursor, converted in the skin by sunlight. Like all other hormones, Vitamin D enters the nucleus of the cell and binds to the DNA where it gives a message to the DNA to manufacture proteins.

Vitamin D And Multiple Sclerosis.

A review by Dr. Brown reported that Vitamin D supplementation prevented the development and progression of experimental autoimmune encephalitis, an animal model of MS, in mice. A large, prospective, cohort study found that vitamin D supplementation was associated with a 40% reduction in the risk of developing MS. Four small, noncontrolled studies suggested that vitamin D supplementation may decrease exacerbation of MS symptoms.*(20)* MRI studies of multiple sclerosis lesions show improvement during summer months and worsening during winter months suggesting a Vitamin D link.*(36)*

Vitamin D and Cancer

A four-year clinical *trial*, involving 1,200 women found those taking the vitamin had about a 60-per-cent reduction in cancer incidence, compared with those who didn't take it, a drop so large — twice the impact on cancer attributed to smoking — it almost looks like a typographical error. The study was done by professor of medicine Robert Heaney of Creighton University in Nebraska and was published in June 2007 American Journal of Clinical Nutrition.*(37)*

Vitamin D and Total Mortality

A 2007 meta-analysis review of 18 studies showed a reduction in all cause mortality of about 10% in people supplementing with commonly used doses of Vitamin D.*(39)*

Vitamin D Supplementation for Adults

The RDA in America is only 400 IU per day, yet current research suggests that our daily Vitamin D requirement is closer to 4,000 to 5,000 IU. Twenty minutes of Sun exposure will give us ten to twenty thousand IU of Vitamin D.

Adult Supplementation with Carlson's Cod Liver Oil can provide Vitamin D along with Vitamin A . However, for an intake of 5,000 IU vitamin D per day, inexpensive Vitamin D3 capsules are widely available for about 5 cents a day.

Vitamin D Testing at the Lab

Optimal serum 25-hydroxyvitamin D values are above 40 ng/ml. Below 40 ng/ml is called Vitamin D insufficiency, and below 20 ng/ml is deficiency.

Conclusion

Our health care system is in crisis. We are spending billions on expensive procedures like coronary artery bypass and organ transplantation, yet measurements of health are lower than other countries that spend less. In terms of getting more bang for your health care buck, Vitamin D testing and supplementation for the population is one solution which is guaranteed to improve overall health of the population at a ridiculously low cost. The cost saving in reduced cancer rates, and lower osteoporotic fracture rates would be enormous, and we would all enjoy improved health. My goal as a physician in our community is to improve the health of our community, and Vitamin D testing and supplementation is one way to achieve that goal with no adverse side effects and enormous cost savings.

References Chapter 3

(1) http://www.vitamind-veith.ms-diet.org/
Prospects for Vitamin D Nutrition. Vitamin D and Human Evolution Clinical relevance of higher vitamin D intakes, Toxicology of Vitamin D Reinhold Vieth, Pathology and Laboratory Medicine, Mount Sinai Hospital, and Laboratory Medicine and Pathobiology, University of Toronto Calgary AB, Oct 13 2005. Highly recommended Web Cast video presentation on Vitamin D by Dr. Vieth

(1A) http://wildhorse.insinc.com/directms13oct2005/
another link to this same video presentation on Vitamin D by Dr. Vieth

(2) http://articles.mercola.com/sites/articles/archive/2004/04/03/vitamin-d-grant.aspx
Valuable Insights Into the Importance of Vitamin D and Sun on Mercola.com, Interview with William B. Grant, Ph.D.

(3) *http://www.sunarc.org/*
Satellite Maps, Cancer mortality rates and multiple sclerosis prevalence rates for U.S. states compared to UVB doses for July, William B. Grant, Ph.D.

(4) *http://www.sunarc.org/embryms1.htm*
Vitamin D Supplementation in the Fight Against Multiple Sclerosis, Ashton F. Embry, Ph.D. 2004, Journal of Orthomolecular Medicine, v.19, p. 27-38.

(5) *http://www.vitamindcouncil.org/*
Vitamin D Council, John Cannell MD Web Site: Understanding Cholecalciferol Vitamin D

(5A) *http://www.vitamindcouncil.org/PDFs/CME-clinicalImportanceVitD.pdf*
Excellent review article on Vitamin D by John Cannell MD full PDF File Clinical Importance of Vitamin D: A Paradigm Shift. Biotics Research Newsletter.

(6) *http://www.vitamindcouncil.org/bestNewsArticles.shtml*
Listing of the best Vitamin D articles on the internet posted by John Cannell Vitamin D Council.

(7) *http://www.knowledgeofhealth.com/*
Cancer Defeated: Vitamin D Pill For All. Economical Pill Would Cut Cancer Rates In Half. Bill Sardi Knowledge of Health Blog

(8) *http://www.lewrockwell.com/sardi/sardi70.html*
Just One Pill Away, by Bill Sardi, review of Vitamin D on Lew Rockwell.

(9) *http://www.medicalnewstoday.com/articles/24941.php*
Medical News Today. Healthcare Professionals Ignore Vitamin D Deficiency Epidemic by John Cannell MD

(10) *http://articles.mercola.com/sites/articles/archive/2006/10/26/beware-of-most-prescription-vitamin-d-supplements.aspx*
Beware of prescription Vitamin D supplements, info from Mercola

(11) *http://articles.mercola.com/sites/articles/archive/2004/02/28/vitamin-d-part-twenty.aspx*
Vitamin D Lowers inflammation by John Cannell MD on Mercola.com

(12) *http://lpi.oregonstate.edu/infocenter/vitamins/vitaminD/index.html*
Linus Pauling Institute on Vitamin D

(13) *http://lpi.oregonstate.edu/infocenter/vitamins/vitaminD/drefs.html*
Linus Pauling Institute Vit D References with Links.

(15) *http://www.clltopics.org/VitaminD3/EssentialforHealth.htm*
Chronic Lymphocytic Leukemia Web Site: CLL topics: vitamin D is quite cytotoxic to CLL cells?

(16) *http://www.ajcn.org/cgi/content/full/69/5/842*
Vieth, Reinhold. Vitamin D supplementation, 25-hydroxyvitamin D concentrations, and safety. American Journal of Clinical Nutrition, Vol. 69, No. 5, 842-856, May 1999

(17) *http://cebp.aacrjournals.org/cgi/content/abstract/16/3/422*
Vieth, Reinhold, Vitamin D and Reduced Risk of Breast Cancer: A Population-Based Case-Control Study. Cancer Epidemiology Biomarkers & Prevention 16, 422-429, March 1, 2007.

(18) *http://www.ajcn.org/cgi/content/full/73/2/288*
Veith R, Chan P-C R, MacFarlane G D. "Efficacy and safety of vitamin D3 intake exceeding the lowest adverse effect level." Am J Clin Nutr 2001; 71: 288-294

(19) *http://jama.ama-assn.org/cgi/content/abstract/296/23/2832*
Munger, Levin,. Hollis, PhD Howard, Ascherio, Serum 25-Hydroxyvitamin D Levels and Risk of Multiple Sclerosis JAMA. 2006;296:2832-2838 Epidemiological and experimental evidence suggests that high levels of vitamin D, a potent immunomodulator, may decrease the risk of multiple sclerosis.

(20) *http://www.theannals.com/cgi/content/abstract/40/6/1158*
Brown, Sherrill J, The Role of Vitamin D in Multiple Sclerosis , DRUG INFORMATION ROUNDS, The Annals of Pharmacotherapy: Vol. 40, No. 6, pp. 1158-1161. DOI 10.1345/aph.1G513

(21) *http://www.ajcn.org/cgi/reprint/76/1/3.pdf*
Michael F Holick, Editorial: Too little vitamin D in premenopausal women: why should we care? Am J Clin Nutr 2002;76:3–4.

(22) *http://www.ajcn.org/cgi/content/full/79/3/362*
Michael F Holick, Vitamin D: importance in the prevention of cancers, type 1 diabetes, heart disease, and osteoporosis American Journal of Clinical Nutrition, Vol. 79, No. 3, 362-371, March 2004

(23) *http://www.ajcn.org/cgi/content/full/80/6/1678S*
Holick , Michael F VITAMIN D AND HEALTH IN THE 21ST CENTURY: BONE AND BEYOND, Sunlight and vitamin D for bone health and prevention of autoimmune diseases, cancers, and cardiovascular disease American Journal of Clinical Nutrition, Vol. 80, No. 6, 1678S-1688S, December 2004. Excellent full text article review.

(24) *http://books.google.com/books?id=FvH7ySek6yAC&pg=PA3&lpg=PA3&dq=michael+f+holick+vitamin+d&source=web&ots=4OzEEZCiX2&sig=pkZAqXRlKtNB-YtwdXxt2HfSXWI#PPR6,M1*
Vitamin D Analogs in Cancer Prevention and Therapy By Jorg Reichrath, M. Friedrich, Chapter by Michael Holick Vitamin D in Book Online:

(25) *http://jn.nutrition.org/cgi/content/abstract/130/11/2648*
1,25-Dihydroxycholecalciferol Prevents and Ameliorates Symptoms of Experimental Murine Inflammatory Bowel Disease. Journal of Nutrition. 2000;130:2648-2652. Margherita T. Cantorna, Carey Munsick, Candace Bemiss and Brett D. Mahon

(26) *http://jn.nutrition.org/cgi/content/full/135/11/2739S*
Holick, Michael F, The Influence of Vitamin D on Bone Health Across the Life Cycle, The Vitamin D Epidemic and its Health Consequences J. Nutr. 135:2739S-2748S, November 2005

(27) *http://www.westonaprice.org/basicnutrition/vitamindmiracle.html*
The Miracle of Vitamin D by By Krispin Sullivan, CN on Weston Price Web Site.

(28) *http://app2.capitalreach.com/esp1204/servlet/tc?cn=asbmr&c=10169&s=20343&e=*
6950
Webcasts : Contemporary Diagnosis and Treatment of Vitamin D-Related Disorders, American Society for Bone and Mineral Disorders.

(29) *http://www.ncbi.nlm.nih.gov/pubmed/2572900*
Garland CF, Comstock GW, et al. "Serum 25-hydroxyvitamin D and colon cancer: eight-year prospective study," Lancet 1989; 2(8,673: 1,176-1,178

(30) *http://www.pubmedcentral.nih.gov/articlerender.fcgi?artid=151071*
http://jn.nutrition.org/cgi/content/abstract/130/11/2648
Regulation of renin expression and blood pressure by vitamin D3 Curt D. Sigmund, J Clin Invest. 2002 July 15; 110(2): 155–156.

(31) *http://www.ncbi.nlm.nih.gov/pubmed/11705562*
Intake of vitamin D and risk of type 1 diabetes: a birth-cohort study. Lancet 2001; 358(9,292): 1,500-1,5003. Hypponen E, Laara E, Reunanen A, Jarvelin MR, Virtanen SM.

(32) *http://www.ncbi.nlm.nih.gov/pubmed/12800453*
The effect of vitamin D3 on insulin secretion and peripheral insulin sensitivity in type 2 diabetic patients. Int J Clin Pract 2003; 57(4): 258-61. Borissova AM, Tankova T, Kirilov G, Dakovska L, Kovacheva R.

(33) http://jcem.endojournals.org/cgi/content/full/86/4/1633
Pfeifer M et al. "Effects of a short-term vitamin D3 and calcium supplementation on blood pressure and parathyroid hormone levels in elderly women." J Clin Endocrinol Metab 2001; 86: 1,633-1,637

(34) http://www.ncbi.nlm.nih.gov/pubmed/2643969
Lind L et al. "Reduction of blood pressure during long-term treatment with active vitamin D (alphacalcidol) is dependent on plasma renin activity and calcium status. A double-blind, placebo-controlled study." Am J Hypertens 1989; 2: 20-25

(35) http://www.ncbi.nlm.nih.gov/pubmed/8541004
Lind L et al. "Vitamin D is related to blood pressure and other cardiovascular risk factors in middle-aged men." Am J Hypertens 1995; 2: 20-25

(36) http://www.ncbi.nlm.nih.gov/pubmed/10939587
Embry AF, Snowdon LR, Vieth R.Ann Neurol. 2000 Aug;48(2):271-2. Vitamin D and seasonal fluctuations of gadolinium-enhancing magnetic resonance imaging lesions in multiple sclerosis.

(36A) http://www.theglobeandmail.com/servlet/story/RTGAM.20070428.wxvitamin28/BNStory/specialScienceandHealth/home
Vitamin D casts cancer prevention in new light by MARTIN MITTELSTAEDT, From Saturday's Globe and Mail, April 28, 2007

(37) http://www.ajcn.org/cgi/content/abstract/85/6/1586
Vitamin D and calcium supplementation reduces cancer risk: results of a randomized trial. American Journal of Clinical Nutrition, Vol. 85, No. 6, 1586-1591, June 2007 Joan M Lappe, Dianne Travers-Gustafson, K Michael Davies, Robert R Recker and Robert P Heaney.

(38) http://en.wikipedia.org/wiki/Vitamin_D
Wikipedia Vitamin D Page with Links

(39) http://archinte.ama-assn.org/cgi/content/full/167/16/1730
Vitamin D Supplementation and Total Mortality A Meta-analysis of Randomized Controlled Trials Philippe Autier, MD; Sara Gandini, PhD Arch Intern Med. 2007;167:1730-1737. Conclusions Intake of ordinary doses of vitamin D supplements seems to be associated with decreases in total mortality rates.

Chapter Four Iodine

Breast Cancer Prevention and Iodine Supplementation

A good friend of ours just went through an ordeal with breast cancer and asked for advice. The incidence of breast cancer has increased to 1 in 8 women, with 4,000 new cases weekly. My friend asked me if there be a preventive measure which is safe, cheap and widely available that has been overlooked? The answer is **YES,** and it's the essential mineral, **Iodine,** which was added to table salt in 1924 as part of a national program to prevent Goiter. It turns out that this same Iodine in table salt is the key to breast cancer prevention as proposed by the following list of prestigious doctors: Guy Abraham, MD *(1)*, Robert Derry MD PHD *(2) (3)*, David Brownstein MD *(4)(5)*, George Flechas MD *(6)(20)*, and Donald Miller, M.D. *(7)(8)*

Our Diet is Iodine Deficient

The problem is that we have been told to avoid table salt because it causes high blood pressure, so dietary intake of iodine has dropped to low levels, and we have a generalized iodine deficiency in the population. Currently 15% of the US adult female population is classified by the World Health Organization (WHO) as iodine deficient. *(9)* We consume a large quantity of salt in processed food, however, the salt in processed foods is not iodized salt. Unfortunately iodized table salt is not a reliable way to supplement with Iodine; it makes sense to use an Iodine supplement.

The RDA for Iodine is too Low for Optimal Health

According to Guy Abraham MD, our dietary intake of Iodine is too low, set at 150 mcg by the government RDA. Dr. Guy Abraham tells us that a healthier level of Iodine intake would be 100 times greater at 12.5 mg, which is the average Iodine intake for Japan, and this higher Iodine intake could explain why the Japanese have the lowest rates of breast, prostate and thyroid cancer.

How Safe is Iodine Supplementation?

Iodine is very safe. Iodine is the only trace element that can be ingested safely in amounts up to 100,000 times the RDA. For example, potassium iodide has been prescribed safely to large numbers pulmonary (COPD) patients in amounts up to 6 grams per day or several years. This potassium iodide is a well known treatment for COPD which helps mobilize lung secretions.*(18)* The FDA has officially stated that Iodine supplementation is safe and actually recommends 165 mg of Iodine for adults in case of Radiation Emergency to protect the population from thyroid cancer. *(17)* "Iodine allergy" is a misnomer since this name applies to allergy to iodinated radiographic contrast agents, and not to elemental iodine which is quite different. *(10)* There can be no allergy to elemental iodine, as this is an essential mineral.

Iodine Deficiency causes Fibrocystic Breast Disease, Breast Cancer and Thyroid Cancer

Iodine, a well known topical antiseptic and antimicrobial agent, also directly kills cancer cells and serves as the key player in our body's surveillance system for removing abnormal pre-cancer cells. There is considerable medical research to support this statement. Dr. B.A. Eskin published 80 papers over 30 years researching iodine and breast cancer, and he reports that iodine deficiency causes breast cancer and thyroid cancer in humans and animals.*(11)(12)* Iodine deficiency is also known to cause a pre-cancerous condition called fibrocystic breast disease. *(13)* Ghent published a paper in 1993 which showed iodine supplementation works quite well to reverse and resolve fibrocystic changes of the breast, and this is again the subject of a current clinical study.*(14)(15)*

Despite its obvious potential, not much has been done with Iodine treatment over the past 40 years in the United States. Since iodine isn't patentable and is therefore unlikely to be profitable to market, there is no money to fund studies for "FDA approval". However, FDA approval is not required since Iodine is already an additive to table salt at the supermarket. The topical antiseptic Povidone Iodine is available over-the-counter (OTC) at the grocery or drugstore.

Iodine Deficiency Diseases

As an interventional radiologist working in the hospital for 25 years, a large part of my job was evaluating thyroid abnormalities, nodules, and cysts with ultrasound, radionuclide scans, and needle biopsy. Although it was obvious these common thyroid abnormalities were due to iodine deficiency, I often wondered why none of the patients ever received iodine supplementation. The obvious answer is Iodine supplementation is ignored by mainstream medicine.

During my previous career as a radiologist, a part of my day was devoted to reading mammograms and breast ultrasound exams which showed many nodules and cysts. Fibrocystic breast disease was quite common, and these women would return for needle aspiration procedure of the many breast cysts, and needle biopsy of the benign solid nodules. Many of these ladies had recurring cyst aspiration procedures because the medical system had no other useful treatment to offer them. Well, as we have just discussed, we now know there is a very useful medical treatment, namely, Iodine supplementation which not only resolves breast cysts and fibrocystic breast disease, it also resolves ovarian cysts and thyroid cysts. Actually Iodine supplementation has always been available, but again this is ignored by mainstream medicine, and hospital based physicians are unaware of it.

Which Iodine Supplement ?

There are many Iodine supplements. Lugol's Solution has been used for many years. A new form is the 12.5 mg Iodoral tablet from Optimox.*(16)* This is the iodine supplement tablet made by Dr. Guy Abraham, a former professor of obstetrics and gynecology at UCLA who started "The Iodine Project" in 1997, and engaged two family practice physicians, Jorge Flechas and David Brownstein to carry out clinical studies of the hypothesis that the body needs 12.5 mg of iodine a day. More than 4,000 patients in this project consumed Iodine supplements from 12 to 50 mg per day, and in those with diabetes, up to 100 mg a day. They reported their findings that Iodine does indeed reverse fibrocystic disease; diabetic patients require less insulin; hypothyroid patients require less thyroid medication; symptoms of fibromyalgia resolve, and patients with migraine headaches stop having them.

The Nobel laureate Dr. Albert Szent Györgi (1893–1986), the physician who discovered vitamin C, used Iodine freely in his medical practice. The standard dose of potassium iodide given in those days was 1 gram, which contains 770 mg of iodine.

Dr. Albert Szent Györgi writes: "When I was a medical student, iodine in the form of KI (Potassium Iodide) was the universal medicine. Nobody knew what it did, but it did something and did something good. We students used to sum up the situation in this little rhyme: **If ye don't know where, what, and why Prescribe ye then K and I"**

Iodoral is available without a prescription as a nutritional supplement from VRP (Vitamin Research Products).*(21)* A bottle of 90 tablets is about 25 dollars plus shipping.*(21)* Visit the hypothyroidism page on my web site for more thyroid related information.*(22)* See David Brownstein's Book on Iodine*(4)*, and The Iodine Group for more information.*(19)* Even though Iodoral is available without a prescription, I recommend you work closely with a knowledgeable physician.

References for Chapter 4

(1) http://www.optimox.com/pics/Iodine/opt_Research_I.shtml
Publications by Guy Abraham MD on Iodine references at Optimox.com

(2) http://www.amazon.com/Breast-Cancer-Iodine-Prevent-Survive/dp/1552128849
The book, Breast Cancer and Iodine : How to Prevent and How to Survive Breast Cancer by Dr. David Derry M.D., Ph.D.

(3) http://thyroid.about.com/library/derry/bl1a.htm
Dr. David Derry Answers Reader Questions Brought to you by Mary Shomon, Your Thyroid Guide. Discussion of Iodine as Breast Cancer Prevention

(4) *http://www.drbrownstein.com/singleproduct.asp?id=787*
Iodine: Why You Need It, Why You Can't Live Without It (2nd Edition) by David Brownstein MD, Book.

(5) *http://www.optimox.com/pics/Iodine/IOD-09/IOD_09.htm*
Clinical Experience with Inorganic Non-radioactive Iodine/Iodide by David Brownstein, M.D.

(6) *www.optimox.com/pics/Iodine/IOD-10/IOD_10.htm*
Orthoiodosupplementation in a Primary Care Practice by Jorge D. Flechas, M.D.

(7) *http://www.lewrockwell.com/miller/miller20.html*
Iodine for Health by Donald W. Miller, Jr., MD on Lew Rockwell Blog

(8) *http://www.donaldmiller.com/Iodine%20Talk.doc*
Iodine in Health and Civil Defense Presented at the 24th Annual Meeting of Doctors of Disaster Preparedness at Portland State University, August 6, 2006 by Donald W. Miller, Jr., M.D.

(9) *http://www.ncbi.nlm.nih.gov/pubmed/8979164*
Int J Vitam Nutr Res. 1996;66(4):350-62. Total diet study: estimated dietary intakes of nutritional elements, 1982-1991.Pennington JA, Schoen SA. Center for Food Safety and Applied Nutrition, U.S. Food and Drug Administration, Washington, DC 20204, USA.

(10) *http://www.optimox.com/pics/Iodine/pdfs/IOD01.pdf*
Optimum Levels of Iodine for Greatest Mental and Physical Health by Guy E. Abraham, MD, Jorge D. Flechas, MD, and John C. Hakala, RPh THE ORIGINAL INTERNIST September 2002 page 5. Effect of daily ingestion of a tablet containing 5 mg iodine and 7.5 mg iodide as the potassium salt, for a period of 3 months, on the results of thyroid function tests and thyroid volume by ultrasonometry in ten euthyroid Caucasian women See Table 7.

(11) *http://cancerres.aacrjournals.org/cgi/reprint/35/9/2332*
Bernard A. Eskin et al. Rat mammary gland atypia produced by iodine blockade with perchlorate. Cancer Res. 1975 Sep;35(9):2332-9

(12) *http://cancerres.aacrjournals.org/cgi/reprint/46/2/877*
Dietary Iodine Deficiency as a Tumor Promoter and Carcinogen in Male F344/NCr Rats Masato Ohshima and Jerrold M. Ward. Cancer Research 46, 877-883, February 1, 1986

(13) *http://content.nejm.org/cgi/content/full/353/3/229*
Benign Breast Disease and the Risk of Breast Cancer. Hartmann, Lynn C. N Engl J Med Volume 353;3:229-237 July 21, 2005

(14) *http://www.ncbi.nlm.nih.gov/pubmed/8221402*
Ghent,W.R., Eskin,B.A., Low,D.A., Hill, L.P.. Iodine replacement in fibrocystic disease of the breast. Can J Surg 1993; 36:453-460.

(15) *http://clinicaltrials.gov/ct/show/NCT00237523?order=1*
Clinical Trial for Iodine treatment of Fibrocystic Breast Disease, Study for Treatment of Moderate or Severe, Periodic, "Cyclic", Breast Pain. Symbollon Pharmaceuticals Clinical Trials.gov Identifier: NCT00237523

(16) *http://www.optimox.com/pics/Iodine/opt_Iodoral.htm*
Iodoral from Optimox

(17) *http://www.fda.gov/cder/guidance/4825fnl.htm*
Guidance on Potassium Iodide as a Thyroid Blocking Agent in Radiation Emergencies, U.S. Department of Health and Human Services, Food and Drug Administration, Center for Drug Evaluation and Research (CDER), December 2001

(18) *http://www.ncbi.nlm.nih.gov/pubmed/5395878*
Bernecker C. Acta Allergol. 1969 Sep;24(3):216-25. Intermittent therapy with potassium iodide in chronic obstructive disease of the airways. A review of 10 years' experience.

(19) *http://iodine4health.com/index.htm*
The Iodine Group

(20) *http://cypress.he.net/~bigmacnc/drflechas/index.htm/iodine.htm*
George Flechas MD Web Site

(21) *http://www.vrp.com/ProductPage.aspx?ProdID=9139&zType=1*
VRP Vitamin Research Products Offers Iodoral Online, no prescription needed.

(22) *http://www.drdach.com/wst_page10.html*
Hypothyroidism Jeffrey Dach MD web site

Chapter Five

Vitamin B12 Deficiency, the Epidemic of Misdiagnosis

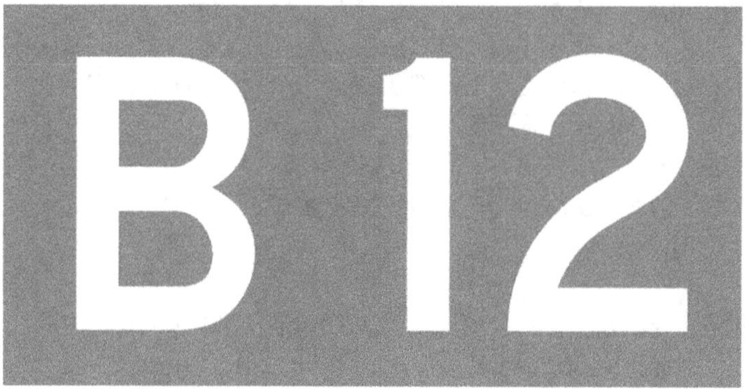

A good friend of ours, otherwise healthy, had the sudden onset of severe leg pain which baffled her doctors who could not explain it. After many months of suffering and no relief from many different medications and treatments, she tried inexpensive vitamin B12 injections, which gave her complete relief. Occasionally the pain returns and reminds her that it is time for another B12 injection. The injections are simple to do, with a syringe and tiny needle, the B12 is injected under the skin twice a week. I found this B12 story interesting, and there are many more B12 stories of misdiagnosis in the book, "Could it Be B12, An Epidemic of Misdiagnoses?" by Sally M. Pacholok R.N. and Jeffrey J Stuart D.O.*(1)*

How Common is B12 Deficiency?

Vitamin B12 deficiency is estimated to affect 10%-15% of individuals over the age of 60. *(2)* A recent study in Israel of elderly hospitalized patients found 40% had low or borderline serum B12 levels.*(3)* Vegetarians are another group with inadequate dietary B12 intake, since much of our B12 comes from meat consumption. A recent study showed 50% of long term vegetarians have B12 deficiency, with decreased serum B12 levels and elevated homocysteine levels.*(4)(5)*

What Causes B12 Deficiency?

B12 is a huge molecule and absorption depends on many cofactors, so that it is quite possible to take adequate amounts of B12 in the diet, and still have a B12 deficiency. Absorption of B12 requires gastric acid, so anything which reduces gastric acid production such as gastric surgery, atrophic gastritis, or antacid drugs could produce B12 deficiency. The very popular antacid drug Prilosec (omeprazole) has been clearly shown to decrease B12 absorption.*(6)(7)* Other antacid pills such as Prevacid, Protonix, Zantac, Nexium, Aciphex, Zantec, Tagamet, Pepcid, Maalox, and Mylanta reduce gastric acid, inhibit B12 absorption and may produce B12 deficiency. Drugs such as *Metformin* and other diabetes drugs can cause B12 deficiency. The anesthetic agent, Nitrous Oxide, or "laughing gas", used in dental or surgical procedures causes B12 deficiency.*(8)(9)(10)*

Pernicious anemia is the second most common cause of B12 deficiency. This is an autoimmune disease with loss of Intrinsic Factor, in which antibodies damage the stomach lining interrupting the B12 absorption mechanism.

Other people at risk for B12 deficiency include vegetarians, people with eating disorders such as bulimia and anorexia, inflammatory bowel disease with malabsorption (crohn's). Auto-immune diseases such as Hashimoto's thyroiditis may be associated with B12 deficiency (pernicious anemia). In addition, Miller has identified genetic defects in which transport proteins are absent or deficient causing B12 deficiency.*(11)*

Symptoms Which Might Indicate a B12 Deficiency

Vitamin B12 deficiency can cause unusual neurological symptoms such as tremor, gait disturbance, severe pain, and can mimic MS (multiple sclerosis) or even Parkinson's Syndrome. The physical signs and symptoms can often mimic other diseases and the diagnosis is frequently missed. An excellent book on the topic is: Could it Be B12? An Epidemic of Misdiagnosis by Sally M. Pacholok, R.N. and Jeffrey J Stuart, D.O. *(1)* B12 deficiency damages the myelin sheath around the nerve fibers, this is a soft fatty insulating material which is also damaged in demyelinating diseases such as multiple sclerosis.

Mental Changes:

B12 deficiency may cause the following mental changes: Irritability, apathy, sleepiness, paranoia, personality changes, depression (including post-partum depression), memory loss, dementia, cognitive dysfunction or deterioration, fuzzy thinking, psychosis, dementia, hallucinations, violent behavior, autistic behavior in children, developmental delay.

Neurological Signs and Symptoms of B12 Deficiency:

B12 deficiency may cause abnormal sensations (pain, tingling, and/or numbness of legs, arms trunk or anywhere), diminished sense of touch, pain or temperature (may mimic diabetic neuropathy Charcot foot), loss of position sense, weakness, clumsiness, tremor, any symptoms which may mimic Parkinson's or multiple sclerosis, spasticity of muscles, incontinence, paralysis, vision changes, damage to optic nerve (optic neuritis).

Vascular Problems:

Atherosclerotic vascular disease is increased by B12 deficiency including; Coronary artery disease, TIAs, CVA, heart attack, heart failure, claudication, all associated with elevated homocysteine levels caused by B12 deficiency.

Megaloblastic Anemia (enlarged red blood cells with anemia)

In this type of anemia, the red blood cells are fewer in number, yet they are larger in diameter (this large size is called megaloblastic and is measured on the CBC with the mean corpuscular volume, MCV). The anemia can cause fatigue, and weakness.

Increased Cancer Risk from B12 Deficiency

Cervical Dysplasia and increased risk for other dysplasias and cancers is associated with B12 deficiency. B12 supplementation is part of our cancer prevention program.

Testing for the Diagnosis of B12 Deficiency

Most doctors do not routinely do the serum B12 blood test which may be unreliable or diffucult to interpret because of the wide reference range.*(12)* A more accurate screening test called the methyl malonate test has been devised.*(13)(15)(16)* The substance, Methyl Malonate is elevated in the urine, and in the serum in patients with B12 deficiency. We have added this test to our standard panel, so everyone will be routinely screened with both the serum B12 level and the methyl malonate test. If the B12 level is low in spite of oral or sublingual B12 supplements, inexpensive B12 injections can be taken at home. Recent work by Kuzminski showed that daily 2 mg. oral B12 serves as well as monthly 1 mg intramuscular B12 injections.*(14)* We also test for Serum Homocysteine which is elevated in B12 deficiency, and of course the standard serum B12 test is also included in our panel. It is important to discover B12 deficiency early, since nerve damage can be irreversible if not discovered right away.

All references are hyperlinked at www.jeffreydach.com and www.naturalmedicine101.com.

References Chapter 5

(1) http://www.amazon.com/Could-Be-B12-Epidemic-Misdiagnoses/dp/1884956467
Could It Be B12?: An Epidemic of Misdiagnoses (Paperback) by Sally M. Pacholok, Jeffrey J. Stuart

(2) http://arjournals.annualreviews.org/doi/abs/10.1146/annurev.nutr.19.1.357
Annual Review of Nutrition Vol. 19: 357-377 (Volume publication date July 1999) (doi:10.1146/annurev.nutr.19.1.357) VITAMIN B12 DEFICIENCY IN THE ELDERLY , H.W. Baik and R.M. Russell USDA Human Nutrition Research Center on Aging at Tufts University

(3) http://www.ncbi.nlm.nih.gov/pubmed/11426294
J Nutr Health Aging. 2001;5(2):124-7.High prevalence and impact of subnormal serum vitamin B12 levels in Israeli elders admitted to a geriatric hospital. Shahar A, Feiglin L, Shahar DR, Levy S, Seligsohn U.

(4) http://www.ajcn.org/cgi/content/full/70/3/626S#SEC4
Cobalamin studies on 2 total vegetarian (vegan) families. Milton G Crane, UD Register, and Richard Lukens. Weimar Institute, Weimar, CA, and the Department of Medicine and School of Public Health, Loma Linda University, CA. Funded by Donald and Barbara Cox and the Callicott-Register fund.

(5) http://www.ncbi.nlm.nih.gov/pubmed/12011576?dopt=Abstract
Ann Nutr Metab. 2002;46(2):73-9.Effect of vegetarian diet on homocysteine levels. Bissoli L, Di Francesco V, Ballarin A, Mandragona R, Trespidi R, Brocco G, Caruso B, Bosello O, Zamboni M.

(6) http://www.ncbi.nlm.nih.gov/pubmed/10369631
Ann Pharmacother. 1999 May;33(5):641-3.Omeprazole and vitamin B12 deficiency. Bradford GS, Taylor CT. Birmingham Baptist Medical Center

(7) http://www.ucpress.edu/books/pages/10083/10083.ch08.php
Merrill Goozner The $800 Million Pill The Truth behind the Cost of New Drugs Chapter 8, Me Too, Story of the Drug Industry in America 1930 to 2000, Prolosic, Nexium. H Pulori, etc. Patents for living things 1980- oil eating bacteria Merrill Goozner is former Chief Economics Correspondent at the Chicago Tribune.

(8) http://www.ncbi.nlm.nih.gov/pubmed/3949064
Int J Biochem. 1986;18(2):199-202.Nitrous oxide induced vitamin B12 deficiency: measurement of methylation reactions in the fruit bat (Rousettus aegyptiacus). McLoughlin JL, Cantrill RC.

(9) http://www.aafp.org/afp/20040115/letters.html
Letters to the Editor Use of Metformin Is a Cause of Vitamin B12 Deficiency DAVID R. BUVAT, M.D. January 15, 2004 AAFP

(10) http://www.aafp.org/afp/20030301/979.pdf
Vitamin B12 Deficiency. Robert C. Oh, David L. Brown. AAFP March 1, 2003. VOL 67, No5.

(11) http://bloodjournal.hematologylibrary.org/cgi/reprint/100/2/718.pdf
Transcobalamin II 775G-C polymorphism and indices of vitamin B12 status in healthy older adults. Blood 2002 100: 718-720. Joshua W. Miller et al

(12) *http://www.clinchem.org/cgi/content/abstract/52/2/278*
Measurement of Total Vitamin B12 and Holotranscobalamin, Singly and in Combination, in Screening for Metabolic Vitamin B12 Deficiency . Joshua W. Miller et al. Clinical Chemistry. 2006;52:278-285.

(13) *http://www.ajcn.org/cgi/reprint/20/6/573.pdf*
Vitamin B12 Deficiency with Emphasis on Methylmalonic Acid as a Diagnostic Aid. Lewis A. Barness, M.D. AJCN Vol 20, No. 6, June, 1967, Ill. p 573

(14) *http://bloodjournal.hematologylibrary.org/cgi/content/full/92/4/1191*
Effective Treatment of Cobalamin Deficiency With Oral Cobalamin By Antoinette M. Kuzminski et al. Blood, Vol. 92 No. 4 (August 15), 1998: pp. 1191-1198

(15) *http://www.b12.com/*
The Norman Clinical Laboratory,an excellent web site devoted to B12 and Methyl Malonic Acid testing with many references. Dr. Norman is the medical pioneer credited with the original methyl malonate work.

(16) *http://www.clinchem.org/cgi/content/full/50/8/1482*
Urinary Methylmalonic Acid Test May Have Greater Value than the Total Homocysteine Assay for Screening Elderly Individuals for Cobalamin Deficiency. Clinical Chemistry. 2004;50:1482-1483. Letter to the Editor, Eric J. Norman Norman Clinical Laboratory, Inc., 1044 Sunwood Ct., Cincinnati, OH 45231

(17) *http://lpi.oregonstate.edu/infocenter/vitamins/vitaminB12/*
B12 information page at the Linus Pauling Institute, with excellent list of references with links.

(18) *http://www.westonaprice.org/basicnutrition/vitaminb12.html*
Vitamin B12: Vital Nutrient for Good Health By Sally Fallon and Mary G. Enig, PhD At Weston Price Foundation

(19) *http://forums.wrongdiagnosis.com/showthread.php?t=9948*
Sally Pacholok, R.N. Health Forum Message Board where you can read her messages and post your own message.

(20) *http://www.postgradmed.com/issues/2001/07_01/dharmarajan.shtml*
Approaches to vitamin B12 deficiency, Early treatment may prevent devastating complications. T. S. Dharmarajan, MD; Edward P. Norkus, PhD. VOL 110 NO 1 JULY 2001 POSTGRADUATE MEDICINE

(21) *http://www.ajcn.org/cgi/content/full/84/6/1259*
American Journal of Clinical Nutrition, Vol. 84, No. 6, 1259-1260, December 2006 Assessing the association between vitamin B-12 status and cognitive function in older adults. Joshua W Miller.

(22) http://adc.bmj.com/cgi/content/abstract/77/2/137
Arch Dis Child 1997;77:137-139 (August) Persistence of neurological damage induced by dietary vitamin B-12 deficiency in infancy, Ursula von Schenck, Christine Bender-Götze, Berthold Koletzko

Chapter 6

Glucosamine for Arthritis, The NIH GAIT Study *(1)(2)*

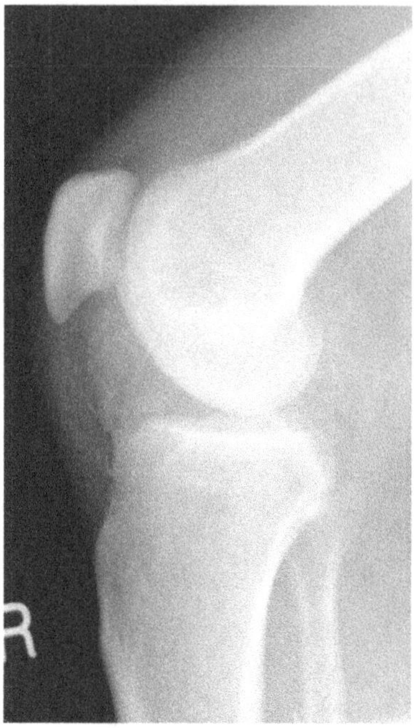

Xray of knee

You may have seen the news story in the media about the results of the NIH GAIT study which examined glucosamine and chondroitin for arthritis pain. As usual, the New York Times and the rest of the media got the story wrong.*(4)* These articles would have you discard the glucosamine and chondroitin as being ineffective for knee pain. However, on closer study, the NIH GAIT study showed that Glucosamine and Chondroitin was actually effective.*(3)* Having no adverse side effects, these are two popular nutritional supplements for osteoarthritis. Annual glucosamine sales have increased considerably over the last 10 years, increasing from 1 million dollars a year in 1995 to 700 million dollars a year in 2005.

Glucosamine Was More Effective than Celebrex

Contrary to the New York Times report, the NIH Gait study actually showed that in patients with **moderate-to-severe knee-pain**, the combination of the two supplements (glucosamine and chondroitin) **was more effective than both Celebrex and a placebo**. The glucosamine-chondroitin combination significantly reduced pain in 79 percent of those who received it. Celebrex significantly reduced pain in 69 percent of the recipients and the placebo in 54 percent.*(1)(2)(15)* The correct conclusion is the less costly glucosamine and chondroitin combination is more effective than Celebrex in cases of moderate to severe knee pain.*(3)(15)*

Financial Ties to the Drug Industry Lead to Biased Results

How is it possible for the New York Times to write the wrong story? Could it be possible that the authors of the New England Journal reporting the GAIT findings were biased in favor of the drug Celebrex, and against the supplements?*(15)* Jay Gordon MD raises this question in his article, "Did You Understand the Arthritis Study? I Did."*(16)* Dr Gordon points out that the authors received financial rewards from the makers of the arthritis drug, Celebrex. This conflict of interests biased the authors to spin the results in favor of the drug and against glusosamine. Dr. Gordon compiled a list of financial ties between the drug makers and the authors of the GAIT Study.

Financial Ties to the Drug Industry

Drs. Bingham, Brandt, Clegg, Hooper, and Schnitzer received consulting fees or served on advisory boards for McNeil Consumer and Specialty Pharmaceuticals.
Drs. Brandt, Moskowitz, Schnitzer, and Schumacher received consulting fees or served on advisory boards for Pfizer.
Dr. Brandt reports equity interests in Pfizer.
Drs. Moskowitz and Weisman report lecture fees from Pfizer.
Dr. Brandt reports lecture fees from McNeil Consumer and Specialty Pharmaceuticals, and royalties from books related to osteoarthritis.
Drs. Bingham, Clegg, Hooper, Jackson, Molitor, Sawitzke, and Schnitzer, had grant support from Pfizer.
Dr. Bingham reports grant support from McNeil Consumer and Specialty Pharmaceuticals.
Dr. Moskowitz reports having served as an expert consultant for Pfizer.

What is Glucosamine and Chondroitin?

Glucosamine and chondroitin sulfate are substances found naturally in the body. Glucosamine is a form of amino sugar that is used for cartilage formation and repair. Chondroitin sulfate is part of a large protein molecule (proteoglycan) that gives cartilage elasticity. Both glucosamine and chondroitin sulfate are sold as dietary or nutritional supplements available at the health food store without the need for a prescription. Glucosamine is a less expensive and safer alternative to NSAID pain pills, commonly prescribed for arthritis pain.***(14)***

Safety of Glucosamine/Chondroitin Compared to the Safety of NSAIDS, Adverse Side Effects of Celebrex

The media stories on the GAIT Study also fail to mention the fact that Glucosamine and Chondroitin have **no adverse side effects**, while Celebrex causes gastric bleeding, ulceration and **death**. This is an important distinction. Celebrex is a NSAID pain pill. NSAID drugs are similar to aspirin, ibuprofen, and naproxen. It has been estimated conservatively that 16,500 NSAID-related deaths occur among patients with rheumatoid arthritis or osteoarthritis every year in the United States.

Deaths Reported from Celebrex

On 4/20/99, The Wall Street Journal reported that celecoxib (Celebrex) has been linked to 10 deaths and 11 cases of gastrointestinal hemorrhages. Five of the 10 who died suffered from gastrointestinal bleeding or ulcers.*(5)(6)* On December 17, 2004, Pfizer publicly announced that patients taking Celebrex may have an elevated risk of suffering heart attack and stroke. The National Cancer Institute designed a study to research the effects of Celebrex on cancer. This Pfizer-sponsored study was suspended after preliminary evidence showed that clinical trial patients who were taking 400 to 800 milligrams of Celebrex were two and a half times more likely to suffer from heart attack or cardiovascular stroke than patients in the control group.*(17)*

Celebrex No Safer than the Older NSAIDS

An editorial published in the British Medical Journal reports that COX-2 selective painkillers (Like Celebrex and Vioxx) are no safer on your stomach than traditional painkillers.*(7)* When COX-2 drugs like Celebrex were introduced to the market, their makers claimed these drugs were as effective and much safer than the older NSAID drugs. In other words, they were easier on the stomach. Older NSAIDs, such as Aleve and Naproxen, are known to cause adverse gastrointestinal side effects like ulcers and bleeding. The authors of this BMJ editorial say that the original studies were flawed and that the new COX-2 drugs like Celebrex and Vioxx are just as dangerous as older NSAID drugs.*(7)(8)*

Annual Death Rate for NSAIDS

The following references provide the estimated annual death rate from NSAIDs (Nonsteroidal anti-inflammatory drugs including aspirin, ibuprofen, naproxen, diclofenac, ketoprofen, and tiaprofenic acid.) How many of these deaths are due to Celebrex vs. the other NSAIDs? Compare this number of deaths to ZERO deaths from glucosamine and chondroitin. Each year, there are an estimated 103,000 hospitalizations and **16,500 deaths** in the United States attributed to complications from NSAID-associated gastric ulcers.*(9)(10)* Another medical report says there are **7,600 deaths and 76,000 hospitalizations** in the United States annually from NSAID drug adverse side effects, mostly gastric bleeding. (NSAIDs include aspirin, ibuprofen, naproxen, diclofenac, ketoprofen, and tiaprofenic acid.) Compare this number of deaths to ZERO deaths from glucosamine and chondroitin.*(11)(12)* According to November 2004 Congressional testimony by Dr. David Graham, associate director for science and medicine in the FDA's Office of Drug Safety, there were 160,000 heart attacks and as many as 55,000 patients may have died as a result of taking Vioxx. *(13)*

Glucosamine and Chondroitin is a SAFER ALTERNATIVE to NSAIDS

The entire point of the above is to demonstrate the safety profile of glucosamine and chondroitin as compared to the dangers of NSAIDS. Glucosamine and chondroitin are nutritional supplements available without a prescription at the vitamin store, most drugstores, and grocery stores.

References are hyperlinked at www.jeffreydach.com and www.naturalmedicine101.com.

References Chapter 6

(1) *http://nccam.nih.gov/research/results/gait/qa.htm*
NIH GAIT STUDY

(2) *http://nccam.nih.gov/research/results/gait/*
NIH GAIT STUDY RESULTS

(3) *http://www.drtheo.com/news/*
The Glucosamine/Chondroitin Arthritis Intervention Trial (GAIT)
Results, Commentary and Analysis by (Jason Theodosakis, MD, MS, MPH, FACPM) Member of the Study's Oversight Steering Committee

(4) *http://www.nytimes.com/2006/02/23/health/23arthritis.html?ex=1298350800&en=8f65c5d34299201d&ei=5088&partner=rssnyt&emc=rss*
Supplements Fail to Stop Arthritis Pain, Study Says By GINA KOLATA New York Times February 23, 2006

(5) *http://implants.clic.net/tony/Corner/H/0401.html*
April 20, 1999 Monsanto's Superaspirin Celebrex Has Been Linked to Several Deaths By ROCHELLE SHARPE Staff Reporter of THE WALL STREET JOURNAL WASHINGTON

(6) *http://www.hopkins-arthritis.org/arthritis-news/1999/comments.html*
John Hopkins Arthritis Information Web Site: On 4/20/99, The Wall Street Journal reported that celecoxib (Celebrex) has been linked to 10 deaths and 11 cases of gastrointestinal hemorrhages. Five (four men age 45-88 and one woman age 75) of the 10 who died suffered from gastrointestinal bleeding or ulcers.

(7) *http://bmj.bmjjournals.com/cgi/content/full/324/7349/1287*
BMJ 2002;324:1287-1288 (1 June) Editorials. Are selective COX 2 inhibitors superior to traditional non steroidal anti-inflammatory drugs? Adequate analysis of the CLASS trial indicates that this may not be the case. Peter Jüni, Anne WS Rutjes, Paul A Dieppe.

(8) *http://www.adrugrecall.com/celebrex/celebrex.html*
Celebrex arthritis drug entered the U.S. marketed in January 1999. The FDA began to send Celebrex manufacture, Pharmacia, warnings that the agency was concerned with

the promotional advertisements that were misrepresenting the safety of Celebrex. FDA letter to the drug company on April 6, 2000.

(9) *http://www.medicalnewstoday.com/articles/40105.php*
NEXIUM(R) Shown To Reduce Gastric Ulcers In At-Risk Patients Using Long-Term NSAIDs Each year, there are an estimated 103,000 hospitalizations and 16,500 deaths in the United States attributed to complications from NSAID-associated gastric ulcers.(5) Among the elderly, NSAID use accounts for nearly one third of gastric-ulcer-related hospitalizations,(6) with an associated four-fold increased risk of death.(7)

(10) *https://content.nejm.org/cgi/content/extract/341/18/1397*
Wolfe M, Lichtenstein R, Singh G. Gastrointestinal toxicity of nonsteroidal anti-inflammatory drugs. N Engl J Med 1999;340:1888-1899.

(11) *http://www.annals.org/cgi/content/full/127/6/429*
Unnecessary Prescribing of NSAIDs and the Management of NSAID-Related Gastropathy in Medical Practice by Robyn Tamblyn, PhD; Laeora Berkson, MD, 15 September 1997, Volume 127 Issue 6, Pages 429-438

(12) *http://gut.bmj.com/cgi/reprint/52/4/600.pdf*
Non-steroidal anti-inflammatory drugs: overall risks and management. Complementary roles for COX-2 inhibitors and proton pump inhibitors by C J Hawkey, M J S Langman Gut 2003;52:600-608

(13) *http://www.senate.gov/~finance/hearings/testimony/2004test/111804dgtest.pdf*
David Graham Senate Testimony November 2004. Dr. Eric Topol at the Cleveland Clinic recently estimated up to 160,000 cases of heart attacks and strokes due to Vioxx, in an article published in the New England Journal of Medicine

(14) *http://ww2.arthritis.org/conditions/alttherapies/Glucosamine.asp*
What are Glucosamine and Chondroitin Sulfate? Arthritis Foundation

(15) *http://content.nejm.org/cgi/content/short/354/8/795*
Volume 354:795-808 February 23, 2006 Number 8
Glucosamine, Chondroitin Sulfate, and the Two in Combination for Painful Knee Osteoarthritis. Daniel O. Clegg, M.D et al.

(16) *http://www.huffingtonpost.com/jay-gordon/did-you-understand-the-ar_b_16399.html*
Jay Gordon, MD Did You Understand the Arthritis Study? I Did. February 26, 2006 Huffington Post.

(17) *http://www.nih.gov/news/pr/dec2004/od-17Q&A.htm*
NIH Halts Use of COX-2 Inhibitor in Large Cancer Prevention Trial

Section Two

Disease Mongering by the Drug Companies

This section deals with the topic of disease mongering by the drug companies with the SSRI drugs for depression, statin drugs for high cholesterol, and other drugs for restless leg syndrome. The Bisphosphonate drugs for osteoporosis are discussed in a later section.

Disease Mongering, a practice used to sell drugs and increase corporate profits, relies heavily on television advertising. With the advent of the internet revolution with web sites and blogs which satirize and ridicule disease mongering advertisements, this practice will be recognized as counter-productive and will eventually be abandoned.

Chapter Seven Restless Leg

Disease Mongering for Restless Leg Syndrome

A textbook example of disease mongering by the pharmaceutical industry is the case of Requip for Restless Leg Syndrome. Requip is a powerful drug for Parkinson's Disease. Requip is also used to treat movement disorders caused by anti-psychotic drugs for mental patients (such as Prolixin and Haldol). Mirapex is similar to Requip. Adverse side effects of Requip includes *compulsive gambling and hypersexual behavior.*(*1*)

Magnesium Deficiency Causes Restless Legs

Magnesium deficiency causes muscle cramps at night and is the most common cause of Restless Leg Syndrome. (*2*) Sixty Eight Per Cent (68%) of Americans are Magnesium deficient, according to the *USDA Agricultural Research Service.(3)* Restless Leg Syndrome, or leg muscle cramping during sleep is not a reason for powerful Parkinson's drugs. Inexpensive magnesium supplementation usually resolves the problem. Using a drug like Requip instead of supplementing for magnesium deficiency is the height of lunacy, and would be comical if it wasn't tragic. This is typical drug mongering indicative of a broken medical system.

Magnesium Deficiency, Not Requip Deficiency

In a medical study by Hornyack, Restless Leg Syndrome (RLS) significantly improved after supplementing with magnesium (about 300 mg each evening for four to six weeks).(*4*) Another study by Popoviciu showed that magnesium deficiency causes neuromuscular excitability and impaired sleep.(*5*) Another study by Bartel showed IV Magnesium to be curative for Restless Leg Syndrome when IV magnesium was incidentally given to pregnant women as a treatment for eclampsia.(*6*) Magnesium supplementation is especially important for diabetic patients with insulin resistance.(*7*) There are many more studies in the medical literature showing the connection between magnesium deficiency and restless legs at night, muscle cramps and muscle pain. We have found in our experience that oral magnesium supplementation works quite well, resolving the problem promptly in most cases.

What is Disease Mongering?

Step One: Create an Illusory Disease called a "Syndrome"

Disease mongering is a marketing program that creates the illusion of disease where in fact, there is none. Instead a real disease, the marketing program uses a symptom or a "risk factor" to create fear in the mass market.

Another example of disease mongering in shown in a later chapter *on Bisphosphonate drugs* (Fosamax, Actonel and Boniva), with Sally Field as television spokeswomen.*(8)* These Sally Field ads create the fear of a real disease called osteoporosis in millions of women who have a lesser diagnosis called osteopenia. Fracture rates actually increase in this Osteopenia group when they take bisphosphonates.

A true disease requires definite pathologic markers that clearly differentiate normal from abnormal. Examples of a real diseases are heart disease in which arteries are blocked, cancer in which abnormal cells invade and can be identified on biopsy, and hypothyroidism in which there are typical symptoms and lab values.

Step Two: Market the New Illusory Disease

To popularize the new illusory disease condition, a pretend grassroots organization is created such as the Restless Legs Syndrome Foundation, a questionable organization sponsored with money from the GlaxoSmithKline (GSK) and Boehringer Ingelheim, makers of the RLS drugs. This is called creative marketing.

Step Three: Create A Marketing Gimmick called "Awareness Week"

In order to make the "worried well" fear they have the new syndrome and need the drug, RLS Awareness Week was invented, and supports groups set up to offer a symptom check list so the masses could self-diagnose themselves as victims and 'sufferers' of the illusory disease.

Step Four: Direct to Consumer Advertising

DTC Television ads imply that your doctor missed your symptoms and failed to diagnose your new syndrome called "Restless Leg". The ads are not required to be truthful and instead may convey misleading, false or incomplete information. *Thirty Nine Special Interest Groups* have asked Congress to ban DTC drug advertising.*(9)*

Where are the Responsible Prescribing Physicians?

Moira Dolan, MD of the Medical Accountability Network says the following:

> "The Restless Legs Syndrome campaign includes all of the essential ingredients for successful disease mongering. Annual Mirapex (Boehringer) sales are over $324 million and Glaxo's Requip makes over $500 million a year. The astounding transparency of the whole-cloth invention of RLS for the sales of the corresponding drugs reflects poorly on the prescribing physician. It represents a gross abdication of

the responsibility of doctors to act as advocates and at least sentient information managers for their patients." *(10)* endquote Dr Dolan.

How to Make Money in the Drug Industry

Identify a nutritional deficiency in the population (such as magnesium deficiency), create a new syndrome caused by the nutritional deficiency (such as Restless Leg), and then start a disease mongering campaign to convince the masses to take an expensive, dangerous, powerful drug (Requip and Mirapex) instead of an inexpensive mineral such as magnesium, that actually solves the problem. This template can be copied and repeated many times over, and it is.

References Chapter 7

(1) http://news.nationalgeographic.com/news/2005/07/0712_050712_parkinsons.html

Compulsive Gambling, Sex Linked to Parkinson's Drugs Stefan Lovgren for National Geographic News July 12, 2005

(2) http://www.pubmedcentral.nih.gov/articlerender.fcgi?tool=pmcentrez&artid=2146789

Can Fam Physician. 1996 July; 42: 1348–1351. Muscle cramps and magnesium deficiency: case reports.D. L. Bilbey and V. M. Prabhakaran

(3) http://www.ars.usda.gov/Services/docs.htm?docid=11219

USDA Agricultural Research Service,Percentage of individuals meeting DRI - Magnesium - 32 per cent

(4) http://www.ncbi.nlm.nih.gov/pubmed/9703590.

Magnesium therapy for periodic leg movements-related insomnia and restless legs syndrome: an open pilot study.Hornyak M et al. Sleep. 1998 Aug 1;21(5):501-5

(5) http://www.ncbi.nlm.nih.gov/pubmed/8363978.

Clinical, EEG, electromyographic and polysomnographic studies in restless legs syndrome caused by magnesium deficiency. Popoviciu L et al. Rom J Neurol Psychiatry. 1993 Jan-Mar;31(1):55-61

(6) http://www.aasmnet.org/JCSM/Articles/020213.pdf

Intravenous Magnesium Sulfate May Relieve Restless Legs Syndrome in Pregnancy Sharon Bartel; Sarah Zallek, M.D. Journal of Clinical Sleep Medicine, Vol. 2, No. 2, 2006

(7) http://www.ias.ac.in/currsci/dec252002/1456.pdf

Magnesium deficiency and diabetes mellitus. Chetan P. Hans, R. Sialy and Devi D. Bansal CURRENT SCIENCE, VOL. 83, NO. 12, 25 DECEMBER 2002.

(8) *http://jeffreydach.com/2008/03/09/bisphosphonates-for-osteoporosis-a-closer-look-at-the-data-by-jeffrey-dach-md.aspx*
Bisphosphonates for Osteoporosis, A Closer Look at the Data by Jeffrey Dach MD

(9) *http://www.czommercialalert.org/news/news-releases/2006/05/39-health-seniors-groups-call-on-congress-to-end-to-dtc-prescription-drug-ads*
NEWS RELEASE May 24th, 2006 39 Health & Seniors Groups Call on Congress to End to DTC Prescription Drug Ads. Gary Ruskin, executive director of Commercial Alert.

(10) *http://www.medicalaccountability.net/essay_RLS.html*
Selling Drugs and Disease, the Case of the Restless Leg Syndrome By Moira Terese Dolan, M.D. of the Medical Acountablilty Network

Aditional References

Television Ads, Videos

(11) *http://www.requip.com/tv_commercial.html*
Requip TV comercial

(12) *http://blogs.consumerreports.org/health/2007/11/finally-an-anti.html*
November 01, 2007 Finally, an antidote to TV drug ads consumer reports Jamie Hirsch evaluates the Requip Ad.

(13) *http://www.youtube.com/results?search_query=requip&search_type=*
Requip videos on U-tube

(14) *http://www.dailycomedy.com/videos/567*
Comedy video discussing requip reatless leg and their marketing

Disease Mongering

(15) *http://medicine.plosjournals.org/perlserv?request=get-document&doi=10.1371/journal.pmed.0030170*
Giving Legs to Restless Legs: A Case Study of How the Media Helps Make People Sick Steven Woloshin*, Lisa M. Schwartz

(16) *http://www.pbs.org/kcet/wiredscience/story/76-the_business_of_disease.html*
The Business of Disease from Wired Science

(17) *http://www.consumerreports.org/cro/health-fitness/health-care/medical-ripoffs-11-07/requip-commercial/requip-commercial.htm*
What the ad doesn't tell you Excerpts from a Requip ad, deconstructed, Consumer Reports.

(18) *http://www.knowledgeofhealth.com/report.asp?story=Disease+Mongering+and +the+American+Health+Movement*
Bill Sardi on Disease mongering

(19) *http://www.bmj.com/cgi/content/full/324/7342/886*
Selling sickness: the pharmaceutical industry and disease mongering Commentary: Medicalisation of risk factors, Selling sickness: the pharmaceutical industry and disease mongering Ray Moynihan, journalist, Iona Heath, general practitioner, David Henry, professor of clinical pharmacology. BMJ 2002;324:886-891 (13 April)

(20) *http://www.diseasemongering.org/downloads/abstracts.pdf*
ABSTRACTS FROM THE INAUGURAL CONFERENCE ON DISEASE MONGERING

(21) *http://jeffreydach.com/2008/03/09/bisphosphonates-for-osteoporosis-a-closer-look-at-the-data-by-jeffrey-dach-md.aspx*
Bisphosphonates for Osteoporosis, A Closer Look at the Data by Jeffrey Dach MD

(22) *http://www.yourlawyer.com/topics/overview/requip*
Suffered from Requip Side Effects? Lawyer wants to litigate.

(23) *http://www.cbsnews.com/stories/2007/04/05/health/webmd/main2650648.shtml?*
source=RSSattr=Health_2650648
24-Hour Parkinson's Drug: Longer Relief? Longer-Acting Requip May Reduce Need For Commonly Used Levodopa April 5, 2007. CBS News.

(24) *http://deliverrants.blogspot.com/2006/08/we-have-nothing-to-fear-but-pharmas.html*
Blogger Comment: WE HAVE NOTHING TO FEAR BUT PHARMAS THEMSELVES I was watching TV the other night and saw a commercial for some new medication for something that sounded serious ... "RLS"! They went on to explain that RLS was "restless leg syndrome." WHAT?

(25) *http://us.gsk.com/products/assets/us_requip.pdf*
REQUIP Web Site: (ropinirole hydrochloride) Tablets REQUIP (ropinirole hydrochloride) is an orally administered non-ergoline dopamine agonist.It is the hydrochloride salt of 4-[2-(dipropylamino)ethyl]-1,3-dihydro-2H-indol-2-one monohydrochloride and has an empirical formula of C16H24N2O•HCl. The molecular weight is 296.84 (260.38 as the free base).

(26) *http://www.mirapex.com/*
Mirapex web site

(27) *http://www.rls.org/*
Restless Leg Foundation Web Site

Magnesium Treats Restless Leg Syndrome

(28) http://www.purecaps.com/healthnotes.asp?org=pureencaps&ContentID=1255009
Treatable causes of restless leg syndrome, Pure Encapsulations Newsletter

(29) http://www.consumerlab.com/tnp.asp?siteid=consumerlab&docid=/tnp/pg000817
Consumer Labs Restless Leg Syndrome Treated with Magnesium

(30) http://www.springerlink.com/content/u51346w213147836/
Magnesium depletion in patients on long-term chlorthalidone therapy for essential hypertension.

(31) http://www.mgwater.com/
Magnesium Information Web Site

(32) http://www.mbschachter.com/importance_of_magnesium_to_human.htm
The Importance of Magnesium to Human Nutrition by Michael B. Schachter M.D., F.A.C.A.M. **Genetic Marker for Restless Leg Syndrome:** Financed by Drug Companies to Market Requip. This is a rare marker affecting a small number of people. Magnesium Deficiency is far more common. This is a blatant misuse of genetics.

(33) http://brain.oxfordjournals.org/cgi/content/full/126/6/1485
Brain, Vol. 126, No. 6, 1485-1492, June 2003 Autosomal dominant restless legs syndrome maps on chromosome 14q, Maria Teresa Bonati1, Luigi Ferini-Strambi2, Paolo Aridon, Alessandro Oldani2, Marco Zucconi and Giorgio Casari Human Molecular Genetics Unit.

Magnesium Deficiency

(34) http://www.pubmedcentral.nih.gov/pagerender.fcgi?artid=1345822&pageindex=1#page
A clinical approach to common electrolyte problems: 4. Hypomagnesemia. C Berkelhammer and R A Bear. Can Med Assoc J. 1985 February 15; 132(4): 360–368.

(35) http://www.ncbi.nlm.nih.gov/pubmed/8264519
Clinical manifestations of magnesium deficiency.Abbott LG, Rude RK. Miner Electrolyte Metab. 1993;19(4-5):314-22.

(36) http://www.ncbi.nlm.nih.gov/pubmed/7977315
Magnesium deficiency: pathophysiologic and clinical overview. Am J Kidney Dis. 1995 Jun;25(6):973.

(37) *http://www.ncbi.nlm.nih.gov/pubmed/6499696*
Drugs. 1984 Oct;28 Suppl 1:143-50. Magnesium deficiency. Causes and clinical implications.

(38) *http://www.ncbi.nlm.nih.gov/pubmed/14977544*
Front Biosci. 2004 May 1;9:1278-93. Magnesium in clinical medicine.

(39) *http://www.ncbi.nlm.nih.gov/pubmed/17402291*
High fructose consumption combined with low dietary magnesium intake may increase the incidence of the metabolic syndrome by inducing inflammation. Rayssiguier Y, Gueux E, Nowacki W, Rock E, Mazur A. Magnes Res. 2006 Dec;19(4):237-43.

(40) *http://www.ncbi.nlm.nih.gov/pubmed/7020347*
Magnesium deficiency. Etiology and clinical spectrum.Flink EB. Acta Med Scand Suppl. 1981;647:125-37.

(41) *http://www.ncbi.nlm.nih.gov/pubmed/7922443*
Should we supplement magnesium in critically ill patients? Olerich MA, Rude RK. New Horiz. 1994 May;2(2):186-92.

(42) *http://www.ncbi.nlm.nih.gov/pubmed/3282851*
Magnesium metabolism in health and disease.Elin RJ.Clinical Pathology Department, National Institutes of Health, Bethesda, Maryland

Videos

(43) *http://blogs.consumerreports.org/health/2007/11/finally-an-anti.html*
Blog entry for Consumer Reports video discusses disease mongering in the Requip Video Ad

(44) *http://www.youtube.com/watch?v=pDvm-5Sochs*
This is the video for the Consumer Reports Video on Requip

(45) *http://www.youtube.com/watch?v=PL3G1MngqK4*
This is the original Requip Ad video in U tube.

Chapter Eight SSRI

Paxil, Prozac and SSRI Induced Suicide

Rush Hospital in Chicago, Internship Years

In 1977, a first year intern at Rush Hospital in Chicago earned an annual salary of $10,000, a minuscule amount, even in those days. By 1978, having survived the internship experience, I was a cocky young MD who could handle anything. Needing the money, I eagerly took a job moonlighting as the Emergency Room doctor in a small hospital in Kankakee, Illinois. This was before the days of Board Certification in Emergency Room Medicine, and my internship made me imminently qualified. The fact that my dad was a doctor on the hospital staff also helped.

Internship

One vivid memory of the weekend ER moonlighting experience was one in which the young doc from the previous shift rushed past me on the way out the door in a hurry. Upon entering the ER, I was supplied with a clipboard and stethoscope, and directed to the examining room. The first patient was an 11 year old boy lying dead on the examining table with his head tilted to the side. Apparently his parents came home to discover he had hung himself in the closet, and they rushed the boy into the ER clinging to the hope that it wasn't too late for resuscitation. The ER staff had been unable to revive him. It was at this point I realized that the previous doctor had left me with the unpalatable task of informing the grief stricken parents that their son was dead, a task which clearly was one of the worst experiences of my medical career and of my life.

Cymbalta Drug Study Induces Suicide

Sharing a similar burden of unspeakable grief were the parents of 19 year old Traci Johnson, a normally healthy, 19-year-old with no history of depression. She needed money for college, and signed on as a participant for $150 a day in a Lilly drug trial for "urinary stress incontinence" which involved the SSRI drug, Cymbalta. Four weeks after starting on the drug, she hung herself with a scarf in the shower room. David Shaffer, an Eli Lilly Spokesman in Indianapolis, admitted that five test subjects including Traci committed suicide while in the drug study. None of the subjects were depressed before entering the study. Remember, the study was testing a urinary tract problem, not depression. *(1)(2)(3)(4)(5)*

FDA Black Box Warning

This story is not an isolated event. As of this date, there are at least 1,400 similar stories of SSRI induced suicide and violence including 18 school shootings, 41 road rage tragedies, and 110 murder-suicides.*(6)* In reply, the FDA issued an SSRI-Suicide advisory on March 22, 2004, and a "black box" suicide warning label for all SSRI drugs as of January 2005. In 2002, 11 million prescriptions for SSRI drugs were given to children, 2.7 million of them to children under 12 years.*(7)(8)(9)(10)*

Common Findings in Patients on SSRI's

SSRI drugs are so prevalent in the population that many patients come through my office with the obvious signs of exhaustion, insomnia and agitation. They may have purple rings under the eyes, and they usually have hyper-active reflexes. The involuntary facial movements, tics, and mouth and tongue movements are common, and when observed in the general population, these are tell-tale signs of adverse drug effects. For example, when observing nationally televised political speeches, the figures in the background may demonstrate involuntary facial movements indicating long term SSRI drug usage.*(11)* These movements are called "Tardive Dyskinesia", including rhythmic involuntary movements of the tongue, face, mouth, or jaw and frequent poking out of the tongue, chewing, puckering, or blowing out of the cheeks.

Adverse Side Effects

Tardive dyskinesia is a dreaded complication of anti-psychotic medications such as prolixin and haldol, in the past associated with institutionalized patients. Tardive dyskinesia is actually an iatrogenic form of Parkinson's disease with a tremor upon initiation of voluntary motion and the classic pill rolling hand tremor. In its early stages, the SSRI induced dyskinesia effect can be subtle. For example, years back, a previous tennis opponent exhibited signs of SSRI drug use. I noticed he could easily hit a winning angled shot into the corner, but completely lost his coordination from the intentional effort of the serve which went wild. He later disclosed he had been taking an SSRI drug for many years. Anyone concerned about maintaining fine motor coordination should be aware of this side effect.*(11)*

Listening to Prozac

In the early 90's, Peter Kramer's book, Listening to Prozac, suggested that Prozac and other SSRI drugs were safe, non-habit forming and even suitable for only mild social phobias. *(12)* Kramer also speculated that this SSRI drug invites a future possibility of "cosmetic psychopharmacology", in which the patient becomes more confident, articulate and less bashful and shy while on the drug. Prozac would produce a "more socially confident" personality. In those days, my doctor colleagues would laud the SSRI drugs they were taking, and those who couldn't take them made excuses. The surgeons couldn't take the SSRI drugs because it caused a tremor which interfered with eye hand coordination and impaired their ability to operate.

Hidden Dangers of SSRIs

Of course, we know now the hidden dangers of the SSRI antidepressants that experts like David Healy (Let them Eat Prozac), Joseph Glenmullen (Prozac Backlash) and Peter R. Breggin (Talking Back to Prozac) have been writing about for years.*(13)(14)(15)(16)* Not only do the SSRI drugs cause akathesia, a form of agitation which drives people to commit suicide, they also cause sexual dysfunction (impotence), tremor, involuntary body and facial movements, tardive dyskinesia, and hyperactive reflexes indicating a hyperactive nervous system. The SSRI induced loss of sexual function may be irreversible even after discontinuation of the drug.*(17)(18)(19)(20)*

Akasthesia, Suicide and Self Harm from SSRI Drugs

As pointed out by David Healy, the SSRI drugs (selective serotonin reuptake inhibitors) are by no means selective in their actions on brain neurotransmitter systems. Imagine a pinball let loose in the pinball machine. Most of the time, the pinball hits the correct bumpers and lights up the scoreboard. However, in a small percentage of patients the pinball bounces around affecting the wrong neurotransmitter systems in the brain, causing the machine to go "tilt". These are the "akasthesia", agitation cases estimated by the FDA to affect 1 in 50 patients, some of these inflicting self harm or committing suicide.*(7)* The drug companies who finance the research have simply avoided the question of why this happens. For example, what are the preliminary lab tests to identify the subpopulation at risk for these adverse effects? We don't know. Currently the only test is a trial of the SSRI medication to find out. As pointed out by Healy during FDA testimony, we track postal parcels 100 times better than we track adverse side effects from SSRI drugs.

University of Illinois Medical School

I started medical school at the University of Illinois in Chicago in 1972. Robert Mendelsohn (author of Confessions of a Medical Heretic) was my adviser and I spent a few evenings at his dinner table learning things about the institution of medicine not safely repeated to anyone if I wished to continue medical school.*(1)(2)*

After a full year listening to basic science lectures and taking exams, our class was released into the hospital wards to start clerkships. This involved making rounds with the intern and resident team examining patients and doing the "scut work" which maintained the University teaching hospital.*(3)* Doing rounds was a daily ritual, and we methodically worked our way up and down the long corridors which had the distinctive smell of alcohol and pseudomonas.

Clerkship Rotations

My first rotation was internal medicine, and we saw the usual litany of diseases: diabetes, rheumatoid arthritis, GI bleeding, congestive heart failure, cancer, and various bacterial and viral infections. After examining each patient, we convened in the hallway wearing our long white coats and stethoscopes as in a football huddle to discuss the diagnosis and treatment. Actually, the discussion was between the intern and resident, while the rest of us listened in. The two of them routinely had a running debate punctuated by brief forays into the rooms to examine patients. Both of them were armed with a pocket notebook inscribed with references to the medical literature, brandished in support of their arguments and decisions regarding testing or treatment. On a good day, I endeared myself to the intern by starting a difficult I.V., or by making a diagnostic coup like homonymous hemianopsia or acute intermittent porphyria.

Fraud and Misconduct in SSRI Research

In those days, the medical literature was rock solid truth and trustworthy beyond question. It was inconceivable to us that any doctor would ever falsify or distort the results of a medical study or research. After all, people's lives were hanging in the balance. This gradually changed over time. I am not sure when awareness of problems with the medical literature emerged and it became sadly obvious that much of medical science is up for sale. After this revelation, I became skeptical and I now tend to believe the data more than the written conclusions of any medical study. A recent example of this fraudulent conduct in medical research is given in the BBC documentary on the SSRI drug Seroxat (Paxil) and pediatric prescriptions.*(4)(5)*

Minimal Benefit in Children

We have previously discussed the adverse risks of SSRI drugs including agitation, suicidal or violent behavior, movement disorders, and chemical dependency in adults.*(6)* We might imagine their "side effects" in children are no less, but what about their efficacy? Surely they must be magic pills against a debilitating "illness" to risk such terrible consequences. However, Jon Jureidini in a comprehensive review of the available data found only minimal benefit from the SSRI drugs in children. He writes," The magnitude of benefit is unlikely to be sufficient to justify risking those harms, so confidently recommending these drugs as a treatment option, let alone as first line treatment, would be inappropriate."*(7)*

A Dirty Little Secret

According to Irving Kirsch in Prevention & Treatment, "there is now unanimous agreement that the mean difference between response to antidepressant drugs and response to inert placebo is very small. It is so small that, despite sample sizes involving hundreds of participants, 57% of the trials funded by the pharmaceutical industry failed to show a significant difference between drug and placebo. Most of these negative data **were not** published and were accessible only by gaining access to US Food and Drug Administration (FDA) documents. The small difference between the drug response and the placebo response has been a "dirty little secret". It was not known to the general public, depressed patients, or even their physicians".*(8)(19)(20)*

Manipulating the Data

Various methods were used to manipulate the results of SSRI drug studies to insure a favorable outcome:

1) Responders to the placebo are eliminated at the beginning of the study. (This is called placebo washout)
2) Benzodiazepine sedatives were given to mask the SSRI induced agitation.
3) Unfavorable drug studies are buried in the file cabinet and not disclosed to the public.
4) Miscoding suicidal events as "emotional lability", and homicidal events as "aggression" to hide suicidal events from regulators.
5) False attribution of suicide to the placebo arm.
6) Hiring ghost writers to make the medical articles more favorable.
7) Cash settlements for SSRI drug litigants serving to seal the court records and hide unfavorable drug studies from the public.

Using these and other gimmicks, the drug industry managed to gain FDA approval for the SSRI class of drugs.

Halt the Waiver System at the FDA

Since the FDA approval is the foundation of our medical system, the first step in restoring integrity to the FDA is to halt the "waiver system" which gives doctors immunity from prosecution for conflicts of interest. This waiver system allows doctors to deliberate on FDA advisory committees while receiving money from the drug industry, a conflict of interest that is also a federal crime *(9)(10)*.

Direct to Consumer Advertising

Direct to consumer advertising of SSRI drugs presents the message that depression is a disease caused by a chemical imbalance in the brain, namely a deficiency of serotonin, which is cured by the SSRI drug.*(12)* Unfortunately, the serotonin deficiency concept as presented by the direct to consumer advertising is poorly supported by medical science *(13)*. A naturally occurring amino acid, tryptophan is the metabolic precursor to serotonin in the brain. It is well known that brain serotonin can be increased safely with ingestion of a food supplement, tryptophan and 5-HTP, available at the health food store. Why risk the adverse side effects of SSRI drugs when a safer alternative is available?*(14)*

The True Utility of SSRI Drugs

According to drug company advertising, the unfortunate soul who loses his job, gets divorced or experiences the grief of a death in the family now has a "disease" caused by a chemical imbalance which requires him to be prescribed an SSRI drug. This is not a description of a disease state. This is a description of a life event which makes anyone depressed, and the treatment is the support of friends and family through a difficult time. Perhaps the depressed individual bears inner turmoil of unresolved conflicts with work or family, and the SSRI drug "numbs" the individual to this unbearable inner conflict, allowing continuation of the job or unhappy home. Perhaps this is the true utility of SSRI drugs in our society.

Drugging of Our Children

We have known about SSRI drug induced suicide since Teicher's landmark article in 1990 *(15)*. Where is the overpowering sense of public outrage that should have banned these drugs in children years ago? The drug industry, the FDA and the medical profession continue the widespread drugging of our children with addictive toxic placebos in an uncanny similarity to the classic Lucas film THX 1138, a science fictional remake of Orwell's 1984 which paints a totalitarian world of enslaved citizens controlled by drugs *(16)(17)*.

Sacrifice of Isaac

Child sacrifice is an important theme of the three major, monotheistic religions *(18)*. Abraham's intended sacrifice of Isaac took place at the "Dome of the Rock" on the temple mount, near the "Wailing Wall" in the old city of Jerusalem. Isaac's life was spared at the last minute by an angel who ordered Abraham to spare Isaac and sacrifice a ram instead. We know today's Abrahams and Issacs well enough, but the horizon seems frighteningly devoid of any signs of angels.

References For Chapter 8

(1) http://www.antidepressantsfacts.com/Traci-Johnson-19-duloxetine2.htmPosted on Tue, Feb. 10, 2004 Woman testing depression drug kills herself, by Gloria Campisi, Knight Ridder Newspapers

(2) http://www.antidepressantsfacts.com/Traci-Johnson-19-duloxetine3.htm Suicide brings changes to Lilly drug trials By J.K. Wall and John TuohyFebruary 11, 2004

(3) *http://www.antidepressantsfacts.com/Traci-Johnson-19-duloxetine4.htmWed,*
Feb. 11, 2004 Bucks woman found dead in Ind. laboratory Traci R. Johnson was found at clinic where she was part of testing for a new drug by Walter F. Naedele Inquirer Staff Writer

(4) *http://www.antidepressantsfacts.com/2004-02-12-Philad-Traci-Johnson.htm*
Thu, Feb. 12, 2004 Drug test altered in wake of suicide By Walter F. Naedele Inquirer Staff Writer

(5) *http://query.nytimes.com/gst/fullpage.html?sec=health&res=9C03E5D8133AF931A25751C0A9629C8B63*
Student, 19, in Trial of New Antidepressant Commits Suicide By Gardiner Harris Published: February 12, 2004

(6) *http://www.ssristories.com/*
SSRI Stories Antidepressant Nightmares

(7) *http://www.fda.gov/cder/drug/antidepressants/default.htm*
FDA - Antidepressant Use in Children, Adolescents, and Adults.

(8) *http://content.apa.org/psycarticles/browse/?UseCanonicalURLs=1&pg=33&iss=1&vol=5&jrn=pre&Printable=1*
Antidepressants and placebos: Secrets, revelations, and unanswered questions. July 15, 2002.

(9) *http://www.commondreams.org/headlines/092500-01.htm*
Published on Monday, September 25, 2000 in USA Today, FDA Advisers Tied To Industry,by Dennis Cauchon,.

(10) *http://www.senate.gov/~finance/hearings/testimony/2004test/111804dgtest.pdf*
Testimony of David J. Graham, MD, MPH, November 18, 2004,

(11) *http://barnesworld.blogs.com/barnes_world/2007/01/jeffrey_dach_on.html*
Jeffrey Dach on Lipitor and "The Dracula of Modern Technology" Jan 3 2007

(12) *http://www.zoloft.com/zoloft/zoloft.portal?_nfpb=true&_pageLabel=depr_causes*
Zoloft web site, "Scientists believe that it could be linked with an imbalance of a chemical in the brain called serotonin. If this imbalance happens, it can affect the way people feel."

(13) *http://medicine.plosjournals.org/perlserv/?request=get-document&doi=10.1371/journal.pmed.0020392*
Serotonin and Depression: A Disconnect between the Advertisements and the Scientific Literature. Jeffrey R. Lacasse, Jonathan Leo

(14) *http://www.thorne.com/altmedrev/.fulltext/5/1/64.pdf*
Use of Neurotransmitter Precursors for Treatment of Depression by Stephen Meyers, MS, Thorne Research

(15) *http://www.ncbi.nlm.nih.gov/pubmed/2301661?dopt=AbstractPlus*
Emergence of intense suicidal preoccupation during fluoxetine treatment. Teicher MH, Glod C, Cole JO. Department of Psychiatry, Harvard Medical School, MA.

(16) *http://www.lucasfilm.com/films/other/thx1138.html*
THX-1138 Population controlled by a government controlled sedating drug program

(17) *http://www.thx1138movie.com/*
THX-1138 Movie trailer

(18) *http://198.62.75.1/www1/ofm/sbf/dialogue/symp95.html*
March 16-17, 1995 - Symposium on The Sacrifice of Isaac in the Three Monotheistic Religions

(19) *http://medicine.plosjournals.org/perlserv/?request=get-document&doi=10.1371/journal.pmed.0050045*
Initial Severity and Antidepressant Benefits: A Meta-Analysis of Data Submitted to the Food and Drug Administration. Irving Kirsch et al.

(20) *http://www.bmj.com/cgi/content/full/336/7643/516*
BMJ 2008;336:516-517 (8 March)

(21) *http://en.wikipedia.org/wiki/Selective_serotonin_reuptake_inhibitor*
SSRI's Wikipedia: Prozac, Lexepro, Zoloft, Effexor, Wellbutrin, Cymbalta, Paxil, citalopram

Chapter Nine

Lipitor and the Dracula of Modern Technology

Perhaps you have seen the Direct-to-Consumer TV and print advertisements with Robert Jarvik, the inventor of the Jarvik Heart, speaking on behalf of the Pfizer's anti-cholesterol drug, Lipitor. With 13 billion dollars in sales last year, Lipitor was the best selling statin drug, the best selling drug in the world, and most prescribed drug in the U.S.

Jarvik first came to the attention of a media circus in 1982 with the implantation of his Jarvik-7 artificial heart into the chest of Seattle dentist, Barney Clark. Although the artificial heart continued to beat, Barney Clark died of multi-organ failure 112 days after the operation, tethered to a dishwasher sized air compressor. The heart device acted as a blender which chewed up the blood cells. Recipients of the Jarvik-7 suffered horribly for months, finally succumbing to infections, strokes, convulsions and immune system failure with progressive decline in T cells, thus making the Jarvik-7 another cause of HIV negative AIDS. *(1)(2)*

During the ensuing media coverage, the New York Times dubbed the Jarvik Heart the "Dracula of Medical Technology".*(3)(4)* Jarvik-7 patients had the Kevorkian option of assisted suicide, a small on-off button which allowed the mechanical heart to be stopped when too unbearable. About 90 people received the Jarvik heart before it was banned. The FDA recently approved a revised mechanical heart September 5, 2006 for heart transplant candidates, intended for temporary humanitarian use to prolong the terminal patient while awaiting a suitable donor.*(5)*

Why Select Jarvik?

Why would Pfizer select an MD like Jarvik as spokesman for their Direct to Consumer (DTC) campaign? Jarvik himself doesn't have the strongest of professional credentials, and apparently had difficulty gaining admission to a US medical school. Instead, he enrolled for the first two years at the University of Bologna in Italy, later returning for the MD degree at the University of Utah.*(6)* Jarvik never did an internship or residency, and never actually practiced medicine. And the heart device had been invented by somebody else, Paul Winchell, the ventriloquist, who assigned the patent to the University.*(7)* Why does Jarvik's "Dracula of Medical Technology" make him an expert on statin drugs?

Eight controlled clinical *trials* have shown that statin drugs cause Coenzyme Q10 depletion by inhibition of HMG-CoA reductase, which is the rate limiting step in cholesterol and Coenzyme Q-10 biosynthesis.*(8)* Coenzyme Q10 serves in the mitochondria as an electron carrier to cytochrome oxidase, the major system for cellular energy production. Heart muscle requires high levels of Co-Q10. Side effects of Co-Q10 deficiency include muscle wasting, muscle pain, heart failure, neuropathy, amnesia, and cognitive dysfunction.*(9)* Deaths from heart failure have doubled nationwide since the introduction of statin drugs in 1987.*(10)* Statin induced heart failure can be prevented by supplementing with Co Enzyme Q10, a form of intervention considerably less expensive and less traumatic than an artificial heart operation followed by cardiac transplantation.

Duane Graveline MD, a Better Spokesman

Perhaps Jarvik is not the best choice for the Lipitor campaign which has had mixed reviews.*(11)* Instead of Jarvik, a more convincing yet unlikely spokesman would be the popular Duane Graveline MD MPH, a former NASA astronaut, and author who was started on Lipitor during an annual astronaut physical at the Johnson Space Center, and 6 weeks later had an episode of transient global amnesia, a sudden form of total memory loss described in his book.*(12)(13)* Graveline points out that 50 percent of the dry weight of the cerebral cortex is made of cholesterol, an important substance for memory and cerebral function.

Graveline also points out that statins are useful for secondary prevention of heart disease in patients with significant pre-existing coronary artery disease, however the benefit is independent of cholesterol response during statin use.*(14)* Contrary to the secondary prevention findings, no statin primary prevention study has ever shown a benefit in terms of all cause mortality in healthy men and women with only an elevated serum cholesterol, and no known coronary artery disease. Patients with known heart disease are customarily placed on statin drugs by the medical system with no need for direct to consumer (DTC) advertising to this group. DTC ads for Lipitor are clearly directed at the larger group of untreated primary prevention patients, for which there is no benefit in terms of all cause mortality.*(15)*

The J-Lit study actually showed higher mortality at the lowest serum cholesterol (both total and LDL-C), a paradox called the J-Shaped Curve.*(16)* The highest mortality was found at the lowest total cholesterol of 160 mg/dl, and lowest mortality at serum cholesterol around 240 mg /ml, exactly the opposite one would expect if cholesterol lowering was beneficial for health. The authors state that the increased mortality at the lower cholesterol levels was due to increased cancer. Another statin trial, CARE (Cholesterol And Recurrent Events), showed 1500 % increase in breast cancer among women in the statin treated group, explained as merely a statistical aberration.*(17)* This is disputed by Uffe Ravnskov who feels that the difference is significant, and points to rodent studies showing statin drugs cause cancer in animals.*(18)(19)*

The Honolulu Heart Study of elderly patients showed the lowest serum cholesterol predicted the highest mortality.*(20)* A study by Krumholz found lack of association between cholesterol and coronary heart disease mortality and morbidity in persons older than 70 years.*(21)* Jenkins (BMJ) states that no statin drug study has ever shown an all cause mortality benefit for women.*(22)*

The Jarvik-Lipitor ad campaign is a perfect example of why prescription drug ads are dishonest, do not promote public health, increase unnecessary prescriptions, increase costs to taxpayers, and can be harmful or deadly to patients. New Zealand and the US are the only two industrialized nations to allow direct-to-consumer advertising for prescription drugs. Here in the USA, thirty nine public interest groups have proposed congressional legislation to ban DTC prescription drug ads.*(23)(24)*

Mary Enig and Uffe Ravnskov, Better Spokesmen

Two more unlikely spokesmen for the Lipitor ad campaign include Mary Enig and Uffe Ravnskov. Should either one be selected as Lipitor spokesman, I myself would run down to the corner drug store to buy up the drug. It seems unlikely that even Pfizer's deep pockets could ever induce them to recant their opposing position on the cholesterol theory of heart disease. Mary G. Enig writes, "hypercholesterolemia is the health issue of the 21st century. It is actually an invented disease, a problem that emerged when health professionals learned how to measure cholesterol levels in the blood".(25) *Uffe* Ravnskov MD PhD, who can easily be regarded as the "Peter Duesberg" of the Lipid Hypothesis, is spokesman for Thincs, The International Network of Cholesterol Skeptics, and author of "The Cholesterol Myths, Exposing the Fallacy That Saturated Fat and Cholesterol Cause Heart Disease". His controversial ideas have angered loyal cholesterol theory supporters in Finland who demonstrated by burning his book on live television.*(26)*

During a condolence call to a dear friend who just lost her mom to Alzheimer's, the conversation touched on her mom's mental decline in a nursing home, and I mentioned that sometimes treatment for B12 deficiency or hypothyroidism can help. They had already tried that to no avail. We chatted about her mom's life and the reason for the cognitive decline. Apparently, her mom had been taking Lipitor for 15 years, and had a few initial episodes of transient global amnesia, followed by progressive dementia, and later her death was attributed, in retrospect, to the drug. How many demented nursing home patients will suffer from the adverse side effects of statin drugs? We will never know. People experiencing adverse side effects from statin drugs may share their experiences in Internet discussion groups.*(27)* One such Internet Discussion Board has 3800 messages.*(28)*

References for Chapter 9

(1) http://www.ncbi.nlm.nih.gov/pubmed/3261735?dopt=Abstract
Wellhausen SR, Ward RA, Johnson GS, DeVries WC. Immunologic complications of long-term implantation of a total artificial heart. J Clin Immunol. 1988 Jul;8(4):307-18. PMID: 3261735

(2) *http://www.ncbi.nlm.nih.gov/pubmed/3566584?dopt=AbstractPlus*
Stelzer GT, Ward RA, Wellhausen SR, McLeish KR, Johnson GS, DeVries WC. Alterations in select immunologic parameters following total artificial heart implantation. Artif Organs. 1987 Feb;11(1):52-62.

(3) *http://query.nytimes.com/gst/fullpage.html?res=940DE7DB143CF935A25756C0A96E948260*
The Dracula of Medical Technology Published: May 16, 1988 New York Times

(4) *www.time.com/time/magazine/article/0,9171,44039,00.html*
Time Magazine, Reviving Artificial Hearts Sunday, Apr. 30, 2000 By MICHAEL D. LEMONICK

(5) *http://www.fda.gov/bbs/topics/NEWS/2006/NEW01443.html*
FDA Approves First Totally Implanted Permanent Artificial Heart for Humanitarian Uses P06-125 September 5, 2006

(6) *http://www.bookrags.com/biography/robert-k-jarvik-woh/*
Robert K. Jarvik Biography

(7) *http://www.paulwinchell.com/artificialheart.htm*
Paul Winchell's story, inventing and patenting the first artificial heart.

(8) *http://www.fda.gov/ohrms/dockets/dailys/02/May02/052902/02p-0244-cp00001-02-Exhibit_A-vol1.pdf*
The clinical use of HMG CoA-reductase inhibitors (statins) and the associated depletion of the essential co-factor coenzyme Q10, by Peter H. Langsjoen, M.D.

(9) *http://www.tga.gov.au/adr/aadrb/aadr0504.htm*
Australian Adverse Drug Reactions Bulletin Volume 24, Number 2, April 2005

(10) *http://library.thinkquest.org/27533/facts.html*
September 1996, National Heart, Lung, and Blood Institute, National Institutes of Health NIH,Data Fact Sheet,

(11) *http://www.msnbc.msn.com/id/16039753/*
Is this celebrity doctor's TV ad right for you? Despite past failures, Dr. Robert Jarvik succeeds hawking statin drug Lipitor By Robert Bazell, Chief science and health correspondent, NBC News, March. 1, 2007

(12) *http://www.spacedoc.net/*
Duane Graveline MD SpaceDoc,Statin Drug Side Effects, Transient Global Amnesia

(13) *http://www.spacedoc.net/lipitor_thief_of_memory.html*
Lipitor Thief of Memory, the Book by Duane Graveline MD

(14) *http://www.ncbi.nlm.nih.gov/pubmed/12446061?dopt=AbstractPlus*
Allen Maycock CA, Muhlestein JB, Horne BD, Carlquist JF, Bair TL, Pearson RR, Li Q, Anderson JL; Intermountain Heart Collaborative Study. Statin therapy is associated with reduced mortality across all age groups of individuals with significant coronary disease, including very elderly patients. J Am Coll Cardiol. 2002 Nov 20;40(10):1777-85.

(15) *http://www.cmaj.ca/cgi/content/full/173/10/1207-a*
CMAJ November 8, 2005; 173 (10). Letters, Questioning the benefits of statins, Eddie Vos and Colin P. Rose, Sutton, Que.; Cardiologist, McGill University, Montréal, Que.

(16) *http://www.jstage.jst.go.jp/article/circj/66/12/1096/_pdf*
J-Lit Study, Large Scale Cohort Study of the Relationship Between Serum Cholesterol Concentration and Coronary Events With Low-Dose Simvastatin Therapy in Japanese Patients With Hypercholesterolemia and Coronary Heart Disease Secondary Prevention Cohort Study of the Japan Lipid Intervention Trial (J-LIT)

(17) *http://www.annals.org/cgi/content/full/131/2/155-b*
Cholesterol Lowering in Older Patients Sandra J. Lewis, MD; Frank Sacks, MD; and Eugene Braunwald, MD 20 July 1999 | Volume 131 Issue 2 | Pages 155-156

(18) *http://www.thincs.org/unpublic.UR3.htm*
Uffe Ravnskov, MD, PhD, Letter to the editor of Lancet, sent 10. December 2002, Evidence that statin treatment causes cancer

(19) *http://www.ncbi.nlm.nih.gov/pubmed/8531288?dopt=Abstract*
Newman TB, Hulley SB. Carcinogenicity of lipid-lowering drugs. JAMA. 1996 Jan 3;275(1):55-60. Review.

(20) *http://www.ncbi.nlm.nih.gov/pubmed/11502313?dopt=AbstractPlus*
Schatz IJ, Masaki K, Yano K, Chen R, Rodriguez BL, Curb JD. Cholesterol and all-cause mortality in elderly people from the Honolulu Heart Program: a cohort study. Lancet. 2001 Aug 4;358(9279):351-5.

(21) *http://jama.ama-assn.org/cgi/content/abstract/272/17/1335?ijkey=d2fe4b0874ba7917*
Lack of association between cholesterol and coronary heart disease mortality and morbidity and all-cause mortality in persons older than 70 years. H. M. Krumholz et al. JAMA Vol. 272 No. 17, November 2, 1994

(22) *http://www.bmj.com/cgi/content/full/327/7420/933-b*
Letter Might money spent on statins be better spent? Arnold J Jenkins. BMJ 2003;327:933 (18 October),

(23) *http://www.commercialalert.org/news/news-releases/2006/05/39-health-seniors-groups-call-on-congress-to-end-to-dtc-prescription-drug-ads*
39 Health & Seniors Groups Call on Congress to End to DTC Prescription Drug Ads

(24) *http://www.commercialalert.org/phpa.pdf*
Public Health Protection Act. We call on Congress to enact the Public Health Protection Act to prohibit direct-to-consumer marketing of prescription drugs.

(25) *http://www.westonaprice.org/moderndiseases/statin.html*
Dangers of Statin Drugs: What You Haven't Been Told About Popular Cholesterol-Lowering Medicines By Sally Fallon and Mary G. Enig, PhD

(26) *http://www.ravnskov.nu/uffe.htm*
The Cholesterol Myths by Uffe Ravnskov, MD, PhD

(27) *http://search.yahoo.com/search?p=lipitor+message+boards&fr=yfp-t-501&toggle=1&cop=mss&ei=UTF-8*
Message Boards for Statins

(28) *http://mb.rxlist.com/rxboard/lipitor.pl?*
Lipitor Message Board, adverse events

(29) *qjmed.oxfordjournals.org/cgi/content/full/96/12/927*
QJ Med 2003; 96: 927-934; High cholesterol may protect against infections and atherosclerosis U. Ravnskov I

Chapter 10

Cholesterol Lowering Statin Drugs for Women, Just Say No

A Woman on Crestor With Leg Muscle Pain

Sally, a 56 year old retired real estate agent, came to see me in the office with the chief complaint of hot flashes, night sweats, mood disturbance and weight gain which are all fairly typical post-menopausal symptoms. In addition, she also had leg pain for the past 3 months, which prevented exercising. Lumbar Spine MRI Scan to evaluate the leg pain showed only a bulging disk and was otherwise negative. About 6 months ago, Sally's cholesterol was 245, and her cardiologist prescribed a cholesterol lowering statin drug, Crestor. Sally has no history of heart disease, does not smoke, eats a healthy diet, and takes a few vitamins, and doesn't supplement with CoEnzyme Q-10.

I explained to Sally that her leg pain was a well known adverse side effect of Crestor, a valid reason for stopping the drug. The leg muscle pain is caused by Statin Drug depletion of Co-Enzyme Q 10, which is important for energy production in the muscle cells. I suggested to Sally that she supplement with CO-enzyme Q-10, and strongly recommended stopping the statin drug.

What is the definition of elevated cholesterol?

When I was a medical student in 1976, normal cholesterol was 240. However, this was changed in 1993 to the new guidelines.

New Cholesterol Guidelines in 1993

above 240: high
200-240: borderline high
below 200: desirable

The cholesterol guidelines were revised downward to 200 by a committee of nine doctors, eight of whom were receiving money from statin drug companies, a blatant conflict of interests. In addition, there was no science behind this revision. *(1)(2)(3)*

A 2006 paper in the Annals of Internal Medicine (October 3, 2006; 145 (7):520-530) argues that there is **NO EVIDENCE** to support the target numbers outlined by the Cholesterol Guidelines panel, challenging the mainstream medical belief that lower cholesterol levels are always better. "This paper is not arguing that there is strong evidence against the LDL targets, but rather that there's **no evidence** for them," said Dr. Rodney A. Hayward, a study author. A 2004 petition letter to the NIH by 30 prominent MD's complains about the faulty Cholesterol Guidelines and asks for a revision.*(41)*

The laboratory will flag any cholesterol test results above 200 as abnormal. In reality a cholesterol reading above 200 and below 240 is normal. If above 240, then nutritional supplements containing niacin, omega 3 oils, and plant sterols are used to bring it down to 240.(*4*) As discussed in a later chapter, other lipoprotein parameters are more important risk factors than total cholesterol, such as the LDL particle size and number, and Lipoprotein (a) (little A) which are available on the more sophisticated lipoprotein analysis (VAP and NMR) rendering the conventional cholesterol panel obsolete..

Mary Enig says:

> "Blood cholesterol levels between 200 and 240 mg/dl are normal. These levels have always been normal. In older women, serum cholesterol levels greatly above these numbers are also quite normal, and in fact they have been shown to be associated with longevity. Since 1984, however, in the United States and other parts of the western world, these normal numbers have been treated as if they were an indication of a disease in progress or a potential for disease in the future."(*4*)

Contrary to the stated guidelines, my opinion is that a cholesterol of 240 is normal and compatible with good health.

Medical Terrorism through Drug Company Advertising:

Drug company advertising strikes fear into the hearts of the public with the message, "You will die unless you lower your cholesterol." The reality is that in patients with no pre-existing heart disease, there is **no mortality benefit** from lowering cholesterol with statin drugs. Analyzing data from five statin drug studies (4S, WOSCOPS, CARE, TEXCAPS/AFCAPS and LIPID), Peter R Jackson found a **1% increase in mortality after 10 years** on statin drugs for primary prevention.*(38)*

Women should just say NO to Statin Drugs.

The truth is that NO woman should ever be given Lipitor or any other statin drug for elevated cholesterol. Dr. Rose says, "There are no statin trials with even the slightest hint of a mortality benefit in women and women should be told so".*(5)*. In other words, **statin drugs don't work for women.** Let me repeat that so this is very clear: No female should ever take a statin drug to lower cholesterol for primary prevention of heart disease. They don't work for women. Women who take Lipitor or any other statin drug to lower cholesterol do not live any longer than women who don't take the drug. There is no benefit in terms of prolonging your life for women.

Adverse Side Effects of Statin Drugs:

On the other hand, there are plenty of adverse side effects which include muscle pain, cognitive impairment, neuropathy, congestive heart failure, transient global amnesia, dementia, cancer and erectile dysfunction (impotence). Read about Statin Drug adverse side effects on internet message boards. Many of the adverse side effects are thought to be caused by Co-Enzyme Q10 depletion.

Why do Cardiologists Give Statin Drugs to Women?

Why do cardiologists and mainstream doctors continue to prescribe statins to women? It is very simple. They succumb to the drug company "spin" from the drug reps and the medical journals which are slanted in favor of statins. In addition, the mainstream doctors succumb to patient's demands and expectations for the drugs after seeing the celebrity TV ads.

Are You Still Not Convinced?

Mary Enig writes, "No study has shown a significant reduction in mortality in women treated with statins. The University of British Columbia Therapeutics Initiative came to the same conclusion, with the finding that statins offer no benefit to women for prevention of heart disease." *(6)(7)*

Are you still not convinced that women should NOT take Statin Drugs? Don't take my word for it. Take the word of Judith Walsh MD who wrote this in JAMA, 4 years ago in an article entitled, Treatment of Hyperlipidemia in Women: "For women without cardiovascular disease, lipid lowering does not affect total or CHD (Cardiovascular Heart Disease) mortality. Lipid lowering may reduce CHD events, but current evidence is insufficient to determine this conclusively. For women with known cardiovascular disease, treatment of hyperlipidemia is effective in reducing CHD events, CHD mortality, nonfatal myocardial infarction, and revascularization, **but it does not affect total mortality**." *(8)*

Translation: Cholesterol lowering with statin drugs does not reduce total mortality in women, **PERIOD.** It doesn't reduce mortality in women without heart disease, called primary prevention. It doesn't reduce mortality in women with heart disease, called secondary prevention.

Still not convinced? then read this article by Malcolm McKendrick, a doctor in England, in the British Medical Journal, May 2007, entitled: "Should Women be Offered Cholesterol Lowering Drugs? **NO** ".*(8A)* "To date, none of the large trials of secondary prevention with statins has shown a reduction in overall mortality in women. Perhaps more critically, the primary prevention trials have shown neither an overall mortality benefit, nor even a reduction in cardiovascular end points in women. This raises the important question whether women should be prescribed statins at all. I believe that the answer is clearly no."*(8A)*

Note: Secondary prevention means women with known heart disease. Primary prevention means women without known heart disease.

Still not convinced? Then read this June 2007 article by Electra Kaczorowski, of the National Women's Health Network *(9)* "There is currently no indication that women of any age or any risk level will benefit from taking statins to prevent CHD and other heart conditions – yet this is precisely how statins are being marketed to women. "*(9)*

Still not convinced? Are statin drugs good for anybody? Read this review article by Joel Kauffman PhD, Dec 2003, in which the best statin trial results (the HPS simvastatin study) had an absolute reduction of all cause death rate of 0.38% per year. Yet this performance was inferior to the less expensive alternatives of buffered aspirin or Omega-3 oils.*(10)*

Quote: "The most favorable (statin) trial with seemingly impeccable reporting and minimal financial conflict of interest was the Heart Protection Study (HPS), on simvastatin for 5 years, in which secondary prevention in men (86% of patients) of any unwanted vascular event gave a RR = 0.76 (5.5% absolute, 1.1% per year), and an all-cause death rate drop of 0.38% per year. (Lancet 2002; 360:7-22) Since this performance is inferior to that of either Bufferin in men or omega-3 fatty acid supplements, both of which have lesser side-effects, and are far less expensive, the logic of prescribing simvastatin seems faulty."*(10)*

Still not convinced? Then read this article by Harriett Rosenberg from Women and Health Protection from June 2007, Do Cholesterol Lowering Drugs Benefit Women ?*(11)* Evidence for Caution: Women and statin use By Harriet Rosenberg Danielle Allard Women and Health Protection June 2007

Quote: "Our review of these fields identifies a troubling disjuncture between the widespread use of statin medication for women and the evidence base for that usage. What we found instead was evidence for caution." Endquote Harriett Rosenberg.

Still not convinced? Not only are statin drugs a failure for women, they also should never be prescribed to the elderly. Mortality in the elderly goes up as cholesterol goes down. Read this Letter to the Editor by Eddie Vos.*(12)*

Quote: "Regarding women, two 2004 analysis found no reduction in deaths from statin over placebo. In actual patient outcomes, the J-LIT study in 41,801 hypercholesterolemic Japanese (2/3rds women) found mortality in the 2 lowest on-statin cholesterol categories 2-3 times higher; its authors cautioned about 'hyperresponders' to statin. The 4S study ended with 3 more dead women on statin vs. placebo, and another 'successful' study, HPS, found no significant mortality benefit in women." See article for references.

Still not convinced? Then read this article by Bill Sardi, Who Will Tell the People? It Isn't Cholesterol ! *(13)* "If physicians were truly honest with their patients, there probably would be very few people being treated for primary prevention with a statin drug."

Still not convinced? Then read this Jan 2007 Lancet article by Harvard trained MD, John Abramson, "Are lipid-lowering guidelines Evidence-Based?".*(14)*

Quote:" No studies have shown statin cholesterol-lowering drugs to be effective neither for women at any age, nor for men 69 years of age or older, who do not already have heart disease or diabetes. Better than 50 adults have to take a cholesterol-lowering drug for 1 patient to avoid a mortal heart attack, and that figure only applies to high-risk patients. There is a vanishing benefit to lowering cholesterol for healthy adults." [Lancet 2007; 369:168-169]. John Abramson MD. Dr. John Abramson joins with 30 more eminent MD's in a Sept 2004 letter to the NIH calling for a complete revision of the faulty cholesterol treatment guidelines.

Still not convinced? Then read this e-book by Shane Ellison, "The Hidden Truth About Cholesterol-Lowering Drugs!" by Shane Ellison, MS, Organic Chemistry.*(15)*

"Among healthy people, statin drugs do not prevent early death from heart disease, despite their cholesterol lowering effects. This is because there is no correlation or relationship between low cholesterol and the progression of atherosclerosis – the number one cause of heart disease. Repeat that sentence. This became abundantly clear with the statin drug trials." Endquote Shane Ellison.

The New York Times Questions the Value of Lowering Cholesterol with Statin Drugs !!

In a surprise turnaround, The New York Times questions the value of treating cholesterol with statin drugs in this article, "New Questions on Treating Cholesterol", By ALEX BERENSON, New York Times January 17, 2008.*(16)*

"In the last 13 months, however, the failures of two important clinical trials have thrown that hypothesis into question. (that cholesterol lowering is beneficial). First, Pfizer stopped development of its experimental cholesterol drug torcetrapib in December 2006, when a trial involving 15,000 patients showed that the medicine caused heart attacks and strokes. That trial — somewhat unusual in that it was conducted before Pfizer sought F.D.A. approval — also showed that torcetrapib lowered LDL cholesterol while raising HDL, or good cholesterol. Torcetrapib's failure, Dr. Taylor said, shows that lowering cholesterol alone does not prove a drug will benefit patients. Then, on Monday, Merck and Schering-Plough announced that Vytorin, which combines Zetia with Zocor, had failed to reduce the growth of fatty arterial plaque in a trial of 720 patients. In fact, patients taking Vytorin actually had more plaque growth than those who took Zocor alone. Despite those drawbacks, that trial, called Enhance, also showed that patients on Vytorin had lower LDL levels than those on Zocor alone. For the second time in just over a year, a clinical trial found that LDL reduction did not translate into measurable medical benefits." endquote from Alex Berenson New York Times (*16*)

Business Week Questions the Benefit of Lowering Cholesterol with Statin Drugs !! *(17)*

In an historic turnaround, Business Week's Jan 28, 2008 cover story asks the heretical question, **"Do Cholesterol Drugs Do Any Good?** Research suggests that, except among high-risk heart patients, the benefits of statins such as Lipitor are overstated." Astonishingly, Business Week makes the following statements: "Current evidence supports **ignoring** LDL cholesterol altogether" and "Cholesterol lowering is **not** the reason for the benefit of statins".*(17)*

Investigation by John Dingell's House Committee and New York Attorney General Andrew Cuomo

Senator John Dingell's House Committee of Energy and Commerce has recently (2008) subpoenaed both Merck and Pfizer. Merck's subpoena investigates the Vytorin - Enhance scandal, and Pfizer's subpoena investigates the Jarvik-Lipitor Celebrity Ads. Dingell wants to know why Jarvik was selected as spokesman for Lipitor even though Jarvik was never licensed to practiced medicine. John Dingell is the Democratic Representative from Michigan and Chairman of the House Committee on Energy and Commerce

The Attorney General Andrew Cuomo has a few questions: The Enhance Vytorin scandal has prompted New York Attorney General Andrew Cuomo to issue a subpoena to Merck & Co and Schering-Plough Corp to investigate the allegations of deceitful marketing and insider trading.

The Vytorin Enhance Data showed no benefit for the Zetia/Zocor combination compared to Zocor alone. This created a scandal because of the late registration of the Enhance study, and accusations of insider trading, dumping stock in advance of the unfavorable results. *Merck and Schering sat on the results* of an unfavorable study for almost two years. They claim they haven't peeked at the data, but Schering President Carrie Cox dumped 28 Million worth of stock back in the spring of 2007.

Two recent drug trials, ENHANCE and Torcetrapib showed no health benefit of lowering LDL cholesterol. Dr Steven Nissen, cardiologist at Cleveland Clinic, said this of the Merck Enhance-Vytorin data:

"ENHANCE (Vytorin) results were a big surprise and a big disappointment. The data show no benefit for ezetimibe (Zetia) on top of simvastatin (Zocor). In fact, the data on both the rate of progression of atherosclerosis and cardiovascular events are trending in the wrong direction. This is a pretty clear failure. Physicians should now stop using ezetimibe or Vytorin except as a last resort. The drug doesn't work".

The results of the ENHANCE had to be released because now all trials must be pre-registered with the government because of new FDA rules Sept 2007. In the old days it would have been buried. *(22B)*

The following quote about Vytorin-Enhance from Bill Sardi at LewRockwell.com is illuminating.(*18*)

> "The revelation that statin cholesterol drugs may be of little or no benefit, as revealed in a lengthy cover story in January 28 issue of Business Week (BW) magazine, begs the question: how did this misdirection go on for so long?
> As the BW article pointed out, statin drugs "are the best-selling medicines in history, used by more than 13 million Americans and an additional 12 million patients around the world, producing $27.8 billion in sales in 2006."
> How can anyone question the benefits of such a drug, asks BW, when they are "thought to be so essential that, according to the official government guidelines from the National Cholesterol Education Program (NCEP), 40 million Americans should be taking them. Some researchers have even suggested – half-jokingly – that the medications should be put in the water supply, like fluoride for teeth. And it's almost impossible to avoid reminders from the industry that the drugs are vital. A current TV and newspaper campaign for one statin drug, as endorsed by Dr. Robert Jarvik, artificial heart inventor, proclaims that this drug 'reduces the risk of heart attack by 36%...in patients with multiple risk factors for heart disease'."

Statin Drug Ruse Revealed:

But the cholesterol/statin drug ruse finally unraveled when, after two years of foot dragging delays to release data from a large study involving Zetia, a cholesterol-lowering drug that inhibits cholesterol absorption from foods, and Vytorin, which is a combination of Zetia plus Zocor, the latter a statin drug that inhibits formation of cholesterol in the liver, revealed no health benefits.

Even though this drug combo lowered circulating cholesterol numbers better than either drug alone, it did not reduce plaque formation in arteries and did not confer a projected reduction in mortality.

In fact, an earlier review published last year in the British journal Lancet by Drs. John Abramson of Harvard Medical School and James M. Wright MD of the University of British Columbia, could find no evidence for a reduction in cardiac mortality in a combined review of all published statin drug studies. [The Lancet 2007; 369:168–169]

Falsifying the numbers:

The Business Week report says statin drugs benefit only 1 in 100 users, but they claim to reduce the risk of a non-mortal heart attack by 36%. But that figure is a relative number, not a hard one. About 3% of patients taking an inactive placebo pill will experience a heart attack compared to 2% taking a statin drug, which produces the so-called 30-plus percent risk reduction. **But in hard numbers, this is only a 1% reduced risk.** This type of misleading advertising wouldn't pass Federal Trade Commission guidelines. But public health agencies, serving as free publicity agents for the statin drug manufacturers, repeat the claim to give it a ring of credibility." from Bill Sardi on Lew Rockwell.com.

America Fooled Again - More on the Merck Vytorin/Enhance Scandal: ***(19)(20)***

Merck ran Cholesterol Lowering-Vytorin Television Ads over the course of about a year spending 160 million dollars, allowing a windfall of 1-2 billion dollars on the sale of Vytorin. All this time they knew that the ENHANCE study showed that Vytorin didn't work. Take a look at the TV ads that fooled a nation into spending a fortune for drugs that don't work. They are posted on the internet. The Vytorin Ads have been pulled, so you won't be seeing them on national TV anymore. More stories: Wall Street Journal story, "Congress Investigates Vytorin Ads", by Anna Wilde Mathews: *(22A)* and "Vytorin Ad Shame Taints Entire Marketing Industry Cholesterol Drug's Ad Campaign Turns Into PR Nightmare, Fanning Flames of Public Mistrust of DTC" by Rich Thomaselli Published: January 21, 2008.*(22C)*

Lipitor and the Dracula of Medical Technology

A previous chapter, Lipitor and the Dracula of Medical Technology discussed the Robert Jarvik celebrity ads for Lipitor. About a year after the ads appeared, John

Dingell's House Committee on Energy and Commerce is now investigating the matter. They have issued Subpoenas to Pfizer CEO, Jeffrey B Kindler, asking for information about the Jarvik-Lipitor Ad Materials.*(22)*

Among other things, Chairman John Dingell wants to know why Jarvik takes Lipitor, and why Jarvik appears to be representing a doctor in the Ads, yet has never actually been licensed to practice medicine. Jarvik never actually prescribed Lipitor or any other drug for that matter. In response, Pfizer pulled the Jarvik Lipitor ads (2/25/08) from Television and will not be shown any more.*(40)*

How to Prevent and Reverse Heart Disease without Statins

From the book, Solved: The Riddle of Heart Attacks by Broda O. Barnes, M.D., Ph.D. and Charlotte W. Barnes. Prevention of Heart Attacks: The Key to Progress in Medicine. In 1970, Dr. Broda Barnes had 1,569 patients on natural thyroid hormone who were observed for a total of 8,824 patient years. These patients were compared to similar patients in the Framingham Study. Based on the statistics derived in the Framingham Study, **seventy-two** of Dr. Barnes's patients should have died from heart attacks; however, only **four** patients had done so. This represents a decreased heart attack death rate of 95 percent in patients who received natural thyroid hormone–a truly remarkable finding.

All references are hyperlinked at www.jeffreydach.com and www.naturalmedicine101.com.

References for Chapter 10

(1) http://www.postgradmed.com/issues/2002/08_02/pearlman.shtml
The new cholesterol guidelines, Applying them in clinical practice Brian L. Pearlman, MD, FACP VOL 112 / NO 2 / AUGUST 2002 / POSTGRADUATE MEDICINE

(2) http://hp2010.nhlbihin.net/ncep_slds/atpiii/slide25.htm
The new cholesterol guidelines

(3) http://www.usatoday.com/news/health/2004-10-16-panel-conflict-of-interest_x.htm
USA Today, 2004, Cholesterol guidelines become a morality play the Associated Press

(4) http://www.westonaprice.org/knowyourfats/fats_phony.html
Mary Enig, Cholesterol and Heart Disease-- A Phony Issue

(5) http://www.cmaj.ca/cgi/content/full/173/10/1207-a
Questioning the benefits of statins Eddie Vos and Colin P. Rose , CMAJ • November 8, 2005; 173 (10). doi:10.1503/cmaj.1050120.

(6) *http://www.westonaprice.org/moderndiseases/statin.html*
Dangers of Statin Drugs: What You Haven't Been Told About Popular Cholesterol-Lowering Medicines By Sally Fallon and Mary G. Enig, PhD

(7) *http://www.ti.ubc.ca/pages/letter48.htm*
Therapeutics Initiative, Do Statins have a Role in Primary Prevention?

(8) *http://jama.ama-assn.org/cgi/content/abstract/291/18/2243*
Drug Treatment of Hyperlipidemia in Women Judith M. E. Walsh, MD, MPH; Michael Pignone, MD, MPH JAMA. 2004;291:2243-2252.

(8A) *http://www.bmj.com/cgi/content/full/334/7601/983*
BMJ 2007;334:983 (12 May), doi:10.1136/bmj.39202.397488.AD Should women be offered cholesterol lowering drugs to prevent cardiovascular disease? No Malcolm Kendrick, general practitioner

(9) *http://www.nwhn.org/newsletter/article.cfm?content_id=134*
Women's Health Activist May/ June 2007: Exploring Statins: What Does the Evidence Say? By Electra Kaczorowski, National Women's Health Network

(10) *http://www.recoverymedicine.com/cholesterol_lowering_drug_side_effects.htm*
Statin Drugs: A Critical Review of the Risk/Benefit Clinical Research, Joel M. Kauffman, Ph.D. Professor of Chemistry Emeritus USP Philadelphia, PA, USA 9 Dec 2003

(11) *http://www.whp-apsf.ca/pdf/statinsEvidenceCaution.pdf*
Evidence for Caution: Women and statin use By Harriet Rosenberg Danielle Allard Women and Health Protection June 2007

(12) *http://www.health-heart.org/malpractice.pdf*
LETTER TO THE EDITOR: Statins for women, elderly: Malpractice? Nutrition, Metabolism & Cardiovascular Diseases (2007) 17, e19ee20 Eddie Vos 127 Courser Rd, Sutton (Qc),

(13) *http://www.lewrockwell.com/sardi/sardi69.html*
Who Will Tell the People? It Isn't Cholesterol! by Bill Sardi

(14) *http://overdosedamerica.com/articles.php*
Lancet: Vol 369 January 20, 2007 Are lipid-lowering guidelines evidence-based? J Abramson and JM Wright

(15) *http://www.health-fx.net/eBook.pdf*
The Hidden Truth About Cholesterol-Lowering Drugs, by Shane Ellison, MS, Organic Chemistry

(16) *http://www.nytimes.com/2008/01/17/business/17drug.html*
New Questions on Treating Cholesterol, By ALEX BERENSON, New York Times January 17, 2008

(18) http://www.lewrockwell.com/sardi/sardi79.html
Government Health Agencies Complicit in Cholesterol Ruse by Bill Sardi on Lew Rockwell.com

(19) http://pharmamkting.blogspot.com/2008/01/should-i-stop-taking-zetia.html
Pharma Marketing Blog by **Shaun McIver**, of Streamlogics, Inc discussion of Zetia Enhance trial.

(20) http://blogs.wsj.com/health/2008/01/14/zetia-doesnt-enhance-zocor/
January 14, 2008, 9:11 am Zetia Doesn't Enhance Zocor Posted by Shirley S. Wang Wall Street Journal

(21) http://www.youtube.com/watch?v=kBfWybm0218
Vytorin video AD on You Tube 30 sec, Humorous clothes which look like the food. These adds have been pulled from natiuonal television.

(22) http://energycommerce.house.gov/Press_110/110-ltr.010708.Pfizer.Jarvik.pdf
Letter from John Dingel Mich to CEO of Pfizer asking for records on Jarvik and Lipitor, celebrity endorsement of Lipitor Ads.

(22A) http://blogs.wsj.com/health/2008/01/16/congress-investigates-vytorin-ads/
Wall Street Journal January 16, 2008, 3:44 pm Congress Investigates Vytorin Ads Posted by Anna Wilde Mathews

(23) http://blogs.wsj.com/health/2008/01/07/congress-to-pfizer-why-is-robert-jarvik-the-lipitor-man/
January 7, 2008, Wall Street Journal, Congress to Pfizer: Why is Robert Jarvik the Lipitor Man? Posted by Shirley S. Wang

(24) http://video.search.yahoo.com/video/play?vid=1298285495&vw=g&b=0&pos=4&p= lipitor&fr=yfp-t-501
Lipitor Ad with Robert Jarvik 60 seconds. This ad has been pulled and no longer shown on national television.

(25) http://www.nytimes.com/2008/01/17/business/17drug.html
New Questions on Treating Cholesterol By ALEX BERENSON Published: January 17, 2008

(27) http://www.jpands.org/vol10no3/colpo.pdf
LDL Cholesterol, Bad Cholesterol or Bad Science by Anthony Colpo, Journal of American Physicians and Surgeons Volume 10 Number 3 Fall 2005

(28) http://www.joplink.net/prev/200411/200411_10.pdf
Recurrent Acute Pancreatitis Possibly Induced by Atorvastatin and Rosuvastatin. Is Statin Induced Pancreatitis a Class Effect? JOP. J Pancreas (Online) 2004; 5(6):502-504.

(29) *http://www.cmellc.com/geriatrictimes/g040618.html*
Statin Adverse Effects: Implications for the Elderly by Beatrice A. Golomb, M.D., Ph.D. Geriatric Times May/June 2004 Vol. V Issue 3.

(30) *http://www.bmj.com/cgi/content/full/335/7614/285*
Preventive health care in elderly people needs rethinking, BMJ 2007;335:285-287 (11 August), "Preventive use of statins shows no overall benefit in elderly people as cardiovascular mortality and morbidity are replaced by cancer".

(31) *http://image.thelancet.com/extras/02art8325web.pdf*
Pravastatin in elderly individuals at risk of (PROSPER): a randomised controlled trial. THE LANCET Published online November 19, 2002

(32) *http://www.spacedoc.net/index.html*
SpaceDoc, Duane Graveline MD Author of Statin Drugs Side Effects

(33) *http://www.thincs.org/index.htm*
THINCS The International Society of Cholesterol Sceptics

(34) *http://www.jpands.org/vol12no1/kauffman.pdf*
Misleading Recent Papers on Statin Drugsin Peer-Reviewed Medical Journals Joel M. Kauffman, Ph.D. Journal of American Physicians and Surgeons Volume 12 Number 1 Spring 2007

(35) *http://www.scientificexploration.org/jse/articles/pdf/18.4_bauer.pdf*
Science in the 21st Century: Knowledge Monopolies and Research Cartels HENRY H. BAUER Professor Emeritus of Chemistry & Science Studies Dean Emeritus of Arts & Sciences Virginia Polytechnic Institute & State University / Journal of Scientific Exploration, Vol. 18, No. 4, pp. 643–660, 2004

(36) *http://www.ajronline.org/cgi/reprint/151/4/667*
Radiologic Appearance of the Jarvik Artificial Heart Implant Its Thoracic Complications AJR 151:667-671, October 1988 Laurie L. Fajardo

(37) *http://query.nytimes.com/gst/fullpage.html?res=9A0DE0DC1F3FF93AA15755C0A960948260*
The End of Life: Euthanasia and Morality (Oxford University Press, 1986).] SUICIDE AND EUTHANASIA Barney Clark's key to turn off artificial heart.

(38) *http://www.pubmedcentral.nih.gov/articlerender.fcgi?tool=pubmed&pubmedid=11678788*
Statins for primary prevention: at what coronary risk is safety assured? Peter R Jackson Br J Clin Pharmacol. 2001 October; 52(4): 439–446. For people with no known heart disease (primary prevention), "statin use could be associated with an increase in mortality of 1% in 10 years."

(39) http://www.ncbi.nlm.nih.gov/pubmed/16815382

Statins act like Vitamin D !! Lancet. 2006 Jul 1;368(9529):83-6. Grimes DS. **of vitamin D.** It seems likely that statins activate vitamin D receptors."

(40) http://www.reuters.com/article/governmentFilingsNews/idUSN2525934020080225

Pfizer pulls TV ads with heart expert Jarvik. By Lisa Richwine Mon Feb 25, WASHINGTON (Reuters) - Pfizer Inc said on Monday it was pulling television advertisements for its Lipitor cholesterol drug featuring Dr. Robert Jarvik, inventor of the Jarvik artificial heart, because they created "misimpressions."

(41) http://cspinet.org/new/pdf/finalnihltr.pdf

PETITION TO THE NATIONAL INSTITUTES OF HEALTH SEEKING AN INDEPENDENT REVIEW PANEL TO RE-EVALUATE THE NATIONAL CHOLESTEROL EDUCATION PROGRAM GUIDELINES September 23, 2004

Chapter 11

Protect Your Family from Bad Drugs

Over the last 30 years, 20 per cent of drugs approved by the FDA were later classified as "BAD Drugs", meaning that they were later withdrawn from the market or given a black box warning.*(1)(2)* Why does the FDA approve risky drugs which are finally banned? This question is explored by Daryl Kulakin on his "That's Fit Blog" detailing conflicts of interest in medicine and corruption in medical journals.*(3)* This issue is also explored by Shannon Brownlee in her Washington Monthly article, "Why you can't Trust Medical Journals Anymore".*(4)*

The FDA Can't Protect You From Bad Drugs

David Graham MD, Director of Drug Safety at the FDA uttered his famous phrase during Congressional testimony November 2004 "The FDA is incapable of protecting the American Public against another Vioxx".*(5)(6)(7)(8)*

How can you determine if you are dealing with a BAD DRUG?

Here are the early warning signs of a bad drug:
1) The drug has been recalled or given a black box warning.
2) The drug is in litigation with numerous lawsuits against the drug company.
3) The drug has been banned in other countries.

Listing of Drugs which have black box warnings:

The list of black box warnings includes literally hundreds of drugs, so best to check it on an internet web site list.(*9*)

Partial Listing of Recalled or Banned drugs: Baycol, Bextra, Colchicine, Complete Moisture Plus, Duract, Duragesic, Fentanyl Patch, Ephedra, Fen-Phen, Hismanal, Lotromex, Palladone, Permax, Pondimen, Posicor, Propulsid, Raplon, Raxar, Redux, Renu Moisture Loc Lens Solution, Rezulin, Seldane, Tysabri, Vioxx, Zelnorm.*(10)(11)* Consumer Reports provides their list of risky drugs on their web site.*(12)*

Drug Litigation may be Our Only Protection from Bad Drugs

Do you like lawyers? If you asked me if I liked lawyers, I would laugh and tell you a few lawyer jokes. One of my favorites is, "How do you tell the difference between a lawyer and a sperm? The answer is: the sperm has a one in 10 million chance of becoming a human being". In spite of the jokes, and since the FDA can't protect us, lawyers and drug litigation may be our last protection from bad drugs. Drug litigation by lawyers gives us an early warning sign about a bad drug. Drug litigation can uncover secret information about adverse drug side effects which drug companies hide from the public.*(13)(42)(43)* A computer search for search keywords, unsafe drugs in litigation gave 1.5 Million hits.*(14)*

The following is my short list of drugs currently in litigation.

Avandia and Rezulin, Diabetes Drugs

Avandia (rosiglitazone) by GlaxoSmithKline, is used for adult onset Type 2 diabetes. (thiazolidinedione class of drugs). Avandia causes a 43% higher risk of heart attacks. This is ironic because diabetes causes accelerated heart disease, and controlling diabetes with drugs is supposed to **reduce** incidence of heart attacks, not increase it. *(15)(16)*

Rezulin was used for blood sugar control in patients with adult onset type 2 diabetes. Rezulin has been recalled due to liver toxicity.

Zelnorm for Constipation - Banned

Zelnorm (tegaserod) was FDA approved for irritable bowel syndrome and constipation in women. Novartis agreed to voluntarily suspend sales of Zelnorm March 2007, following reports of adverse side effects such as heart attack and stroke. They then withdrew Zelnorm from the market.

Permax and Dostinex

Permax (pergolide) and **Dostinex** (cabergoline) are used for Parkinson's, restless leg syndrome, and migraine headaches. Other similar drugs have been banned such as the diet drug Fen-phen. Thy are all associated with heart valve problems and leaky valves. Permax currently has a black box warning about this increased risk of heart valve problems. The sale of Permax has been suspended by Valeant.*(17)*

Osteoporosis Drugs Fosamax (Alendronate), Zometa (Zoledronate), Actonel (Risedronate), Boniva (Ibandronate), the Bisphosphonate Osteoporosis Drugs.*(18)*

Fosamax (alendronate)

As of May 13, 2007, hundreds of lawsuits had been filed against Merck alleging Fosamax-induced Necrosis of the Jaw, (ONJ). The first case is set to be tried in late 2008 in New York. *(19)*

Fosamax is Merck's bisphosphonate osteoporosis drug which causes osteonecrosis ONJ of the jaw, an irreversible breakdown of the jawbone, associated with ulcerations in the mouth, non-healing wounds, and osteomyelitis of the jaw. *(19A) (20) (21) (22) (23)*

Warnings have been sent out to all dentists and endodontists: This is the (Endodontists) AAE Position Statement: "Endodontic Implications of Bisphosphonate-Associated Osteonecrosis of the Jaws American Endodontists Association" *(24)*.

The osteoporosis drugs are supposed to make the bones stronger. Again, it is ironic that these drugs cause the jaw bone to literally fall apart, meaning they make the bones weaker, not stronger. Because of this flaw in bone physiology, my opinion is it is likely that this entire class of bisphosphonate drugs will be banned. For more information on these drugs, see my articles on the bisphosphonate drugs.*(52)(53)*

Synthetic Hormones

Prempro manufactured by Wyeth *(25)* is a hormone replacement pill containing the synthetic hormones, Premarin and Provera. Premarin is estrogen from a pregnant horse. Provera is a synthetic progesterone which is chemically altered and is not normally present in the human body or anywhere else in nature. The NIH funded (WHI) Women's Health Initiative Study was terminated early when its data showed that Prempro increased risk of Heart Disease and Breast Cancer.*(26)(27)* Bio-Identical Human Hormones, on the other hand, are NOT associated with increased risk of cancer or heart disease, this increased risk applies only to the synthetic hormones not found in the human body such as Prempro.

Ortho Evra

Ortho Evra (birth control/contraceptive skin patch) by Ortho-McNeil Pharmaceuticals contains synthetic hormones, norelgestromin and ethinyl estradiol, delivered in a transdermal birth control patch. In November 2005, the FDA warned that the product contains higher levels of estrogen than most others and increases risk of blood clots, strokes, and heart attacks.

Depo-Provera

Depo-Provera is a synthetic hormone used for birth control, injected every 3 months. Long term use causes osteoporosis, fractures, spine injuries and hip injuries. A $700 million class action lawsuit was filed against Pfizer in Toronto on behalf of Canadian women who used Depo-Provera and developed osteoporosis. Several lawsuits making the same allegations against Pfizer have been filed in the United States.

Vioxx, Celebrex, Bextra, Cox-2 inhibitor Pain Pills

Vioxx (rofecoxib) by Merck is a pain medication causing adverse reactions such as heart attack, stroke, and sudden cardiac death. In September 2004, Merck voluntarily withdrew Vioxx from the market. Dr. David Graham, Director of Drug Safety at the FDA, said that Vioxx caused up to 160,000 heart attacks and strokes. *(44)(45)* Forty Five Thousand people have sued Merck, and Merk has spent 1 billion on legal fees. Merck's strategy of fighting every case by dragging out the proceedings ended on November 9, 2007, when Merck agreed to pay $4.85 billion to settle all of the court claims.*(51)*

Celebrex: A Cox-2 inhibitor approved for the treatment of rheumatoid arthritis and osteoarthritis, and later approved for familial polyposis (colon polyps). Celebrex may increase the risk of heart attack or stroke.

Bextra (valdecoxib) by Pfizer is similar to Vioxx. Studies have shown adverse reactions with Bextra such as heart attack, stroke, sudden cardiac death, Erythema Multiforme (EM), Stevens-Johnson Syndrome (SJS), and Toxic Epidermal Necrolysis (TEN). Bextra has been banned from Canada.*(28)*

Anti-Cholesterol Statin Drugs, Baychol, Lipitor, Crestor, Zocor

Baycol

Baychol is a statin anti-cholesterol drug which was recalled because muscle damage releases muscle debris into the bloodstream which then clogs up the kidneys and causes renal failure.

Lipitor - Pfizer

Lawsuits were filed in New York against Pfizer claiming that Lipitor (atorvastatin) causes memory loss, peripheral neuropathy, fatigue and muscle damage. Lipitor's labeling warns patients to tell their doctor if they suffer any symptoms of muscle pain or weakness.

More Lipitor litigation against Pfizer was filed on September 28, 2005 in Boston by Hagens Berman Sobol Shapiro claiming Pfizer deceived consumers about the benefits of Lipitor through deceptive marketing and advertising activities. They claimed that billions of Lipitor profits come from patients who do not benefit from the drug.

According to the complaint, Pfizer launched a massive campaign to convince the public that Lipitor is a beneficial treatment for nearly everyone with elevated cholesterol, even though no studies have shown it to be effective for women, or for those over 65 years of age who do not already have heart disease or diabetes. For more information on lipitor, zocor and all the statin anti-cholesterol drugs, see my previous articles on this topic.*(54)(55)*

Crestor

Crestor (rosuvastatin) is a statin anti-cholesterol drug similar to the recalled drug Baycol. Compared to other statins, Crestor has the greatest kidney toxicity, causing muscle breakdown products to clog the kidneys. During clinical trials, patients taking the 80 mg dose of Crestor began to show clogging of the kidneys with the muscle debris. Because of this finding, the 80 mg dosage was discontinued.

Psychiatric Drugs Atypical Antipsychotics, SSRI's etc

Adderall is an an amphetamine by Shire used for ADHD.*(29)* On February 9, 2005, Health Canada suspended the sale of ADDERALL used for Attention Deficit Hyperactivity Disorder (ADHD) in children because of 20 reports of sudden death, fourteen of which occurred in children, and six in adults. There were 12 reports of stroke, two of which occurred in children.

Ritalin

Numerous Ritalin lawsuits against Novartis were filed through the 1990s. Simultaneously, there was a campaign against ADHD medications for children by various interest groups. Starting in 2000, lawsuits were filed against Novartis for fraud in the marketing and over promotion of Ritalin and Attention Deficit Hyperactivity Disorder. The suits alleged that Novartis was conspiring with the APA (American Psychiatric Association) to increase sales of these lucrative drugs by illegally promoting off label use.

Zyprexa and Seroquel

Zyprexa (Olanzapine) and Seroquel are used for schizophrenia and bipolar disorder, dementia, attention deficit hyperactivity disorder (ADHD), gambling addictions, and postpartum depression. Zyprexa and Seroquel cause Tardive Dyskinesia, diabetes, hyperglycemia, pancreatitis, and ketoacidosis. Eli Lilly has already agreed to pay $1.2 billion to settle 28,500 lawsuits. Secret Zyprexa documents have been disclosed to the public by medical heroes at great personal risk *(30)(31)*

Dr. Timothy Scott, author of, "America Fooled: The Truth about Antidepressants, Antipsychotics and How We've Been Deceived, reports a 2005 study that found there are approximately 30,000 children under 5 on these atypical anti-psychotic drugs.

Dr. Fred Baughman, author of "The ADHD Fraud: How Psychiatry Makes "Patients" of Normal Children," reports that 10 million of the 50-million school children in the nation are on one or more psychiatric drugs and states: "This is death by psychiatry." *(32)(33)(34)(35)*

The Children's Hospital of Philadelphia recently found that 19% of children who were newly diagnosed with Type 2 diabetes were being treated with these new atypical anti-psychotic drugs which cause obesity and diabetes *(36)(37)(37A)*

Risperdal (Risperidone) is an anti-psychotic medication by Janssen Pharmaceutical, Johnson & Johnson used for bipolar disorder. Serious side effects: Diabetes, Diabetic Coma, Hyperglycemia, Ketoacidosis, Neuroleptic Malignant Syndrome, Pancreatitis, Stroke, Tardive Diskinesia, Weight Gain, Death.*(38)*

SSRI Antidepressants, Prozac, Zoloft, and Paxil Antidepressant Users v. Eli Lilly, Pfizer, and GlaxoSmithKline *(39)*

Some 200 legal actions have been filed against Eli Lilly, Pfizer, and GlaxoSmithKline, the manufacturers of Prozac (fluoxetine), Zoloft (sertraline), and Paxil (paroxetine) to recover for suicides or homicides by patients. The lawsuits claim that the companies knew about, but hid the documents which showed increased risk of akathisia, a form of agitation causing suicide and violence.

Prozac

Payouts by Lilly estimated to be over $50 million to quietly settle more than 30 of those Prozac lawsuits. *(40)(41)*

Paxil

Paxil causes serious side effects, agitation, violent or suicidal behavior, painful withdrawal and addiction problems. It may cause birth defects in pregnant women. Paxil has been recklessly prescribed to children when it was proven no more effective than a placebo. Both children and adults taking Paxil have demonstrated suicidal tendencies during treatment, while trying to quit and during withdrawal. For more information on SSRI drug adverse side effects and SSRI induced suicide, see a previous chapter on this topic.*(56)*

Strattera

Strattera is used for ADHD in children, teens, and adults, and causes serious liver side effects and jaundice. Strattera may also cause suicidal thoughts in children and teens.

Serzone

Serzone is an anti-depressant which increases the risk of liver failure by 3-4 times.

Acne Drug, Accutane

Accutane (isotretinoin) is Hoffman La Roche's acne drug, an oral drug for severe nodular acne (the bad type of acne that can lead to scarring). Accutane is a synthetic form of vitamin A designed to dry up oil that clog the pores and cause acne. Accutane can cause depression, psychotic symptoms, and rarely suicide attempts. There have been over 142 suicides involving Accutane since 1982. In October 2001, Congressman Bart Stupak's son committed suicide while taking Accutane. Accutane also causes severe birth defects and fetal death. Accutane side effects are, Inflammatory Bowel Disease, Crohn's Disease, Ulcerative Colitis, Birth Defects, Suicide, Psychiatric disorders.

Erectile Dysfunction ED Drugs, Viagra, Levitra, Cialis

Viagra

On May 27, 2005, the FDA reported that Viagra, (by Pfizer) may cause temporary or permanent vision loss, and reported 50 cases of "Viagra blindness". This blindness is due to occlusion of the artery to the eye, causing optic nerve stroke and damage. This severe adverse event affects people with blood vessel problems, like diabetes or hypertension.

Remicade for Inflammatory Bowel Disease

Remicade (Inflixmab) is an immune-suppressing drug by Centocor (Johnson & Johnson) approved for Crohn's disease and Rheumatoid Arthritis. Remicade side effects include; tuberculosis, histoplasmosis, listeria sepsis, invasive fungal infections, lymphoma, pneumocystosis, seizures, multiple sclerosis, lupus, serious infections, heart failure and death. In August 15, 2001 , Remicade was given a Black Box Warning of increased risk of tuberculosis, invasive fungal infections, and other opportunistic infections. On October 18, 2001 a second warning about increased mortality in patients with congestive heart failure.

Antibiotics

Ketek (telithromycin) by Aventis Pharmaceuticals is a ketolide antibiotic causing liver damage, liver disease, liver failure, and worsening myasthenia gravis.

Tequin (gatifloxacin), an antibiotic by Bristol-Myers Squibb Co. which causes hypoglycemia (low blood sugar) and hyperglycemia (high blood sugar), which can lead to coma or seizure and potentially fatal. Tequin was withdrawn from market in 2006 .

Lariam (mefloquine) causes psychiatric symptoms, anxiety, paranoia, depression, hallucinations and psychotic behavior, even long after Mefloquine has been stopped. Suicidal ideation and suicide have been reported

TROVAN , trovafloxacin On June 9, 1999, FDA issued a public health advisory about risks of liver toxicity from Trovan (trovafloxacin)

Diet Pills Fen-Phen

Fen-phen is a combination of fenfluromine and phentermine. Fen-Phen had been approved for many years as an appetite suppressant in the management of obesity. The trouble with this drug combo is that it has been found to cause heart valve disease. American Home Products Corp. offered $3.75 billion last year to settle lawsuits over its fen-phen diet pills, which it yanked from the market in 1997 over health concerns.

Meridia diet pills cause PPH (primary pulmonary hypertension) as well as cardiac valve dysfunction.

Propulsid, Heartburn

Propulsid is a drug approved for patients with severe heartburn or gastro esophageal reflux. Propulsid can cause irregular or abnormal heart rhythms.

Neurontin A 2004 lawsuit alleges that Parke Davis created an illegal promotional campaign to get more patients to use Neurontin which is approved for epilepsy. Disguised as medical education for the doctors or consulting for the company, the promotional campaign included illegal cash kickbacks to physicians and other sales ploys to pump up sales of Neurontin for non-FDA approved uses.

Thimerosal

Thimerosal is used in vaccines as a preservative. Thimerosal degrades into ethyl mercury, a highly toxic form of mercury which causes neurological disorders*(42)*.

Procrit

Procrit increases the blood count, and is used to treat the anemia of chronic kidney failure, HIV, or cancer. Procrit reduces need for blood transfusions. Procrit has caused deaths, non-fatal heart attacks, strokes, heart failure and blood clots in patients with chronic kidney failure receiving higher than recommended doses. Procrit causes accelerated cancer tumor growth and increased risk of death, and may cause blood clots following surgery. An FDA-mandated black box warning has been added to Procrit labeling

Topical Creams for Eczema

Elidel *(*pimecrolimus*)* and **Protopic** *(*tacrolimus*)* are topical creams for eczema, both linked to skin cancer and lymphoma. A black box warning was given 2006.

Disclaimer: It is important to discuss any treatment plan with your personal physician. Do not start or stop a treatment, drug, supplement or lifestyle change based on information from this article. Even if a drug is on a ligation, recall or black box list, any decision to start or stop a drug should be made in consultation with your own doctor, who should help you weigh the comparative risks and benefits to arrive at an informed decision. Some of the drugs given black box warnings are in common use because the benefits are felt to outweigh the risks. These are complex issues that require professional advice.

References Chapter 11

(1) http://jama.ama-assn.org/cgi/content/abstract/287/17/2215
Timing of New Black Box Warnings and Withdrawals for Prescription Medications Karen E. Lasser, MD,MPH; Paul D. Allen, MD,MPH; Steffie J. Woolhandler, MD,MPH; David U. Himmelstein, MD; Sidney M. Wolfe, MD; David H. Bor, MD JAMA. 2002;287:2215-2220.

(2) http://www.citizen.org/publications/release.cfm?ID=7171
Public Citizen on the article in JAMA: Timing of new black box warnings and withdrawals for prescription medications *(*HRG Publication #1618*)*

(3) http://www.thatsfit.com/2006/10/04/why-the-fda-approves-bad-drugs/
Why the FDA Approves Bad Drugs, Thats Fit Blog, Oct 4th 2006 1:00PM by Daryl Kulak

(4) http://www.pnhp.org/news/2008/may/doctors_without_bord.php
Posted on May 20, 2008 Doctors Without Borders: Why you can't trust medical journals anymore. By Shannon Brownlee Washington Monthly

(5) http://www.intelihealth.com/IH/ihtIH/EMIHC267/333/21291/404591?d=dmtICNNews
FDA Called 'Defenseless' Against Bad Drugs, November 18, 2004 Aetna IntelliHealth

(6) http://www.forbes.com/home/sciencesandmedicine/2004/12/13/cx_mh_1213faceoftheyear.html
Pharmaceuticals Face Of The Year: David Graham by Matthew Herper, 12.13.04 Forbes. To hear Graham tell it, this is part of a systemic failure to address drug safety on the part of the FDA, a story that reaches back over the entirety of his 20-year career at the agency.

(7) *http://en.wikipedia.org/wiki/David_Graham_(whistleblower)*
David Graham Wikipedia Whistleblower Biography

(8) *http://www.drug-injury.com/druginjurycom/2005/12/fdas_david_grah.html*
FDA's David Graham Says U.S. Drug Safety System No Better in 2005 Graham Criticizes Agency's Performance During The Year Since Vioxx Recall by Tom Lamb

(9) *http://www.formularyproductions.com/master/showpage.php?dir=blackbox&whichpage=9*
Black Box Warning information researched and published by: Joyce Generali, MS, RPh, FASHP

(10) *http://www.resource4thepeople.com/recalleddrugs/index.html*
Recalled Drugs Listing, Free Recalled Drugs Case Review, Resource 4 the People

(11) *http://www.consumerreports.org/cro/health-fitness/drugs-supplements/common-drugs-hidden-dangers-106/overview/index.htm*
Prescription for trouble Common drugs, hidden dangers. Consumer Reports

(12) *http://www.consumerreports.org/cro/health-fitness/drugs-supplements/common-drugs-hidden-dangers-106/highrisk-drugs/index.htm*
Drug risks the system missed. This table lists the relatively common drugs we've identified as having known or suspected serious risks that were undetected or underestimated when the FDA approved them. Consumer Reports Overview of Risky Drugs

(13) *http://jama.ama-assn.org/cgi/content/full/297/3/308*
The Role of Litigation in Defining Drug Risks Aaron S. Kesselheim, MD, JD; Jerry Avorn, MD JAMA. 2007;297:308-311.

(14) *http://search.yahoo.com/search;_ylt=A0geu.hlv9BGyF4AVTJXNyoA?p=unsafe+drugs+in++litigation&y=Search&fr=*
Yahoo Search of Unsafe Drug Litigation about 1.5 Million hits

(15) *http://www.annals.org/cgi/content/full/0000605-200710160-00182v1*
Uncertain Effects of Rosiglitazone on the Risk for Myocardial Infarction and Cardiovascular Death George A. Diamond, MD; Leon Bax, MSc; and Sanjay Kaul, MD 16 October 2007 | Volume 147 Issue 8

(16) *http://content.nejm.org/cgi/content/full/NEJMp078167*
The Rosiglitazone Story — Lessons from an FDA Advisory Committee Meeting Clifford J. Rosen, M.D. *www.nejm.org* August 8, 2007 (10.1056/NEJMp078167)

(17) *http://www.fda.gov/cder/drug/advisory/pergolide.htm*
FDA Public Health Advisory Pergolide (marketed as Permax)

(18) *http://search.yahoo.com/search;_ylt=A0geu66F981G_FgA2c1XNyoA?p=fosamax+litigation&y=Search&fr=yfp-t-499*
Fosamax Litigation Search Terms

(19) *http://en.wikipedia.org/wiki/Fosamax*
Fosamax on Wikipedia

(19) *http://www.ada.org/prof/resources/topics/osteonecrosis.asp*
Osteonecrosis of Jaw ONJ, ADA

(20) *http://www.ada.org/prof/resources/pubs/jada/reports/report_bisphosphonate.pdf*
American Dental Association on ONJ and fosamax. Dental management of patients receiving oral bisphosphonate therapy Expert panel recommendations American Dental Association Council on Scientific Affairs

(21) *http://www.ada.org/prof/resources/topics/topics_osteonecrosis_consent.pdf*
Obtaining Obtaining Informed Consent Relating to Risks Associated with Oral Bisphosphonate Use

(22) American Association of Oral and Maxillofacial Surgeons Position Paper on Bisphosphonate-Related Osteonecrosis of the Jaws Approved by the Board of Trustees September 25, 2006 "it would appear prudent to consider all patients taking bisphosphonates to be at some risk for ONJ,"

(23) *http://www.aaoms.org/docs/position_papers/osteonecrosis.pdf*
American Association of Oral and Maxillofacial Surgeons Position Paper on Bisphosphonate-Related Osteonecrosis of the Jaws Approved by the Board of Trustees September 25, 2006

(24) *http://www.aae.org/ManagedFiles/pub/0/Pulp/bisphosonatesstatement.pdf*
Endodontic Implications of Bisphosphonate-Associated Osteonecrosis of the Jaws. Bisphosphonates May Put Patients At Risk For Deterioration Of The Jaw, American Association Of Endodontists

(25) *http://www.prempro.com/index.aspx*
Official Prempro web site

(26) *http://www.nhlbi.nih.gov/new/press/02-07-09.htm*
NATIONAL INSTITUTES OF HEALTH National Heart, Lung, and Blood Institute Tuesday, July 9, 2002 NHLBI Stops Trial of *(*Prempro*)* Premarin Plus Progestin Due to Increased Breast Cancer Risk, Lack of Overall Benefit. NIH Press Release Halting WHI PremPro study because of increase cancer and heart disease from synthetic hormones.

(27) *http://classaction.findlaw.com/cases/prempro/*
Prempro litigation, Lawyer WebSite

(28) *http://www.hc-sc.gc.ca/ahc-asc/media/advisories-avis/_2005/2005_134-eng.php*
Health Canada prohibits sale of Bextra in Canada. Advisory 2005-134 December 16, 2005
Following a review of safety information, Health Canada is informing the public that Bextra, an anti-inflammatory drug used to treat arthritis and pain, will not return to the market.

(29) *http://www.hc-sc.gc.ca/ahc-asc/media/advisories-avis/_2005/2005_01-eng.php*
Health Canada suspends the market authorization of ADDERALL XR®, a drug prescribed for Attention Deficit Hyperactivity Disorder (ADHD) in children

(30) *http://www.furiousseasons.com/zyprexadocs.html*
Zyprexa Documents Revealed Furious Seasons BLog Jim Gottstein

(31) *http://reliableanswers.com/med/zyprexa_off_label.asp*
Activists Take on Eli Lilly Over Off-Label Sale of Zyprexa Update May 28, 2007:by Evelyn Pringle

(32) *http://www.lawyersandsettlements.com/articles/00586/zyprexa-injury.html*
Zyprexa Injury Clock Keeps Ticking Away February 2, 2007. By Evelyn Pringle on Zyprexa Litigation

(33) *http://www.redorbit.com/news/health/611198/zyprexa_users_eagerly_await_settlement_payments/index.html?source=r_health*
Zyprexa Users Eagerly Await Settlement Payments August 2006 By Jeff Swiatek, The Indianapolis Star Aug. 10--More than 8,000 users of Eli Lilly and Co.'s top-selling drug should find out this month how much their pain and suffering is worth.

Zyprexa Litigation Settlements

(34) *http://www.iht.com/articles/2007/04/25/business/drug.php*
U.S. drug agency investigating accuracy of Lilly's Zyprexa data, International Herald Tribune By Alex Berenson Published: April 25, 2007

(35) *http://www.scoop.co.nz/stories/HL0701/S00142.htm*
Public Has Right To Know Zyprexa Secrets Monday, 15 January 2007, Evelyn Pringle

(36) *http://ahrp.blogspot.com/2007/02/zyprexa-cat-out-bag-lilly-problems.html*
zyprexa Info at AHRP, Zyprexa Cat out bag: Lilly Problems Getting Liability Insurance and the Chabasinki brief

(37) *http://zyprexa.pbwiki.com/*
Zyprexa Information Web Site

(37A) *http://www.prnewswire.com/mnr/lilly/12241/docs/zFactSheet.pdf*
Zyprexa Lilly Fact Sheet

(38) *http://www.psychsearch.net/lawsuits.html*
State Lawsuits - Atypical Antipsychotics Abilify, Geodon, Risperdal, Seroquel, Zyprexa The TMAP Drugs (Texas Medication Algorithm Project) TMAP and TeenScreen Litigation Information by State

(39) *http://psychrights.org/Litigation/ProzacZoloftPaxilClassActions.htm*
Prozac, Paxil, Zoloft Class Action Litigation, Prozac, Zoloft, and Paxil Antidepressant Users v. Eli Lilly, Pfizer, and GlaxoSmithKline Commonly-Prescribed Antidepressants Are Extremely Dangerous for Some

(40) *http://search.yahoo.com/search;_ylt=A0geu5S6.M1GfXEA0gFXNyoA?p=prozac+litigation&fr=yfp-t-499*
Prozac Litigation Search Keywords 2 million hits

(41) *http://en.wikipedia.org/wiki/Eli_Lily*
E Lily at Wikipedia, In a trial case of SSRI suicide, Eli Lilly was caught corrupting the judicial process by making a deal with the plaintiff's attorney to throw the case, known as the Fentress Case involved a Kentucky man, Joseph Wesbecker, on Prozac, who went to his workplace and opened fire killing 7 people, and injuring 12 others before turning the gun on himself.

Important JAMA and BMJ Articles on Drug Litigation

(42) *http://psychrights.org/Articles/JAMA_role_of_litign_297_3.pdf*
The Role of Litigation in Defining Drug Risks Aaron S. Kesselheim, MD, JD Jerry Avorn, MD JAMA, January 17, 2007—Vol 297, No. 3 page 308.

(43) *http://ahrp.blogspot.com/2007/01/role-of-litigation-in-defining-drug.html* The Role of Litigation in Defining Drug Risks Aaron S. Kesselheim, MD, JD Jerry Avorn, MD JAMA, January 17, 2007—Vol 297, No. 3 page 308. Role of Drug Litigation

(44) *http://www.bmj.com/cgi/reprint/334/7585/120.pdf*
What have we learnt from Vioxx? Harlan M Krumholz, Joseph S Ross, Amos H Presler and David S Egilman BMJ 2007;334;120-123 British Medical Journal

(45) *http://www.bmj.com/cgi/content/full/334/7585/ 120?maxtoshow=&HITS=10&hits=10&RESULTFORMAT=&fulltext=egilman&searchid=1&FIRSTINDEX=0&resourcetype=HWCIT*
What have we learnt from Vioxx? Harlan M Krumholz, Joseph S Ross, Amos H Presler and David S Egilman BMJ 2007;334;120-123 British Medical Journal

Independent Pharma Watch-Dogs and News Sources

(46) *http://www.pharmedout.org/aboutus.htm*
PharmedOut is an independent project run by physicians for physicians and other prescribers. Our goals are to: Document and disseminate information about how pharmaceutical companies influence prescribing. Provide access to unbiased information about drugs. Encourage physicians to choose pharma-free CME. PharmedOut is led by a team of physicians and academics and is contributed to by a diverse group. The Principal Investigator is Adriane Fugh-Berman MD and the Project Manager is Alicia M. Bell MS. Pharmed Out Blog

(47) *http://www.medicalaccountability.net/index.html*
Moira Dolan, MD, Medical Accountability Network provides business healthcare solutions based on principles of integrity in medicine. We consider informed consent as the keystone to responsible health care management. Through advocacy, education and business solutions the M.A.N. seeks to raise the responsibility of all participants affected by medical matters. Medical Accountability Blog

(48) *http://pharmapseudocals.homestead.com/index.html*
PHARMAPSEUDOCAL INDUSTRY, a humorous look at the drug industry

(49) *http://fiddaman.blogspot.com/*
Bob Fiddaman Blog SEROXAT SUFFERERS - STAND UP AND BE COUNTED . Justice for Seroxat/Paxil/Paroxetine users. "For being a one-man wrecking crew, Fiddy gets my first Bruce Lee Award" - Phil Dawdy

(50) *http://icfda.drugawareness.org/home.html*
Dr. Ann Blake Tracy, Executive Director, International Coalition For Drug Awareness *www.drugawareness.org* & author of Prozac: Panacea or Pandora? - Our Serotonin Nightmare Drug. These are a group of physicians, researchers, journalists and concerned citizens dedicated to educating about the dangers posed by many Rx medicines.

Merck Vioxx Settlement Announced

(51) *http://www.cnbc.com/id/21702896/*
By Reuters 09 Nov 2007 Merck has agreed to pay $4.85 billion to settle claims that its painkiller Vioxx caused heart attacks and strokes in thousands.

(52) *http://jeffreydach.com/2007/05/14/fosamax-actonel-osteoporosis-and-toulouse-lautrec-by-jeffrey-dach-md.aspx*
Fosamax, Actonel, Osteoporosis and Toulouse Lautrec by Jeffrey Dach MD

(53) *http://jeffreydach.com/2008/03/09/bisphosphonates-for-osteoporosis-a-closer-look-at-the-data-by-jeffrey-dach-md.aspx*
Bisphosphonates for Osteoporosis, A Closer Look at the Data by Jeffrey Dach MD

(54) *http://jeffreydach.com/2007/05/14/lipitor-and-the-dracula-of-modern-technology-by-jeffrey-dach-md.aspx*
Lipitor and The Dracula of Modern Technology by Jeffrey Dach MD

(55) *http://jeffreydach.com/2008/01/27/cholesterol-lowering-statin-drugs-for-women-just-say-no-by-jeffrey-dach-md.aspx*
Cholesterol Lowering Statin Drugs for Women, Just Say No by Jeffrey Dach MD

(56) *http://jeffreydach.com/2007/05/14/paxil-prozac-and-ssri-induced-suicide-by-jeffrey-dach-md.aspx*
Paxil, Prozac and SSRI Induced Suicide by Jeffrey Dach MD

Section Three

Bioidentical Hormones for Women, Estrogen, Progesterone

Chapter 12

The Safety Of Bio-Identical Hormones

Are Women's Bio-identical hormones safe? Bio-identical hormones exist naturally in the human body, so it is axiomatic that these are safe. However, we are interested in a slightly different question. What is the safety of bio-identical hormones as routinely used in medical practice? Let's try to answer this question.

The Safety of Water compared to Bio-Identical Hormones

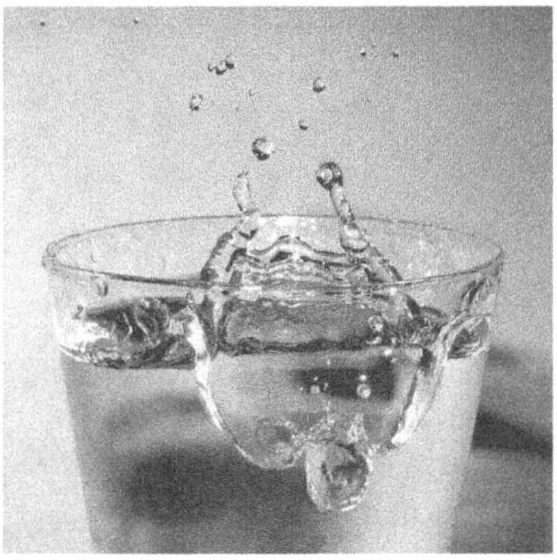

Water is safe, beneficial and required for health. Yet, even so, drinking excess amounts of water causes death from *Fatal Water Intoxication.(1)* Similarly, just like water, bio-identical hormones are safe and beneficial when used at proper dosages. Like excessive water, excessive hormone dosage may result in their own adverse side effects. Excess estrogen, for example, causes fluid retention, breast tenderness, breast enlargement, and disordered mood.

Glass of Water courtesy of Wikimedia Commons

Humans Have Bio-Identical Hormones.

Another answer to the safety question is that bio-identical hormones are found in the human body naturally. Any harmful substance in the human body would impair survival, and over millions of years of evolution would be eliminated by natural selection. This is the basic concept of Darwinian evolution which is accepted by mainstream medical science.

A 50 Million Year Medical Experiment

Consider the following medical experiment, performed over the last 50 million years with the help of our friend, *Darwinian evolution.(2)* Bio-Identical Hormones have been present in the human body for 50 million years, and we humans are still here on the planet. I would consider that a successful medical experiment, wouldn't you?

Either Excess or Deficiency of Anything Can be Harmful

One of our routine labs tests called the Chem Panel measures electrolytes and glucose levels in the blood. The body automatically maintains these within narrow ranges to maintain health. If levels deviate above or below these normal ranges, this causes a serious health disturbance. For example elevated potassium levels causes cardiac arrest. Magnesium deficiency causes muscle spasm and arrhythmia. Excessive amounts of Vitamins A and D are toxic. Hormone levels enjoy a considerably wide range wide range of acceptable limits. Even so, a deficiency or an excess of women's bio-identical hormones can produce adverse symptoms. This is called estrogen deficiency/excess, and progesterone deficiency/excess, and they each have *typical signs and symptoms* easily recognized.*(3)*

Common Signs of Estrogen Deficiency *(4)*

Mental fogginess
Forgetfulness
Depression
Minor anxiety
Mood change
Difficulty falling asleep
Hot flashes
Night sweats
Temperature swings
Day-long fatigue
Reduced stamina
Decreased sense of sexuality
Lessened self-image and attention to appearance
Dry eyes, skin, and vagina
Loss of skin radiance
Feel balanced 2nd part of cycle
Sagging breasts and loss of fullness
Pain with sexual activity
Weight gain
Increased back and joint pain
Episodes of rapid heartbeat
Headaches and migraines
Gastrointestinal discomfort
Constipation

Common Signs of Excess Estrogen *(***takes longer to notice***)*

Breast tenderness or pain
Increased breast size
Water retention, fingers, legs
Impatient, snappy behavior, but with clear mind
Pelvic cramps
Nausea

Common Signs of Progesterone Deficiency

No period at all *(*no ovulation*)*
The period comes infrequently *(*every few months*)*
Heavy and frequent periods *(*large clots, due to buildup in the uterus*)*
Spotting a few days before the period. *(*Progesterone level is dropping*)*
PMS
Cystic breasts
Painful breasts
Breasts with lumps
Most cases of endometriosis, adenomyosis, and fibroids.
Anxiety, irritability, nervousness and water retention

Above list courtesy of *Uzzi Reiss MD OB GYN.(4)*

No Reported Adverse Events from Bio-Identical Hormones

Over-the-counter pain pills *(*NSAIDs*)* such as aspirin, naproxen and ibuprofen are considered fairly safe. After all, you don't need a prescription to buy them, yet they cause an estimated *16,500 deaths* in the US annually, mostly from gastric bleeding.*(5)* Compare this to *no reported adverse events* from bio-identical hormones last year, according to an FDA press conference January 2008.*(6)*

Do Bio-Identical Hormones Cause Breast Cancer ?*(7)*

The answer is no. According to the *French Cohort study*, there is no increase in breast cancer in women using bio-identical hormones.*(8)* However, having said that, *avoiding excess environmental estrogens* as well as excessive estrogen levels from any source, is the key to preventing breast cancer.*(9)* My previous *article* covers our program for breast cancer prevention which includes iodine supplementation, Indole-3-carbinol and fiber. To read about this, see: *Breast Cancer Prevention and Iodine Supplementation by Jeffrey Dach MD.(10)*

Do Bio-Identical Hormones Cause Heart Disease?

Again, the answer is no. A *study of CAT calcium scores* by JoAnn E. Manson in the June 2007 JAMA actually showed less heart disease in the women taking unopposed estrogen (they had hysterectomies and were not given the synthetic progestins).*(11)* These same results had already been published 2 years previously in a calcium score study by Budoff in *J Womens Health 2005.(12)*

A Closer Look at the Women's Health Initiative WHI Study

Understanding the Women's Health Initiative (WHI) study is not difficult, and is very important to answer the question of hormone safety. The WHI study was the large NIH sponsored medical study which compared synthetic hormones to placebo in two large groups of women. The WHI study consisted of two arms. The first arm used the synthetic hormones Premarin and Provera, and the second arm used Premarin alone.*(13)(14)*

What is Premarin and Provera?

Premarin and Provera are not bio-identical hormones. *Premarin* is a hormone obtained from pregnant horses, which contains Equilin, a horse hormone not found in humans.*(15)* *Provera* is a synthetic hormone which is not found anywhere in the natural world (see provera diagram below).*(16)* The Premarin and Provera combination is called PremPro, a synthetic hormone pill commonly prescribed by mainstream medicine. Prempro was the hormone preparation used in the first arm of the WHI study.*(13)*

WHI study First Arm:

The WHI study (first arm published in JAMA 2002) was terminated early because the combination of premarin and provera (Prempro) caused increased breast cancer and heart disease.*(13)* Immediately after this study was published, there was a massive switch by women to bio-identical hormones which resulted in a 4 billion dollar loss for Wyeth, the maker of Prempro. Wyeth is still trying to recoup that money by manipulating the FDA. They want the FDA to ban their competition, the bio-identical hormones or their components.*(36)(37)(38)* Use this easy *tool to email your Congressman* and voice your opposition to Wyeth's attempts to ban estriol and other bio-identical hormones.*(17)* While you are at it, tell your Congressman that synthetic hormones are chemically altered monsters that should be banned.

WHI study second arm:

All the women in the second arm of the WHI study had prior hysterectomies, so they did not need the progestin, provera. Rather, they were only given Premarin (the horse hormone, also called CEE, for Conjugated Equine Estrogen). Unlike the first arm of the study, these women had ***no increase in breast cancer risk***.*(18)* A useful chart showing the data from the *second arm of the WHI* in JAMA 2004*(14)* can be found at *Susan Ott's Bone Physiology* Web Site.*(19)*

Premarin causes endometrial cancer, so the mainstream medical system always gives Provera (progestins) to prevent endometrial cancer, unless of course, the uterus is absent from prior hysterectomy.*(20)*

The WHI Culprit was the Synthetic Progestin (an altered form of Progesterone)

Back to the first arm of the WHI which used Prempro, it is clear from the data that the culprit which caused breast cancer and heart disease was Provera, a synthetic monster hormone. This is nothing new. For years, Provera has been known to cause ***heart disease*** and ***breast cancer***.*(21)(22)(39)*

Provera Proven to Cause Breast Cancer

In fact, medical studies prove that Provera causes breast cancer. In these studies, Primates were treated with either Progesterone or Provera showing that the Provera causes breast cancer, while the Progesterone provides protection from breast cancer.*(22)*

Monster Hormones are Chemically Altered

Chemically altered hormones were used in the WHI study, and are routinely handed out by the medical system. These altered hormones are **monsters** that should never have been approved for marketing to the American people. They should be banned.

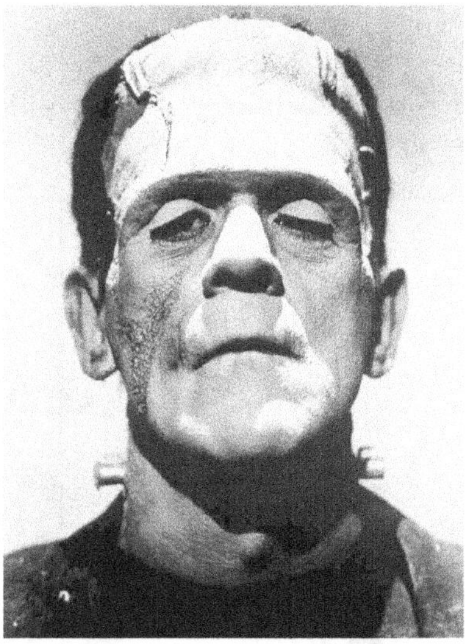

Boris Karloff in Frankenstein 1931 Courtesy of Wikimedia Commons

The Media Says Hormones Cause Cancer and Heart Disease

If bio-identical hormones are so safe, then why do the newspapers say that women's hormones cause breast cancer and heart disease?*(23)* The answer is that the media and the medical profession routinely confuse synthetic chemically altered monster hormones with the bio-identical hormones. The drug companies intentionally create this confusion because they want to hide the fact that synthetic hormones are monsters that should be banned. Chemically altered hormones were made because of a quirk in our legal system which grants patent protection for chemically altered versions of a natural substance. The natural hormones were chemically altered so that they could be patented to protect profits from competition. Naturally occurring bio-identical hormones by law cannot be patented. Examples of monster synthetic hormones are provera, all progestins, and birth control pills which are never found in nature. These are the monster hormones.

Monster Hormones Listed:

Chemically Altered Forms of Progesterone:
Dienogest, Desogestrel, Drospirenone, Dydrogesterone, Ethisterone, Etonogestrel, Ethynodiol diacetate, Gestodene, Gestonorone, Levonorgestrel, Lynestrenol, Medroxyprogesterone, Megestrol, Norelgestromin, Norethisterone, Norethynodrel, Norgestimate, Norgestrel, Norgestrienone, Tibolone
Chemically altered forms of estrogen:
Dienestrol, Diethylstilbestrol, Ethinylestradiol, Fosfestrol, Mestranol
Chemically alered hormones in BCP's Birth Control Pills:
levonorgestrel and ethinyl estradiol [oral contraceptive] *(*ALESSE 28, AVIANE, NORDETTE, SEASONALE, TRIPHASIL, TRIVORA-28*)*; norethindrone and ethinyl estradiol *(*COMBI PATCH, LOESTRIN FE 1/20, NEOCON 1/35, ORTHO-NOVUM 7/7/7, OVCON 35*)*; norgestimate and ethinyl estradiol *(*ORTHO-CYCLEN, ORTHOTRI-CYCLEN, TRINESSA*)*; norgestrel and ethinyl estradiol *(*LO/OVRAL 28, LOW-OGESTREL*)*, desogestrel and ethinyl estradiol *(*DESOGEN, MIRCETTE, ORTHO-CEPT*)*, drospirenone and ethinyl estradiol *(*YASMIN*)*
Chemically altered forms of testosterone:
Androstanolone, Fluoxymesterone, Mesterolone, Methyltestosterone

How to make a Monster Hormone, Add a Side-Chain

Chemical Structure of progesterone *(*left*)* and provera *(*right*)* courtesy of Wikimedia. Arrow denotes added medroxy group which alters chemical structure.

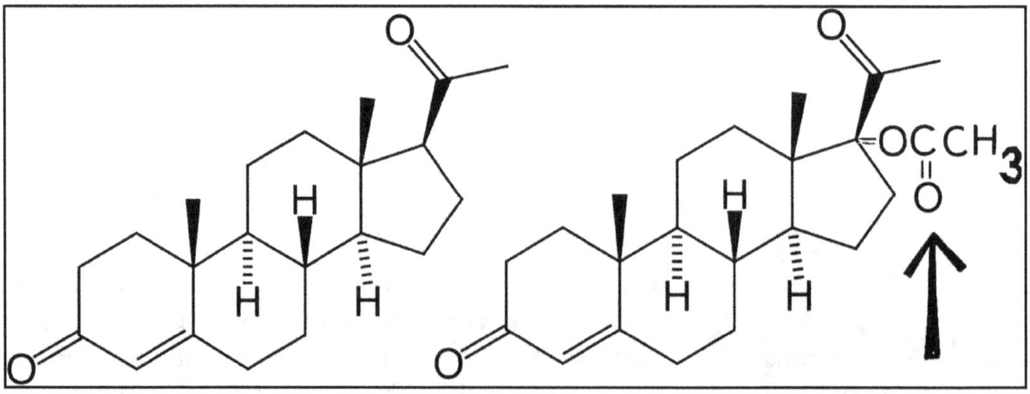

Left Image Progesterone *Right Image Provera (chemically altered form of progesterone)*

Take a good look at human bio-identical **Progesterone** *(*Upper left*)*, and the chemically altered version *(*upper right*)* **Provera** *(*medroxyprogesterone*)*. The added side-chain is indicated by the arrow located on the upper right side of the Provera molecule. This side-chain has been added in order to make a totally new structure that can be patented, and is the only difference with progesterone *(*upper left*)*. In the process of adding this side-chain, a Monster was created. In the opinion of John R Lee MD, "to prescribe a chemically altered version of progesterone called Provera is medical malpractice", and yet this practice is common in mainstream medicine.

An Illustration which Explains the Problem of Synthetic Drugs

Supposing a biochemist working for a drug company has an idea to alter the chemical structure of vitamin C so a patent can be obtained. The biochemist adds a chlorine molecule to the vitamin C carbon ring, and gives is a new name "super-Vitamin C", which is really a chlorinated version of vitamin C. Next they do a one year medical study with 5,000 people taking the chlorinated vitamin C tablet every day, and another 5000 people taking a placebo. After the year is up, they count a .5 per cent incidence of heart disease events in the Super Vitamin C group and a 1.0 percent in the placebo group. FDA approval is easily obtained based on reduction in heart disease events by 50 per cent *(.5 per cent is 50% of 1.0 %)*. The drug company is at liberty to spend million dollars on television advertising designed to rake in millions more for the new heart prevention miracle drug. This absurd scenario is now the norm for our medical system. Why would anyone want to spend money for a monster version of vitamin C when the real thing is available for pennies? Why use a monster hormone when human hormones are available? Compared to their monster counterparts, Bio-Identical Hormones are more effective, have fewer adverse side effects, and are less costly.

High Hormone Levels of Early Pregnancy Confer Protection from Breast Cancer.

During the 16th century in Italy, breast cancer was quite rare. An Italian doctor, *Bernardino Ramazzini,* noted in 1713 the relatively high incidence of breast cancer in nuns and wondered whether this was related to celibate lifestyle.(24) Recent *studies* confirm that early pregnancy and multiple pregnancies confer protection from breast cancer, while no pregnancies *(*as in the nuns*)* leads to increased risk of breast cancer.*(25)* This protection is thought to be conferred by high levels of progesterone. This was confirmed in a *2007 study by Rajkumar* who showed that hormone treatment protected genetically engineered mice from developing breast cancer. *(26)*

Progesterone, the Great Protector

Progesterone is so safe, it is available over the counter without a prescription. In addition, a *deficiency of progesterone* is associated with an increase in breast cancer risk.*(27)* Progesterone is known to be *protective and prevents breast cancer.(28)*

Why Don't Birth Control Pills use Natural Progesterone?

Birth Control Pills, BCP's, are very effective at preventing pregnancy by suppressing ovulation. However, BCP's contain *synthetic hormones* which have *adverse side effects.(29)(30)(31)* To avoid these monster hormones, the IUD *(*intra-uterine device*)* is available. Numerous scientists were involved in the early development of birth control pills: Russell Marker, Percy Lavon Julian, Carl Djerassi, Luis E. Miramontes, George Rosenkranz, Gregory Pincus, Min Chueh Chang, John Rock.*(32)*

In the future of medicine, I predict that progesterone will replace progestins as oral contraception. The bio-identical hormone, Progesterone, will be used in the birth control pills of the future. Early research on contraception was done with progestereone, and research was switched to synthetic progestins to obtain a patent and make a profit. Another consideration was ease of use of the oral tablet, at the time available only as a progestin. Bio-Identical progesterone suppresses ovulation and was the original agent investigated in early research for a contraceptive agent. However, timing and dosages were never officially worked out, so we currently are left with the synthetic birth control pills by default. Again, the IUD can be used instead to avoid the monster hormones. I predict that new research outside the US in the next decade will establish progesterone as the hormone of choice for birth control. Most likely, funding for this research will come from a foreign government agency, in a country with universal health care which has economic incentives to make a healthier pill.

Conclusion

In conclusion, bio-identical hormones used at appropriate dosages are safe, effective, and beneficial for health. On the other hand, chemical alteration of a human hormone creates a monster hormone, which should never be approved for marketing to the American people. These monster hormones are unsafe and should be banned immediately.

Three Excellent Articles on the Safety of BioIdentical Hormones

(1) For a good summary and explanation of the issues, I recommend the article, *The Case for Bioidentical Hormones* by Steven F Hotze MD. 2008.*(33)*

(2) Another excellent article is *The Safety of Bioidentical Hormones — the Data vs. the Hype* by Jacob Teitelbaum, MD From the Townsend Letter June 2007.*(34)*

(3) A third excellent article: *Bioidentical vs. Synthetic HRT, A Review of the Literature* by the *Bio-Identical Hormone Inititiative*, Erika Schwartz MD, David Brownstein MD, Kent Holtorf MD.*(40)(41)*

Recommended Reading: books by John R Lee MD *(35)*

What Your Doctor May Not Tell You About Menopause: The Breakthrough Book on Natural Progesterone *(Warner Books, 1996)(35)*

What Your Doctor May Not Tell You About Premenopause: Balance Your Hormones and Your Life from Thirty to Fifty *(Warner Books, 1999)(35)*

What Your Doctor May Not Tell You About Breast Cancer: How Hormone Balance Can Help Save Your Life, *(Warner Books, 2002)(35)*

References *(*All references are hyperlinked at www.jeffreydach.com and www.naturalmedicine101.com.*)*

(1) http://www.pubmedcentral.nih.gov/articlerender.fcgi?artid=1770067
Fatal water intoxication. D J Farrell1 and L Bower. J Clin Pathol. 2003 October; 56*(*10*)*: 803–804.

(2) http://en.wikipedia.org/wiki/Charles_Darwin
Charles Darwin, theory of natural selection.

(3) http://www.johnleemd.com/store/premenstrual_syndrome.html
Excerpted From: WHAT YOUR DOCTOR MAY NOT TELL YOU ABOUT BREAST CANCER: Balance Your Hormones and Your Life from Thirty to Fifty. PHYSIOLOGICAL EFFECTS OF ESTROGEN AND PROGESTERONE. How Hormone Balance Can Help Save Your Life. by John R. Lee, M.D., David Zava, Ph.D. and Virginia Hopkins. Warner Books 2002

(4) http://www.uzzireissmd.com/book_naturalhormone.html
Natural Hormone Balance for Women: Look Younger, Feel Stronger, and Live Life with Exuberance. by Uzzi Reiss MD

(5) http://www.drtheo.com/news/NSAIDs.pdf
Medical Progress. p 1888. June 17, 1999 The New England Journal of Medicine GASTROINTESTINAL TOXICITY OF NONSTEROIDAL ANTIINFLAMMATORY DRUGS M. MICHAEL WOLFE , M.D., DAVID R. LICHTENSTEIN, M.D.,AND GURKIRPAL SINGH, M.D.

(6) http://www.fda.gov/bbs/transcripts/transcript010908.pdf
Transcript of FDA Press Conference on FDA Actions on Bio-Identical Hormones FTS HHS FDA Susan Cruzan January 9, 2008

(7) http://www.womentowomen.com/breasthealth/estrogenbreastcancer.aspx
Causes of Brea6t Cancer- the Estrogen Controversy, Dixie Mills MD

(8) http://www.ncbi.nlm.nih.gov/pubmed/12626212
Climacteric. 2002 Dec;5*(*4*)*:332-40. Combined hormone replacement therapy and risk of breast cancer in a French cohort study of 3175 women.de Lignières B et al. French Cohort Study.

(9) http://www.johnleemd.com/store/cancer_progest.html
Breast Cancer Book Intro. WHAT YOUR DOCTOR MAY NOT TELL YOU ABOUT BREAST CANCER. How Hormone Balance Can Help Save Your Life By John R. Lee, M.D., David Zava Ph.D., and Virginia Hopkins INTRODUCTION

(10) http://jeffreydach.com/2007/05/05/jeffreydachdrdachiodine.aspx
Breast Cancer Prevention and Iodine Supplementation by Jeffrey Dach MD

(11) http://content.nejm.org/cgi/content/short/356/25/2591
Estrogen Therapy and Coronary-Artery Calcification. NEJM Volume 356:2591-2602 June 21, 2007 Number 25. JoAnn E. Manson, M.D., et al.

(12) http://www.ncbi.nlm.nih.gov/pubmed/15989413
J Womens Health (Larchmt). 2005 Jun;14(5):410-7. Effects of hormone replacement on progression of coronary calcium as measured by electron beam tomography.Budoff MJ, et al.

(13) http://jama.ama-assn.org/cgi/content/abstract/288/3/321
Risks and Benefits of Estrogen Plus Progestin in Healthy Postmenopausal Women Principal Results From the Women's Health Initiative Randomized Controlled Trial Writing Group for the Women's Health Initiative Investigators JAMA. 2002;288:321-333. First Arm.

(14) http://jama.ama-assn.org/cgi/content/full/291/14/1701
Effects of Conjugated Equine Estrogen in Postmenopausal Women With Hysterectomy The Women's Health Initiative Randomized Controlled Trial. JAMA. 2004;291:1701-1712. Second Arm. This is the Second Arm of the Study. Premarin Only.

(15) http://en.wikipedia.org/wiki/Premarin
Premarin From Wikipedia, the free encyclopedia

(16) http://en.wikipedia.org/wiki/Medroxyprogesterone
Provera, Medroxyprogesterone, From Wikipedia, the free encyclopedia

(17) http://homecoalition.org/TakeAction
Take Action. Write a letter to your elected officials using our online advocacy tool. Act now to defend your right to bio-identical hormones! Please contact your congressional representative, senators, and the White House immediately. HOMECoalition.org.

(18) http://jama.ama-assn.org/cgi/content/full/295/14/1647
Effects of Conjugated Equine Estrogens on Breast Cancer and Mammography Screening in Postmenopausal Women With Hysterectomy. Marcia L. Stefanick, PhD et al. for the WHI Investigators. JAMA. 2006;295:1647-1657. Conclusions Treatment with CEE alone for 7.1 years does not increase breast cancer incidence in postmenopausal women with prior hysterectomy.

(19) http://courses.washington.edu/bonephys/opestrogen.html#WHI
Osteoporosis and Bone Physiology, Susan Ott, MD, Associate Professor, Department of Medicine, University of Washington. A Review of the results from the Women's Health Initiative.

(20) http://www.ncbi.nlm.nih.gov/pubmed/3358913
The dose-effect relationship between 'unopposed' oestrogens and endometrial mitotic rate: its central role in explaining and predicting endometrial cancer risk.Key TJ, Pike MC. Br J Cancer. 1988 Feb;57*(2)*:205-12.

(21) http://atvb.ahajournals.org/cgi/content/full/24/7/1171
Should Progestins Be Blamed for the Failure of Hormone Replacement Therapy to Reduce Cardiovascular Events in Randomized Controlled Trials ? Kwang Kon Kohet al. Arteriosclerosis, Thrombosis, and Vascular Biology. 2004;24:1171.

(22) http://www.ncbi.nlm.nih.gov/pubmed/16841178
Effects of estradiol with micronized progesterone or medroxyprogesterone acetate on risk markers for breast cancer in postmenopausal monkeys. Wood CE et al. Breast Cancer Res Treat. 2007 Jan;101*(2)*:125-34.

(23) http://www.time.com/time/magazine/article/0,9171,1002897,00.html
The Truth About Hormones Monday, Jul. 22, 2002 Time Magazine. By CHRISTINE GORMAN AND ALICE PARK.

(24) http://www.ama-assn.org/amednews/2006/04/17/hlsa0417.htm
AMA Medical NEws. Collecting clues: Cancer registries might have an answer. By Kathleen Phalen Tomaselli, AMNews correspondent. April 17, 2006.

(25) http://breast-cancer-research.com/content/7/3/131
The protective role of pregnancy in breast cancer. Jose Russo et al.Breast Cancer Research 2005, 7:131-142doi:10.1186/bcr1029

(26) http://www.pubmedcentral.nih.gov/articlerender.fcgi?tool=pubmed&pubmedid=1725 7424
Hormone-induced protection of mammary tumorigenesis in genetically engineered mouse models. Lakshmanaswamy Rajkumar et al.Breast Cancer Res. 2007; 9*(1)*: R12.

(27) http://aje.oxfordjournals.org/cgi/content/abstract/114/2/209
BREAST CANCER INCIDENCE IN WOMEN WITH A HISTORY OF PROGESTERONE DEFICIENCY . LINDA D. COWAN et al. American Journal of Epidemiology Vol. 114, No. 2: 209-217

(28) http://www.annclinlabsci.org/cgi/content/abstract/28/6/360
Progesterone inhibits growth and induces apoptosis in breast cancer cells: inverse effects on Bcl-2 and p53. B Formby and TS Wiley. Annals of Clinical and Laboratory Science, Vol 28, Issue 6, 360-369

(29) *http://en.wikipedia.org/wiki/Birth_control_pill*
Combined oral contraceptive pill. From Wikipedia, the free encyclopedia. (Redirected from Birth control pill)

(30) *http://www.worstpills.org/results.cfm?disease_id=26*
Oral Contraceptives on Worst Pills.org. Adverse effects of the synthetic hormones in BCP's: headaches, bloating, nausea, irregular bleeding and spotting, breast tenderness, weight gain, or vision changes. high blood pressure, gallbladder disease, liver tumors, depression, and metabolic disorders, such as diabetes. Temporary infertility. blood clots and cancer.

(31) *http://www.jeffreywarber.com/hc%20pages/pillsideeffects.html*
Birth Control Pill Adverse Side Effects by Jeffrey Warber MD

(32) *http://www.quickoverview.com/reproductive/birth-control-pill.html*
History and Development of an effective combined oral contraceptive. People Involved.

(33) *http://www.jpands.org/vol13no2/hotze.pdf*
Point/Counterpoint: The Case for Bioidentical Hormones Steven F. Hotze, M.D.Donald P. Ellsworth, M.D.Journal of American Physicians and Surgeons Volume 13 Number 2 Summer 2008

(34) *http://www.townsendletter.com/June2007/painfree0607.htm*
The Safety of Bioidentical Hormones — the Data vs. the Hype by Jacob Teitelbaum, MD

(35) *http://www.johnleemd.com/store/main_books.html*
Books by John R Lee MD

Wyeth and the FDA

(36) *http//:naturalnews.com/022595.html*
FDA's Assault of Bioidentical Hormones Demonstrates Pro-Pharma Loyalties, Disregard for Consumer Choice Tuesday, February 05, 2008 by: Mike Adams

(37) *http://www.drerika.com/blog?action=viewBlog&blogID=-7512711561726201 13*
February 16, 2008. Women, Doctors Wage Crucial Battle With FDA To Save Bioidentical Hormones From Wyeth's Wrath. A major coalition of informed women and their doctors have launched an all out war on the Federal Drug Administration's (FDA) cynical and corrupt decision to ban compounded hormones containing Estriol.

(38) *http://jeffreydach.com/2008/01/11/fda-declares-war-on-bioidentical-hormones-by-jeffrey-dach-md.aspx*
FDA Declares War on BioIdentical Hormones by Jeffrey Dach MD

Provera and Heart Disease

(39) http://atvb.ahajournals.org/cgi/content/full/17/1/217
Medroxyprogesterone Acetate Antagonizes Inhibitory Effects of Conjugated Equine Estrogens on Coronary Artery Atherosclerosis. Michael R. Adams; Thomas C. Register; Deborah L. Golden; Janice D. Wagner; J. Koudy Williams .Arteriosclerosis, Thrombosis, and Vascular Biology. 1997;17:217-221.

Bio-Identical Hormone Inititiative

(40) http://www.drerika.com/pg/jsp/bhi/bioidentical_vs_synthetic.pdf
Bioidentical vs. Synthetic HRT, A review of the literature

(41) http://www.bioidenticalhormoneinitiative.org/
Bio-Identical Hormone Inititiative, Erika Schwartz MD, David Brownstein MD, Kent Holtorf MD

Additional References

http://www.endfatigue.com/health_articles_f-n/Menapause-safety_effectiveness_bi-oidentical_hormones.html
The Safety and Effectiveness of Bio-Identical Hormones: Natural (Bio-Identical) vs. Synthetic HRT. Kent Holtorf, M.D.

http://www.thorne.com/media/hormones11-3.pdf
A Comprehensive Review of the Safety and Efficacy of Bioidentical Hormones for the Management of Menopause and Related Health Risks. Deborah Moskowitz, ND. Altern Med Rev 2006;11(3):208-223)

http://www.drcranton.com/hrt/hrt_references.htm
Hormone Replacement References linked to the National Library of Medicine (MEDLINE)

http://www.medscape.com/viewarticle/408096_print
Special Article: Addressing Postmenopausal Estrogen Deficiency: A Position Paper of the American Council on Science and Health January 26, 2001 Sander Shapiro, MD Medscape General Medicine 3(1), 2001.

http://www.drerika.com/pg/jsp/general/scientificarchive.jsp
Scientific Literature on Hormones on Dr Erika.com, Dr Erkika Schwartz Web/Blog

http://www.womeninbalance.org/research/
research available women in balance.

Fatal Water Intoxication

http://www.msnbc.msn.com/id/16614865/
Woman dies after water-drinking contest

Synthetic Hormones and Breast Cancer

http://www.nwhn.org/healthinfo/detail.cfm?info_id=9&topic=Fact%20Sheets
Menopause Hormone Therapy and Breast Cancer. National Women's Health Network

http://www.bmj.com/cgi/content/full/310/6979/598/b
BMJ 1995;310:598 (4 March) Letters Risk factors for breast cancer

Chapter 13

FDA Declares War on BioIdentical Hormones

Inept FDA Declares Misguided War on Bio-Identical Hormones, and Promptly Shoots Own Foot

FDA Tries to Protect Wyeth From Financial Losses

Acting as agent for drug maker Wyeth this week, a dysfunctional and inept FDA fired the opening salvo in a misguided war on bio-identical hormones. Using typical Orwellian DoubleSpeak, the FDA issued a series of nonsensical and contradictory statements intended to serve the financial interests Wyeth, maker of synthetic hormones Premarin and Prempro, found to cause cancer and heart disease in the 2002 NIH sponsored Women's Health Initiative Study. Since the study's release, millions of women have switched to the safe and more effective bio-identical hormones, currently prescribed by thousands of physicians, available as FDA approved products at local drug stores and compounding pharmacies. Wyeth has lost market share and suffered financial loss as synthetic hormone profits have declined from 4.4 to 1.2 billion annually from 2001 to 2006.

Wyeth Files a Citizen's Complaint with the FDA

October 2005, in a move to prevent further financial losses, Wyeth filed a Citizen's Complaint with the FDA, requesting the FDA take action against Wyeth's competition, prohibiting compounding pharmacies from providing bio-identical hormones to their patients. More than 66,000 doctors, patients, and pharmacists filed comments in favor of bioidentical hormones and against Wyeth. In spite of this public outcry, Wyeth continues to abuse the FDA to the harm and detriment of millions of women who use bio-identical hormones.

Analysis of the FDA Statements Jan 9, 2008:

Here is an analysis of the recent FDA statements: a comedy of errors, omissions, contradictions, and Orwellian DoubleSpeak. The January 9, 2008 statements can be found at the *FDA website*.

FDA Takes Action Against Compounded Menopause Hormone Therapy *(1)(2)*

Astonishingly, the FDA does not recognize the term, "bio-identical"!

FDA says:

The term "bio-identical" has no defined meaning in any medical or conventional dictionary, and FDA does not recognize the term. Even different medical groups define the term differently. The Endocrine Society, for example, defines "bio-identical" hormones as "compounds that have the exact same chemical and molecular structure as hormones that are produced in the human body," while the American College of Obstetricians and Gynecologists *(*ACOG*)* defines "bio-identical" hormones as "plant-derived hormones that are biochemically similar or identical to those produced by the ovary or body."

My Reply:

The term bioidentical has a *definite meaning* and is *widely used*. The term, bioidentical, means a hormone chemical structure which is identical to that found in the human body. Both the Endocrine Society and ACOG define the term, "bioIdentical", exactly the same, even though the two definitions are worded differently. It is an embarrassment to medical science that the word BioIdentical has to be used at all. All Hormones should have been manufactured as bio-identical hormones. However, because of U.S. patent law which prevents patenting a bioidentical hormone, the drug industry created chemically altered hormones which could be patented and sold at higher profit margins.

Astonishingly, the FDA is UNAWARE of a basic fact of biochemistry !

Astonishingly, the FDA is UNAWARE that identical chemical structures have the same biological effects. This is the basis for all biochemistry. A water molecule, for example, will have the same biologic effect in the body regardless of how it is synthesized, and this is also true for any other chemical, including hormones.

FDA says:

Many compounding pharmacies use Bio-identical as a marketing term to imply that drugs are natural, or have effects identical to those from hormones made by the body. FDA is not aware of credible scientific evidence to support these claims.

My Reply:

Bio-identical hormones are *(*1*)* natural and *(*2*)* have effects identical to hormones made in the body. These are basic axioms of biochemistry, and accepted as basic truth by all of biochemistry, including the following medical textbooks Lehninger Principles of Biochemistry, Guyton Textbook of Medical Physiology, and Williams Textbook of Endocrinology. It is astonishing that the FDA can be UNAWARE of the scientific evidence that is present in every medical textbook, and thousands of Medline references that state that bio-identical hormones ARE natural and DO produce the same effects as human hormones !!

The FDA Does Recognize this basic fact of biochemistry when looking at Synthetic Hormone Structures !

Astonishingly, for the FDA, when it comes to synthetic hormones, all of a sudden, chemical structures that are identical DO have the same biologic effects !!

FDA says:

Compounded products that have identical chemical structures to synthetic hormones can be expected to have the same benefits—and risks— associated with FDA-approved hormone therapy.

My Reply:

This is Orwellian DoubleSpeak again. Compounded natural bio-identical hormones DO NOT have the same chemical structure as synthetic hormones. Compounded hormones are natural and bio-identical, and DO NOT increase risk of increased cancer and heart disease, as was demonstrated for the synthetic hormones in the WHI study. The Women's Health Initiative study published in JAMA July 2002 showed that Provera, a chemically altered form of progesterone causes increased risk of cancer and heart disease, while the natural, human bioidentical progesterone does not. *(5) (6)*

The following two studies show that bio-identical hormones are safe: One is the French Cohort Study which showed that Bio-identical hormone therapy does not cause increased risk of breast cancer.*(3)* The second is the June 2007 NEJM Calcium Score study which showed no increase in heart disease risk with estrogen. *(4)*

The FDA Attacks Saliva Hormone Testing !

FDA says :

Some compounding pharmacies and other promoters of "BHRT" claim that estrogen levels in a person's saliva can be tested by practitioners to help practitioners estimate the amount of hormone a person needs and purportedly to "customize" the hormone therapy for individual patients. There is no scientific basis for using saliva testing to adjust hormone levels. Instead, practitioners should adjust hormone therapy dosages based on a patient's symptoms.

My Reply:

Salivary hormone testing has been done by two large companies for many years, *Diagnos-Techs* and *ZRT*. Both Web Sites list plenty of scientific evidence validating saliva hormone testing. ZRT lists references supporting salivary hormone testing *here* and *here*.

Here is a comment on Saliva Testing by Kenna Stephenson, MD *(50)*

> "Saliva testing has been used in clinical research, including studies conducted at the National Institutes of Health *(*NIH*)* for more than 30 years. Saliva testing has been available to practicing physicians for over a decade, and Medicare and many insurance companies provide reimbursement for its use. Over years of clinical practice, I have found that saliva testing is the most accurate measurement of the body's availability of the steroid hormones cortisol and DHEA and the sex steroid hormones estrogen, progesterone, and testosterone. Saliva testing correctly identifies the level of hormone at the cellular level *(*i.e. the biologically interactive form of the hormone*)*, in contrast to a serum *(*blood*)* test, which measures the level of hormone circulating in the bloodstream."

In addition, salivary hormone testing for cortisol and melatonin is accepted and used by NASA on the astronauts on the space shuttle. *(7)* A PubMed Medline search shows many research studies validating the use of salivary hormone testing.*(8)* Number of medical articles on key word search on Medline: Salivary hormone: 4075, Salivary cortisol: 1478, Salivary estradiol: 177, Salivary progesterone: 317, Salivary testosterone: 428.

The FDA Claims Ignorance of Its Own FDA Approvals !

FDA says:

Some pharmacies promote hormone therapy for men in the form of testosterone to treat a decline in the level of testosterone in older men, sometimes referred to as andropause. There are currently no FDA-approved products for the treatment of andropause. In addition, there are no FDA-approved testosterone drugs for women.

My Reply:

Testosterone insufficiency in older men is associated with increased risk of death over the next 20 years. *(17)* Testosterone has been FDA approved for both men and women for decades. FDA approved testosterone commercial products can be obtained at the corner drugstore. *Androgel* for example, is FDA approved and contains testosterone. *Estra-test* is an FDA approved hormone for women. Estra-Test contains testosterone.

The following is a list of FDA-approved bio-identical hormone commercial products available at the drugstore commonly used to treat menopause and andropause:

FDA Approved Bio-Identical Hormones

Alora (estradiol): FDA approved 1996 - Watson Labs
Climara (estradiol): FDA approved 1994 - Bayer
FemPatch : FDA approved 1997 - Parke Davis
Vivelle-Dot (estradiol): FDA approved 1994 - Novartis
Estraderm: FDA approved 1986 - Novartis
Esclim: FDA approved 1998 - Women's First Healthcare
Estrace (estradiol): FDA approved 1993 -Bristol Myers Squibb
Estring: FDA approved 1996 - Pharmacia UpJohn
Prometrium (natural progesterone): FDA approved 1998 - Solvay
Androgel (natural testosterone): FDA approved 2000 - Unimed Pharmaceuticals
Crinone: FDA approved 1997 - Columbia Labs

FDA approved Estradiol containing products:Estrace, Progynova, estrofem, Alora, Climara, Vivelle, Vivelle-Dot, Menostar, Estraderm TTS Estrasorb Topical, Estrogel, Elestrin, Lunelle Estring, Femring

FDA approved Progesterone products Prometrium, Utrogestan, Minagest, Microgest, CRINONE, PROCHIEVE, Cyclogest

FDA approved testosterone:Testoderm, Androderm, AndroGel

The FDA Tries to Ban Estriol !

Astonishingly, the FDA wants to ban estriol, a popular component of natural hormone therapy for women.

FDA says:

Some compounded "BHRT" drugs contain an estrogen component called estriol. No drug containing estriol has been approved by FDA and the safety and effectiveness of estriol is unknown. Pharmacies may not compound drugs containing estriol unless they have an FDA-sanctioned investigational new drug application.

My Reply:

Like many commonly prescribed drugs *(*e.g. quinine, Phenobarbital, tinidazole*)*, estriol has a monograph from the U.S. Pharmacopeia *(*USP*)*. When Congress passed the FDA Modernization Act in 1997, it clearly indicated that drugs with a USP monograph could be compounded. 50,000 compounding pharmacists, 15,000 doctors and 2 million women have been prescribing, making and using estriol for decades. FDA approval is not required since this is regulated by the states, not the FDA.

Finally, the Truth About Bio-Identical Hormones ! Quoted from the IACP, the International Academy of Compounding Pharmacists web site.*(48)*

Myth 1*)* Bioidentical hormone replacement therapy *(*BHRT*)* is unregulated.

Fact: Bioidentical hormones – like all compounded medications – are made from FDA- and USP-registered materials – the same used by pharmaceutical manufacturers – and their preparation is well regulated by state boards of pharmacy that have responsibility for overseeing all pharmacy practice in each state. Pharmacies that compound medications, including bioidentical hormones, are regulated by state pharmacy boards – similar to the relationship doctors have with state medical boards. In addition, there are also national standards and guidelines for compounded medications. The ingredients and their suppliers are regulated at the federal level by the FDA, with additional oversight provided by the U.S. Pharmacopeia.

Myth 2*)* Compounded bioidentical hormones are unsafe because they aren't FDA-approved.

Fact: Compounded medications are regulated by state boards of pharmacy and are not subject to federal laws designed to regulate mass-produced drugs. This is because they are customized to meet the unique needs of patients based on the specific orders of a physician. The FDA approval process is designed for mass-produced manufactured drugs; it is universally recognized that holding compounded medications to these standards would completely eliminate their availability. Compounded medications are in a similar position as manufactured products prescribed for off-label use, which constitutes about a fifth of all prescriptions. They are not approved by the FDA for such use, and yet it is well accepted that physicians should be able to use their discretion to prescribe medications for off-label use.

Myth 3) Bioidentical hormones are just as risky as manufactured products like Premarin and Prempro.

Fact: There are no studies comparing the two types of therapies, so we cannot make any direct comparisons. The Women's Health Initiative study examined only Premarin and Prempro, which do not use the same ingredients that are used to compound bioidentical hormones. To date there have been no studies that show a link between BHRT and cancer/strokes/heart attack, however the pharmacy community supports and funds studies to better determine the risk profile of BHRT.

A physician is trained and licensed to diagnose disease and to determine appropriate therapy for patients. A physician uses clinical expertise to determine appropriate therapies for patients. Premarin and Prempro may be appropriate for some patients. Bioidentical hormones may be appropriate for others. It is up to doctors to make that determination.

Myth 4) Pharmacists are recklessly promoting BHRT as safe and effective.

Fact: Compounded medicines are a lot like off-label prescriptions: they are not subject to FDA approval and, as a result, cannot be marketed as safe or effective. In fact, the FTC Act, 15 U.S.C. § 41 et seq., prohibits unfair or deceptive acts and practices, including false and unsubstantiated advertising claims. It is already illegal for a pharmacy to make claims without substantiation or to overstate the health benefits of the products they promote.

Myth 5) Bioidentical is a misleading term.

Fact: The chemical structures of bioidentical hormones are identical to those produced by the human body. Because the chemical structure is identical, these hormones are often referred to as bioidentical. Endquote IACP.

Sign a Petition and Join a Boycott

Don't let the financial interests of the drug industry restrict your health freedom, call or email your senator today and voice your outrage at this blatant abuse of the FDA by special interest groups.

References and Links (Hyperlinked at www.jeffreydach.com and www.naturalmedicine101.com)

Listing of medical textbooks stating that bio-identical hormones have the same chemical structure as those in the human body and have the same effect. (all of them):

Lehninger Principles of Biochemistry, Fourth Edition by David L. Nelson (Author), Michael M. Cox (Author)
Textbook of Medical Physiology by Arthur C. Guyton
Williams Textbook of Endocrinology
Basic & Clinical Endocrinology by Francis S. Greenspan
Review of Medical Physiology by Ganong, William F. MD
Endocrinology (5th Edition) by Mac E. Hadley
Endocrine Physiology by Susan Porterfield

(1) January 9, 2008 FDA Takes Action Against Compounded Menopause Hormone Therapy Drugs

(2) Compounded Menopausal Hormone Therapy Questions and Answers

(3) Climacteric. 2002 Dec;5(4):332-40. Combined hormone replacement therapy and risk of breast cancer in a French cohort study of 3175 women. De Lignières B, de Vathaire F, Fournier S, Urbinelli R, Allaert F, Le MG, Kuttenn F. Service d'Endocrinologie et Médecine de la Reproduction, Hôpital Necker, Paris, France.

The French Cohort Study showed that Bio-identical hormone therapy does not cause increased risk of breast cancer.

(4) NEJM Volume 356:2591-2602 June 21, 2007 Number 25 Estrogen Therapy and Coronary-Artery Calcification JoAnn E. Manson, M.D., The NEJM CAT Scan Calcium Score study showed no increase in heart disease risk with estrogen.

(5) Risks and Benefits of Estrogen Plus Progestin in Healthy Postmenopausal Women Principal Results From the Women's Health Initiative Randomized Controlled Trial Writing Group for the Women's Health Initiative Investigators JAMA. 2002;288:321-333.

(6) Effects of Conjugated Equine Estrogen in Postmenopausal Women With Hysterectomy The Women's Health Initiative Randomized Controlled Trial,The Women's Health Initiative Steering Committee,* JAMA. 2004;291:1701-1712.

(7) Assessment Of Sleep Dynamics In A Simulated Space Station Environment Lakshmi Putcha, Ph.D., Ram Nimmagudda, Ph.D., Chantal Rivera, Ph.D.

(8) Entrez pubmed, A simple medline search shows a research studies validating the use of salivary hormone testing.

salivary hormone 4075 articles, Salivary cortisol: 1478 articles, Salivary estradiol 177, Salivary progesterone 317, Salivary testosterone 428

(9) special committee on aging senate Hearings- Bioidentical Hormones: Sound Science or Bad Medicine? April 19, 2007

(10) Bioidentical hormone replacement therapy wikipedia

(11) The Truth about Bioidentical Hormones-IACP

(12) Irresponsible Journalism: BusinessWeek Regurgitates Wyeth's Attacks on Pharmacy Compounding

(13) The Endocrine Society Position Statement Oct 2006 Bio-Identical Hormones

(14) The Endocrine Society Position Statement Oct 2006 Bio-Identical Hormones

(15) Bioidentical Hormones Lack Evidence for Safety and Effectiveness

(16) Low levels of testosterone may increase risk of death in older men Men's Health News Published: Tuesday, 16-Oct-2007, Journal of Clinical Endocrinology & Metabolism (JCEM).

(17) The Journal of Clinical Endocrinology & Metabolism Vol. 93, No. 1 68-75 Low Serum Testosterone and Mortality in Older Men, Gail A. Laughlin Testosterone insufficiency in older men is associated with increased risk of death over the following 20 yr, independent of multiple risk factors and several preexisting health conditions.

(18) DrErika Blasts Wyeth's War on Bioidentical Hormones, Erika Schwartz, MD, Patients' Health Advocate and Leading Expert on Bioidentical Hormones

(19) Wyeth's War on Women and Bioidenticals, Erika Schwartz, MD, Patients' Health Advocate and Leading Expert on Bioidentical Hormones.

(20) Bioidentical Hormones are not snake oil: They are available commercially at your local drugstore with a prescription from your regular MD . Erika Schwartz blog, web site. Erika Schwartz, MD, Patients' Health Advocate and Leading Expert on Bioidentical Hormones

(21) FDA says alternative hormone claims unsupported Wed Jan 9, Reuters news service

(22) Listing of references in the Scientific Literature on validating use of bio-identical hormones, Erika Schwartz, MD, Patients' Health Advocate and Leading Expert on Bioidentical Hormones

(23) Wednesday, Jan. 09, 2008 FDA Asserts New Policy to Restrict Women's Access to Bioidentical Hormones International Academy of Compounding Pharmacists

(24) FDA Asserts New Policy To Restrict Women's Access To Bioidentical Hormones,m edicalnewstoday, 10 Jan 2008

(25) FDA Asserts New Policy to Restrict Women's Access to Bioidentical Hormones Agency Warns Pharmacies Not to Compound Commonly Prescribed Hormone Treatments, Use the Term "Bio-identical" , IACPRX

(26) Tell Congress: Don't Take Away My Compounded Medications! Send a letter to your congressman.

(27) Hot Flash: FDA Warns About BHRT Drugs,January 9th, 2008 2:51 pm By Ed Silverman Pharmalot

(28) E- Book on natural progesterone

(29) Understanding the Controversy:Hormone Testing and Bioidentical Hormones

(30) Vivelle dot, estradiol fda approved

(31) About USP—An Overview Who We Are, The United States Pharmacopeia *(*USP*)* is the official public standards-setting authority for all prescription and over-the-counter medicines, dietary supplements

(32) Estriol listing in USP

(33) Pharmacies Warned About Compounding Estriol, Touting Mixture's Benefits Does the FDA have jurisdiction over these compounding pharmacies?There's a court battle going on right now to determine the answer to that question. Oral arguments are expected tomorrow in the U.S. 5th Circuit Court of Appeals in New Orleans. The fda is appealing a lower court ruling, which found that they do not have jurisdiction over drug preparations produced by compounding pharmacies.

(34) FDA Goes After 'Natural' HRT Claims Compounding Pharmacies Told to Stop Marketing 'Bio-identical Hormone Replacement Therapy'

(35) C.W. (Randy) Randolph, Jr., M.D. As a trained pharmacist and Board Certified practicing gynecologist, web site.

(36) Judge Issues Landmark Decision in Compounding Pharmacy Case Friday, May 26, 2006Midland, Texas, C.W. (Randy) Randolph, Jr., M.D. As a trained pharmacist and Board Certified practicing gynecologist, web site.

(37) Wyeth Pharmaceuticals tries to STOP your access to Bio-Identical Hormone Replacement Therapies (BHRT). BHRT-A BATTLE FOR THE TRUTH, C.W. (Randy) Randolph, Jr., M.D. As a trained pharmacist and Board Certified practicing gynecologist, web site.

(38) Bio-Identical Hormone Drug Information

(39) Wyeth web site

(40) Sepp Hasslberger web site, Wyeth Asks FDA: Prohibit Bio-Identical Hormones, Excellent Summary of Wyeth Activities and War Against BioIdentical Hormones

(41) wyeth earnings report 2006

(42) Wikipedia bio-identical hormone therapy definition

(43) Double speak

references for salivary hormone testing

(44) Salivary testosterone levels in preadolescent children, Daniela Ostatníková1

(45) Pathol Biol (Paris). 2001 Oct;49(8):660-7., Saliva assays in clinical and research biology.Lac G., Département génie biologique,

(46) Patterns of Salivary Estradiol and Progesterone across the Menstrual Cycle, BEATRICE K. GANDARA,a LINDA LERESCHE,a and LLOYD MANCLb

(47) FDA Approves Biex Test to Aid in Identifying Risk of Preterm Labor and Delivery. 5/5/1998 Biex, Inc. announced today the FDA granted marketing approval for the Company's salivary estriol test to help physicians identify risk for spontaneous preterm labor and delivery.

(48) The Truth about Bioidentical Hormones-IACP

(49) WomenInBalance.org NonProfit Advocacy Group for BioIdentical Hormones. They have compiled the currently available science references behind the use of bioidentical hormones for women.

(50) *http://www.womeninbalance.org/pdf/Kenna.pdf*
Kenna Stephenson MD on salivary hormones

Chapter 14

BioIdentical Hormones, Cook Book or Tailor Made?

The following is an exchange with Larry Frieders RPh about Bio-Identical Hormone Therapy. In Letter Number One, Larry asks my opinion about the Wiley Protocol, cycling vs. non-cycling bio-identical hormone therapy. Larry J Frieders RPh is a compounding pharmacist in the Aurora, Illinois.

From: Larry Frieders, R.Ph.
To: Jeffrey Dach
Sent: Wed, August 22, 2007
Subject: BioIdentical Hormones

Good morning Dr. Dach;

I've been approached by some local doctors about getting involved with the WILEY PROTOCOL for hormone replacement. I received a call yesterday from someone who works for Wiley and they've sent their contract materials. I am not completely familiar with the ins and outs, but I am aware that there is some controversy about her approach. There are fees involved, but they don't concern me as much as the protocol. My current information is mostly hearsay - and somewhat tainted.

However, upon review of the materials they sent I get an impression that perhaps Wiley is onto something - particularly as it relates to a method for standardizing hormone replacement. I've been involved with this type of therapy since 1998 and I become more and more dismayed at the wide range of methods and dosing I see. Some prescribers order large doses and others get along with what seems to be miniscule amounts. Some dose EVERY day and others tell me that the only legitimate way is to cycle the dosing - allowing time for receptors to clear.

Then, there's the variety of dosage forms, capsules, suppositories, troches, sublingual drops, transdermal creams, etc. Even when there seems to be some consistency in using a topical, the different bases used are enough to cause me to doubt the integrity of the whole idea of balancing hormones.

About 3 years ago a doctor I know very well threw up his hands in exasperation and stopped prescribing hormone replacement. He said that he was finished until "they" could give him better guidelines for evaluating and prescribing. I scurried to relocate his patients with other doctors. Perhaps Wiley is on the path to helping doctors like that.

You're a specialist in hormone replacement. What are your thoughts about Wiley's approach?

Larry J Frieders, RPh, MMgt, MA
http://www.thecompounder.com/
340 Marshall Ave Unit 100
Aurora, IL 60506
630 859 0333

From: Jeffrey Dach
To: 'Larry Frieders, R.Ph.'
Sent: Thursday, August 23, 2007 3:14 PM

Dear Larry,

I agree, the BHRT *(*Bioidentical Hormone Replacement Therapy*)* field is all over the place. I heard Wiley's presentation at one of the ACAM meetings about 2 years ago, and the major criticism from the audience was that her dosing was too high and causes irregular bleeding. Besides, most patients prefer to avoid the inconvenience of cycling. We don't use it.

My Approach to BHRT

My approach to Bio Identical HRT is fairly straightforward. We start at a low dose and gradually increase until symptoms of hot flashes and night sweats are relieved. Maintenance dose is the lowest with relief of symptoms and good quality of life. Starting dosage for the average 50 year old is 1.25 mg/gram topical Bi-Est daily, and for the average 70 year old is 0.625 Bi-Est daily. Sometimes we even start lower. Dosage is increased gradually if needed for symptom relief.

Of course, we use an extensive baseline lab panel from either Quest or Labcorp and recheck labs at 6 month intervals. Although some authors such as Dr. Vliet have given target areas for the labs published in her books, we don't dogmatically use those, since after trying that we found so much individual patient variation that Dr. Vliet's hormone target ranges are only rough approximations, and in many cases too high. We also initially tried using Dr. Uzi Reiss's recommended hormone formulations and dosages mentioned in his book, and found that these were too high for our patient population for starting dosages. CW Randolph MD, for example, has hormone target areas on blood testing which are considerably lower and seem to be better tolerated.

In terms of hormone testing, there are those who are dogmatic hormone saliva testers and those who are blood testers *(*Reiss, Vliet, Cenegenics etc.*)*. We have tried both ways and have settled on hormone blood testing.

Common Mistakes with BHRT

A common mistake made by many practitioners is to omit giving thyroid which most BHRT patients need in spite of normal labs. We use the thyroflex *(*Daryl Turner*)* to measure reflex time which, in some cases, is a more accurate indicator of thyroid function than is the TSH. We use natural thyroid *(*RLC labs, Western Research Naturethroid*)*. If thyroid is omitted, the patients gain weight and become discouraged with the program. Another common mistake is to omit or ignore Iodine supplementation. We use Iodoral from Optimox *(*Guy Abraham, MD*)*.

We also check serum vitamin B12 and Vitamin D levels. I have observed that patients may not have a good result with BHRT unless vitamin B12 and vitamin D levels are optimized. And you know B12, D, and Iodine are inexpensive. We have uncovered quite a few severe B12 deficient patients missed by conventional docs. This is rewarding because patients immediately improve with nontoxic and inexpensive B12 shots or SL tabs. Excess vitamin D *(*abover 100 ng/ml*)* can cause toxicity, so we monitor serial blood levels of Vitamin D during supplementation.

In my opinion another pitfall is missing the diagnosis of adrenal fatigue often ignored by conventional medicine. We give adrenal supplements in selected cases. Another stumbling block is progesterone excess from topical creams which can manifest in bizarre symptoms and can be difficult to recognize until the cream is stopped and symptoms go away. This may completely discourage the patient at the beginning of the program, so it is best avoided. Progesterone capsules or lozenges seem to avoid the excess problem. On the other hand some women do better with the topical progesterone cream *(*Dr. Lee is a big advocate of the topical progesterone cream at dosage of about 20 mg per day.*)* If we use the topical progesterone, we dose 27 on and 3 days off to prevent excess build up in the subcutaneous fat area.

Topical Progesterone

There are some such experts as Dr. Rami, the hormone specialist at Diagnos-Techs *(*the saliva lab*)* who told me that they have totally given up on using topical progesterone *(*Caps or SL troches are OK*)* because they have run into progesterone excess too many times in their patients *(*mood disturbance such as depression seems to be the major symptom*)*. I spoke to Rami about this and he said he had a consultation with Dr. Lee *(*before he passed away*)* who came to their facility and worked with them on this issue. In spite of the Lee visit, Rami still doesn't advise using topical progesterone. He prefers the caps or lozenges. Rami is very knowledgable and a great intellectual asset, and I am glad he is available for consultation and advice on difficult cases. *(*author's note: Since writing this entry, for the majority of patients, we have switched from troches and capsules to the use of topical progesterone cream with excellent results. Progesterone excess is avoided by taking a monthly 3 day break.*)*

For the first few months starting the program, we may change the route of administration and tweak dosages, so we usually call the patient every two or three weeks for the first few months just to check in on them. This can be time consuming and labor intensive, but needs to be done. Not only do we follow serial labs, we also do a baseline pelvic sonogram and follow endometrial thickness, and keep track of the usual routine annual exams and send out reminders if that stuff needs to get done.

The major points are *(1)* start low and gradually increase over time to relieve symptoms. *(2)* Hormones are just part of an overall evaluation and other issues such as B12, vit D, thyroid, iodine, adrenal are all part of the picture and need to be addressed to get good results.

Please let me know your thoughts on the above and what changes or additions you would make, as I value your opinion. Your newsletter is the greatest, and thanks for thinking of me.

from, Jeffrey Dach, M.D.

From: Larry Frieders, R.Ph.
Sent: Monday, August 27, 2007 4:13 PM
To: Jeffrey Dach

Dear Dr. Dach;

We first got involved with the HRT stuff about 10 years ago and we've been doing our best to let people know about the advantages of using human *(*bioidentical*)* hormones instead of the commercial types *(*the alien substances*)*.

We have devoted most of our attention to saliva testing and helping women who are predominantly plagued by estrogen dominance. This is clearly a widespread problem that is made worse by the chemicals in our environment. The majority of the people we consult with are clearly deficient in progesterone. They benefit dramatically from a small non-prescription dose of progesterone cream. We always recommend using it according to a schedule. Younger women apply 20mg daily from days 13 through 26. Those with more symptoms or nearer to menopause are instructed to apply 20mg once daily from day 1 to 12, then twice daily from 13 to 26, then stopping until day one. If they are not having periods the days are marked with a calendar. For the first few years we suggested retesting *(*saliva*)* in 9 to 12 months. But, as many have seen, saliva testing after using a supplement returns some wild numbers. We concluded that follow-up testing by saliva is a waste of resources.

As I said, most women do well with progesterone - and lifestyle adjustments. Women who have a history of birth control pill use, or who have had a hysterectomy usually need something more than just progesterone. These are a problem for us because we cannot prescribe estrogens or testosterone. Problems? There aren't many doctors around our office who are comfortable prescribing B HRT. I also think that these patients require more time and attention than most "employed" doctors are able to devote.

Back to testing. I think that an initial saliva test is useful. Yet, I am seeing more people going to blood/serum, especially for testosterone levels. I also think that blood/serum tests have a long history and they add a solid degree of comfort for the prescribers.

Almost all of our estrogen doses are less than 1 mg. People who have had prescriptions for larger doses don't seem to have them refilled as regularly as those who are using the lower amounts.

Your observations about thyroid are vital. Too many doctors, though, seem to shy away from those systems. We regularly talk to people who have every hypothyroid symptom in the book, but they have a "normal" TSH. I'd say that most prescribers are uncomfortable ordering thyroid supplements for someone who has a "normal" TSH.

We've been dispensing a thyroid challenge test that consists of 5 strengths of T3 (slow release) and a chart to report temperatures and symptoms. Patients take the doses every 12 hours - increasing and then decreasing strengths according to a schedule. There is usually a place in the doses where the person reports feeling better (or has a higher temp). The doctors use that dose as a starting place for further supplementing.

We have stocked Iodoral since it first became available and it is fairly popular. I remember when almost all table salt was "iodized". Recently I've noticed that it doesn't seem to be the case these days.

FYI... some of my compounding colleagues are starting to use hormones mixed in oil (almond, grape seed, etc) and the doses are in the drop range. They use a calibrated dropper and apply the dose to the wrist - and then rub the wrists together. The claim is that patients appreciate the convenience. Also, some people are reporting that they can adjust their doses by their need. Women seem to be particularly good at knowing when they need a little boost of testosterone or estrogen. I'm hoping that one or two of our local doctors might be interested in trying this approach. Do you have any experience with hormones in topical oils?

Finally, I'm pretty certain that we are not going to get involved with Wiley - the high doses make me nervous - and I agree that most women are not eager to continue having periods into their 60s and beyond. There is one doctor locally who has asked me to get involved. Wiley asks for about $6,000 to get started - and then requires that the pharmacy purchase devices only from her. There is a statement in her patient guide that specifically tells the users to NOT take any medical advice from the pharmacist. She wants me to play along with her protocol but not offer any advice. I think I'd have a difficult time staying silent when someone asks for my input.

I really appreciate your comments about our newsletter.

Regards,
Larry J Frieders, RPh, MMgt, MA
http://www.thecompounder.com/
340 Marshall Ave Unit 100 | Aurora, IL 60506
630 859 0333

From: Jeffrey Dach MD
To: 'Larry Frieders, R.Ph.'
Sent: Tuesday, August 28, 2007 11:20 AM

Dear Larry,

Regarding the estrogen doses all less than 1 mg, is this Bi-Est cream, oral capsules, or Sublingual troches? What form is it?

So far, we haven't used the Oil based drops for hormone administration. I am willing to try it, though, if it offers a benefit. Keep me updated on it. Also, so far, we haven't used a thyroid T3 schedule to determine dosage. We usually start with ½ grain Naturethroid and gradually increase by ½ grain increments every 2 to three weeks until there is relief of symptoms or early symptoms of mild thyroid excess become apparent (palpitations or rapid heart rate at rest), at which point we reduce dosage.

We also monitor reflex time on the thyroflex, and thyroid labs every 12 weeks. The free T3 level is a useful lab measurement. TSH usually drops below 1 with adequate treatment. So far we have been having good results with the NatureThroid from RLC labs, Western Research, so I have no plans to use the compounded T3/ T4 combinations available. Another issue is safety, I feel that the Naturethroid is safer, since after discontinuing, the adverse effects dissipate within 6 hours. I am not sure about the extended release T3, though, and I am hesitant to use it for safety reasons.

Warmest Regards from,
Jeffrey Dach, M.D.

From: Larry Frieders, R.Ph.
To: Jeffrey Dach MD
Sent: Tuesday, August 29, 2007

Dr. Dach,

Dosage forms - almost exclusively topical/transdermal. There are a few doctors who still order oral estrogens in spite of the slight increased risks. I think the research says one thing about risk, but something else happens in practice. Biest seems to be the leader - Triest is practically off the screen. I don't know many prescribers who are still ordering estrone (E1). The ratios range from 50/50 to 90/10. Probably greater than half of our Biest are the 80/20. The 90/10 ratio is out of fashion and 50/50 is running a distant second.

Progesterone capsules are still popular, particularly for younger women who may be having difficulties with PMS. It seems that the metabolites from oral doses are active - actually calming. Some ladies insist on oral progesterone because it helps them relax and sleep. The oral preparations we make are in a slow release formulation - much different from the commercial capsules that are made with peanut oil (Prometrium).

I've not had much luck with any kind of troche - or sublingual drops for that matter. First, hormones are terrible tasting and it is difficult to find a flavor/sweetener that is satisfactory. Second, I find that a LOT of a sublingual dose is actually swallowed. In effect, then, it's an oral dose - or at least a lot of it is an oral dose.

I'm not particular about the version of thyroid. Naturthroid is an excellent commercial product and probably meets most needs. We're ready when someone wants something a little different. The slow release ingredient is methocel and it somewhat retards the dissolution in the gut. It makes some medicines a little easier on the GI lining - probably not a big issue with T3 and T4.

Our most popular T3 preparation is the challenge kit. It consists of 5 different strengths of T3 (from 7.5mcg to 37.5mcg. The patient starts low and takes 1 capsule every 12 hours, changing doses every 2 days on the way up and every 3 days on the way down. The dose at which there's an improvement or a temperature increase is an indication of a place to start dosing. Some people find this useful when they exhibit hypothyroid symptoms without a definitive lab report.

It's a rare doctor who aggressively treat hypothyroid symptoms in the absence of clear TSH values. We think the challenge helps identify low thyroid and points to a starting supplement dose.

If you'd like to use any of my writings, feel free. I haven't written anything that I wouldn't want to see in print elsewhere. Use whatever you think best suits your needs. I'd be delighted to contribute to a book. Just let me know when and point me in the right direction. Will your audience be other practitioners or patients?

Regards, Larry, Larry J Frieders, RPh, MMgt, MA *http://www.thecompounder.com/*
340 Marshall Ave Unit 100, Aurora, IL 60506, 630 859 0333

Section Four

Human Growth Hormone, Testosterone, Thyroid

Chapter 15

Dr. Andrew Weil, AARP, and Human Growth Hormone, HGH

Dr. Andrew Weil Says Human Growth Hormone is "Snake Oil"

Perhaps you have seen the Andrew Weil article entitled, "Dr. Debunker: The Truth About the Fountain of Youth" in the June 2007 AARP magazine which gives retired folks advice about anti-aging and longevity.*(1)* I have considerable respect for Dr. Weil and have followed his work over the years. However, after reading his article, my opinion of Dr. Weil has changed. This article is such poor quality and contains so many factual errors and errors of omission, that it raises serious questions about the author.

Dr. Weil the Debunker omits bioidentical estrogen and progesterone for post menopausal women, and the many health benefits such as reduction in heart disease in women.*(1A)* He also omits testosterone for males with declining testosterone levels. This story was again told by golf star Shawn Micheel in Golf Digest.*(2)* Dr. Debunker omits the multiple medical reports showing that males with low testosterone have a higher mortality.*(3)(4)*

Dr. Debunker also omits low thyroid evaluation, Vitamin B12 levels, vitamin D levels, Vitamin C Supplementation, and Iodine Supplementation, all of which are important for health, well being and longevity for the over 50.*(5)*

Rather than discussing the above important topics, Dr. Debunker concentrates on Human Growth Hormone *(*HGH*)* for adults, warning us that HGH is a form of "snake oil" treatment. Perhaps Dr. Weil could explain the logic of how a patented, FDA approved pharmaceutical drug with proven efficacy can be called "snake oil".*(6)(7)(8)*

The Dr. Debunker article fails to tell us that our hormone levels decline dramatically after age 50, and "by the age of 60 most adults have Growth Hormone levels indistinguishable from those of hypopituitary patients with organic lesions in the pituitary gland."*(9)*

The Dr. Debunker article gives the mistaken impression there is only one single medical publication *(*Rudman NEJM 1990*)* which reports the beneficial effects of growth hormone on the physical parameters of aging.*(10)(11)* In reality there has been over 20 years of research with thousands of medical studies showing benefits from Growth Hormone therapy, and extremely high safety profile. A few of these many medical research studies are listed on the Ron Rothenberg MD Web Site.*(12)*

Benefits of Human Growth Hormone

Benefits of *(*HGH*)* growth hormone include improved body composition, increased muscle and less body fat, improved bone density, improved wound healing, improved cognitive function, and improved sense of well being. Burn victims heal faster with growth hormone and have increased muscle protein synthesis. Patients with Crohn's disease and short bowel syndrome show improved nutritional status with HGH treatment. Cardiac cachexia patients gain weight, get well and leave the hospital. There are studies showing improvement in cognitive function, and improvement in quality of life with HGH. *(13)(14)(15)(16)(17)(18)(19)(20)(21)(22)(23)(24)(25)(26)(27)*

Dr. Debunker mistakenly assumes human growth hormone is given to aging adults to lengthen their years. This couldn't be farther from the truth, and is a straw man argument. This is not the intended use of human growth hormone by anti-aging docs like Ron Rothenberg, MD, a pioneer in Anti-Aging Medicine and Board Certified by the American Academy of Anti-Aging Medicine. Dr. Rothenberg gives the Growth Hormone lectures at the medical meetings, and he treats hundreds of patients with growth hormone therapy at the California Healthspan Institute.*(28)*

Ron Rothenberg MD

Dr. Rothenberg's goal is not to lengthen lifespan; rather it is to improve the **QUALITY** of our lifespan. I spoke with Dr. Rothenberg after his lecture at the medical meeting. I found him to be outgoing and personable fellow, appearing younger than his stated age of 62. He is an avid California surfer, and his favorite surfing photos are posted on his web site.*(29)*

Here is what Dr. Ron Rothenberg says about human growth hormone therapy for adult deficiency:

> "As anti-aging physicians, our goal is to help our patients stay strong and vigorous as long as possible without gradual and protracted deterioration. We know Growth Hormone Replacement Therapy is a proven defense against frailty, and when added to lifestyle, this is our chance to stay stronger and more functional. If we were to stay perfect, why intervene? But since we don't, this is one way to maintain function while we await the genetic and biochemical therapies that will be available in the near future. These patients are happier and healthier. Just ask one."*(30)*

This is good advice for Dr. Andrew Weil the Debunker, who should actually talk to the people over 50 who benefit from human growth hormone therapy as part of a comprehensive wellness program.

Use of Human Growth Hormone is Legal

Dr. Weil the Debunker also makes the grievous factual error in stating that human growth hormone therapy for adult deficiency is illegal. Again this couldn't be farther from the truth. If this were true, the 15,000 members of the American Academy of Anti-Aging Medicine, many of whom are board certified MD's, would already be in jail, a scenario, so ludicrous as to be laughable. In reality, well trained anti-aging physicians perform a complete medical workup including history, physical examination and extensive laboratory testing which includes tests for growth hormone levels *(*such as IGF-1*)*, and then treat for the FDA approved indication of Adult Growth Hormone Deficiency.*(33)* In addition, there is follow up with serial blood testing to ensure safety. Contrary to what Dr. Weil says, I assure you this is *very legal.*

It is certainly true that mainstream medicine differs from the position of the American Academy of Anti-Aging Medicine on the use human growth hormone for aging adults, and this is for political reasons. Growth hormone is expensive, and would bankrupt the health insurance industry and Medicare program. It is also certainly true that human growth hormone is an FDA approved pharmaceutical which has been proven effective, and therefore "snake oil" is hardly an appropriate label.

Avoid Internet Anti-Aging Operations

Of course there are problems. There are hordes of disreputable boiler room operations selling Growth Hormone on the internet without adequate medical supervision. The buyer should beware of these types of operations, beware of purchasing counterfeit drugs, and avoid purchasing Growth Hormone or any other prescription drugs over the phone from strangers. It is highly recommended that you have a close personal relationship with a knowledgeable physician with the proper training to oversee the program and monitor for adverse side effects. *(31)* To find such a physician, use the Doctor's Directory at the American Academy.*(32)* For more information on HGH human growth hormone see my web site.*(33)*

References

(1) www.aarpmagazine.org/health/debunker_fountain_of_youth.html
Dr. Debunker, The Truth About the Fountain of Youth, By Andrew Weil, M.D., May & June 2007, AARP Magazine How to live a healthy, vigorous—and long—life. No gimmicks

(1A) http://content.nejm.org/cgi/content/short/356/25/2591
Estrogen Therapy and Coronary-Artery Calcification NEJM Volume 356:2591-2602 June 21, 2007 Number 25 JoAnn E. Manson, M.D., et al

(2) www.golfdigest.com/features/index.ssf?/features/gd200608callahan.html
A diagnosis of low testosterone helped Micheel turn around his life. "I wasn't myself," he says. By Tom Callahan Golf Digest August 2006

(3) *archinte.ama-assn.org/cgi/content/abstract/166/15/1660*
Low Serum Testosterone and Mortality in Male Veterans Molly M. Shores, MD; Alvin M. Matsumoto, MD; Kevin L. Sloan, MD; Daniel R. Kivlahan, PhD Arch Intern Med. 2006;166:1660-1665.

(4) *www.medicinenet.com/script/main/art.asp?articlekey=81592*
Low Testosterone Levels Linked to Increased Mortality By Jeffrey Perkel HealthDay Reporter

(5) *http://www.jeffreydach.com/*
Jeffrey Dach MD, Blog site.

(6) *www.google.com/patents?id=ylEoAAAAEBAJ&printsec=abstract&zoom=4&dq=human+growth+hormone*
Growth Hormone Patent

(7) *http://www.fda.gov/cder/handbook/develop.htm*
FDA New Drug Development Process:Steps from Test Tube to New Drug Application Review

(8) *www.usatoday.com/news/health/2006-05-31-growth-drug_x.htm*
USA TODAY: FDA approves growth hormone WASHINGTON *(*AP*)*

(9) *content.karger.com/ProdukteDB/produkte.asp?Aktion=ShowAbstract&ArtikelNr=23531&Ausgabe=225980&ProduktNr=224036*
Growth Hormone - Hormone Replacement for the Somatopause? Richard Savine, Peter Sönksen Department of Medicine, St Thomas' Hospital, London, UK, Growth Hormone Research, Vol. 53, Suppl. 3, 2000

(10) *http://content.nejm.org/cgi/content/abstract/323/1/1*
NEJM, Volume 323:1-6 July 5, 1990 Number 1. Effects of human growth hormone in men over 60 years old. D Rudman, AG Feller, HS Nagraj, GA Gergans, PY Lalitha, AF Goldberg, RA Schlenker, L Cohn, IW Rudman, Abstract

(11) *http://content.nejm.org/cgi/content/full/323/1/1*
NEJM, Volume 323:1-6 July 5, 1990 Number 1. Effects of human growth hormone in men over 60 years old. D Rudman, AG Feller, HS Nagraj, GA Gergans, PY Lalitha, AF Goldberg, RA Schlenker, L Cohn, IW Rudman Full article

(12) *http://ehealthspan.com/references/index.html*
Listing of Published Research on Human Growth Hormone, California Healthspan Institute Ron Rothenberg MD

(13) *http://www.pubmedcentral.nih.gov/pagerender.fcgi?tool=pmcentrez&artid=1234282*
Recombinant human growth hormone accelerates wound healing in children with large cutaneous burns. D A Gilpin, R E Barrow, R L Rutan, L Broemeling, and D N Herndon Shriners Burns Institute, Galveston, Texas. Ann Surg. 1994 July; 220*(*1*)*: 19–24.

(14) http://www.pubmedcentral.nih.gov/articlerender.fcgi?tool=pmcentrez&artid=147 9605

Beneficial Effects of Extended Growth Hormone Treatment After Hospital Discharge in Pediatric Burn Patients. Rene Przkora, MD, et al. Ann Surg. 2006 June; 243*(6)*: 796–803.

(15) http://www.pubmedcentral.nih.gov/articlerender.fcgi?tool=pmcentrez&artid=149 3563

Metabolic effects of recombinant human growth hormone in patients receiving parenteral nutrition. T R Ziegler, L S Young, J M Manson, and D W Wilmore Department of Surgery, Harvard Medical School, Boston, Massachusetts. Ann Surg. 1988 July; 208*(1)*: 6–16.

(16) http://www.pubmedcentral.nih.gov/articlerender.fcgi?tool=pmcentrez&artid=166 4832

The effect of recombinant human growth hormone and resistance training on IGF-I mRNA expression in the muscles of elderly men. M Hameed et al. J Physiol. 2004 February 15; 555*(Pt 1)*: 231–240.

(17) http://www.pubmedcentral.nih.gov/articlerender.fcgi?tool=pmcentrez&artid=140 9868

Growth Hormone, Glutamine, and an Optimal Diet Reduces Parenteral Nutrition in Patients With Short Bowel Syndrome A Prospective, Randomized, Placebo-Controlled, Double-Blind Clinical Trial. Theresa A. Byrne et al. Ann Surg. 2005 November; 242*(5)*: 655–661.

(18) http://www.pubmedcentral.nih.gov/articlerender.fcgi?tool=pmcentrez&artid=177 3673

Non-alcoholic steatohepatitis and hepatic steatosis in patients with adult onset growth hormone deficiency. T Ichikawa et al. Gut. 2003 June; 52*(6)*: 914.

(19) http://www.pubmedcentral.nih.gov/articlerender.fcgi?tool=pmcentrez&artid=119 1645

Perioperative growth hormone treatment and functional outcome after major abdominal surgery: a randomized, double-blind, controlled study. P Kissmeyer-Nielsen et al, Ann Surg. 1999 February; 229*(2)*: 298–302.

(20) http://www.pubmedcentral.nih.gov/articlerender.fcgi?tool=pmcentrez&artid=150 1119&rendertype=abstract

The Role of Anabolic Hormones for Wound Healing in Catabolic States. Robert H. Demling, MD et al. J Burns Wounds. 2005; 4: e2.

(21) http://www.pubmedcentral.nih.gov/pagerender.fcgi?artid=1669103&pageindex=1

Cardiac cachexia treated with HGH. P H Sönksen, F Salomon, R Cuneo, M Umpleby, and S Bowes. BMJ. 1991 March 23; 302*(6778)*: 725–726.

(22) *http://www.pubmedcentral.nih.gov/articlerender.fcgi?tool=pmcentrez&artid=507772*
Effects of recombinant human growth hormone on muscle protein turnover in malnourished hemodialysis patients. G Garibotto et al. J Clin Invest. 1997 January 1; 99(1): 97–105.

(23) *http://www.pubmedcentral.nih.gov/articlerender.fcgi?tool=pmcentrez&artid=149 3563*
Metabolic effects of recombinant human growth hormone in patients receiving parenteral nutrition.T R Ziegler et al. Ann Surg. 1988 July; 208(1): 6–16.

(24) *http://www.pubmedcentral.nih.gov/articlerender.fcgi?tool=pmcentrez&artid=111 9467*
BMJ. 2001 January 27; 322(7280): 203. 2001, BMJ Science commentary Insulin-like growth factor and cognitive function Abi Berger, science editor BMJ

(25) *http://www.ncbi.nlm.nih.gov/pubmed/10984257*
Growth hormone, insulin-like growth factor I and cognitive function in adults.van Dam PS et al.Growth Horm IGF Res. 2000 Apr;10 Suppl B:S69-73.

(26) *http://www.ncbi.nlm.nih.gov/pubmed/15094076*
Insulin-like growth factor-I, cognition and brain aging. Van Dam PS et al. Eur J Pharmacol. 2004 Apr 19;490(1-3):87-95.

(27) *http://www.ncbi.nlm.nih.gov/pubmed/15478038*
The role of the somatotropic system in cognition and other cerebral functions. Creyghton WM, van Dam PS et al. Semin Vasc Med. 2004 May;4(2):167-72.

(28) *http://ehealthspan.com/treatment/bios.html*
The Doctor's Biography. Ron Rothenberg, MD, FACEP , Board Certified American Board of Anti-Aging Medicine.

(29) *http://ehealthspan.com/treatment/surf.html*
Short clips Dr. Rothenberg surfing at a "secret spot" south of the border.

(30) *http://ehealthspan.com/treatment/gh-therapy.html*
Adult Growth Hormone Therapy - Clinical Perspectives. Quality of Life Improves with GH Therapy By Ron Rothenberg, MD

(31) *http://www.drdach.com/wst_page16.html*
Jeffrey Dach MD Web Site Human Growth Hormone Page

(32) *http://www.worldhealth.net/directory/dach_jeffrey1*
Doctors Directory American Academy of Anti-Aging Medicine A4M

(33) *http://www.cenegenicsfoundation.org/library/Guidelines_hGH_Rx_on_LH.pdf*
Guidelines for the Diagnosis and Treatment of Adult Growth Hormone Deficiency

Chapter 16

Does Testosterone Cause Prostate Cancer?

What are the Risks and Benefits of Testosterone Therapy

The Nobel Prize in Chemistry was awarded to Butenandt and Ruzicka in 1939 for the synthesis of testosterone *(1)*, which has been the subject of intense medical research for the past seventy years. There are literally massive volumes of medical research studies showing numerous health benefits.*(2-27)*

Appropriate use of testosterone can prevent or reduce the likelihood of osteoporosis, type 2 diabetes, cardio-vascular disease *(CVD)*, obesity, depression, anxiety and the risk of early mortality.*(7)* Health benefits include positive effects on mood, energy levels, verbal fluency, strength, increased muscle size, decreased body fat and increased bone density.*(2-27)* Testosterone restores and enhances male libido, and is a treatment for male sexual dysfunction.*(33)*

The 2007 EPIC study concluded that testosterone level is inversely related to cardiovascular disease risk and all-cause mortality. Thus, low testosterone may be a marker for increased risk of cardiovascular disease.*(35)* A low Testosterone level is linked to reduced cognitive performance and the onset of Alzheimers Disease in elderly men. *(36)(37)*

Testosterone Benefits the Heart

Here are a few studies showing testosterone benefits the heart and circulation.

Dr. Dobrzycki studied men with known coronary artery disease and showed significantly lower levels of testosterone *(J Med Invest 2003)*.*(22)* He also showed low testosterone is associated with reduced pumping ability of the heart.

Dr. C.J. Malkin showed that testosterone therapy reduces risk of death from abnormal heart rhythms *(arrhythmias)*.*(23)* Dr. Malkin also reported that testosterone improves the pumping action of the heart in patients with Congestive Heart Failure,*(24)* and acts as a protective factor against atherosclerosis and plaque formation in arteries. *(J Endocrin 2003)*.

Dr. Eugene Shippen presented an impressive study at a medical meeting, in which testosterone therapy was used to successfully reverse diabetic gangrene of the lower legs and avoid amputation in many of the cases.

For more information on testosterone for aging males, see my testosterone *information page* at www.drdach.com.*(25)*

No Evidence of Adverse Effect on the Prostate

Regarding the hypothetical risk of prostate cancer from testosterone administration, there is no evidence for this in the medical literature. The studies listed below are only three of many in the medical literature reporting no evidence of any adverse effect on the prostate, and no evidence that testosterone causes prostate cancer.

> "It has been part of the conventional medical wisdom for six decades that higher testosterone in some way increases the risk of prostate cancer. This belief is derived largely from the well-documented regression of prostate cancer in the face of surgical or pharmacological castration. However, there is an absence of scientific data supporting the concept that higher testosterone levels are associated with an increased risk of prostate cancer. Specifically, no increased risk of prostate cancer was noted in 1*)* clinical trials of testosterone supplementation, 2*)* longitudinal population-based studies, or 3*)* in a high-risk population of hypogonadal men receiving testosterone treatment. Moreover, hypogonadal men have a substantial rate of biopsy-detectable prostate cancer, suggesting that low testosterone has no protective effect against development of prostate cancer. These results argue against an increased risk of prostate cancer with testosterone replacement therapy." Quoted from: Testosterone replacement therapy and prostate risks: where's the beef? Morgentaler A. Can J Urol. 2006 Feb;13 Suppl 1:40-3. *(28)*

> "No evidence exists that appropriate androgen administration with knowledgeable monitoring carries significant or potentially serious adverse effects on the prostate gland." Monitoring androgen replacement therapy: testosterone and prostate safety by Morales A. J Endocrinol Invest. 2005;28*(*3 Suppl*)*:122-7*(29)*

> "Despite decades of research, there is no compelling evidence that testosterone has a causative role in prostate cancer." Risks of Testosterone-Replacement Therapy and recommendations for Monitoring. N Engl J Med 2004;350:482-92. Rhoden and Morgentaler.*(30)*

For more information, see my web page on *Testosterone Safety and Benefits.(25)*

Is it possible to determine with a questionnaire if one has a low testosterone level? Yes, this is the ADAM Questionnaire which asks about symptoms of low testosterone *(*Androgen Deficiency in the Aging Male*).(43)(44)*

The ADAM Testosterone Questionnaire

1. Do you have a decrease in libido (sex drive)? Yes No

2. Do you have a lack of energy? Yes No

3. Do you have a decrease in strength and/or endurance? Yes No

4. Have you lost height? Yes No

5. Have you noticed a decreased "enjoyment of life" Yes No

6. Are you sad and/or grumpy? Yes No

7. Are your erections less strong? Yes No

8. Have you noticed a recent deterioration in your ability to play sports? Yes No

9. Are you falling asleep after dinner? Yes No

10. Has there been a recent deterioration in your work performance? Yes No

If you answered YES to questions 1 or 7, or any 3 other questions, you may have low testosterone.

The next step is a testosterone blood test to determine your testosterone levels. If low, then testosterone supplementation may be considered. It is important to work closely with a knowledgeable physician who can do a full evaluation, order the appropriate tests, and prescribe treatment.

Testosterone for Dry Eyes in Women

Among other things, some post-menopausal women have a chronic dry eye problem with redness and irritation of the eyes. This is called the evaporative dry eye and is usually a sign of testosterone deficiency, which can be confirmed by blood test for testosterone level, and rapidly resolves with topical testosterone cream in appropriate dosage.*(31)(32)*

References Chapter 16

(1) http://nobelprize.org/nobel_prizes/chemistry/laureates/1939/press.html
The Nobel Prize in Chemistry 1939 Presentation Speech The following account of Butenandt's work has been made.

Benefits of Testosterone

(2) http://www.hms.harvard.edu/news/pressreleases/mcl/0103testosteronereplace.html
Study Suggests Depressed Men May Benefit from Testosterone Replacement Therapy Belmont January 1, 2003

(3) http://www.revolutionhealth.com/healthy-living/mens-health/hot-topics/mens-health-101/testosterone-therapy-men
Testosterone therapy: The answer for aging men? Date updated: April 14, 2006 Content provided by MayoClinic.com Mayo Foundation for Medical Education and Research (MFMER)

(4) http://www.duj.com/Article/Hellstrom2/Hellstrom2.html
Digital Urology Journal. Testosterone Replacement Therapy. Wayne J.G. Hellstrom, M.D. Tulane University Medical Center New Orleans, LA

(5) http://www.medscape.com/viewarticle/556617_print
Testosterone and Ageing: What Have We Learned Since the Institute of Medicine Report and What Lies Ahead? M. M. Miner; A. D. Seftel Int J Clin Pract. 2007;61(4):622-632. 05/21/2007

(6) http://www.aafp.org/afp/20060501/1591.html
Testosterone Treatments: Why, When, and How? American Academy of Family Physicians.May 1, 2006 KATHERINE MARGO, M.D., University of Pennsylvania School of Medicine, Philadelphia, Pennsylvania ROBERT WINN, M.D., Jefferson Medical College, Philadelphia, Pennsylvania

(7) http://www.sciencedaily.com/releases/2006/08/060816083120.htm
Science News Low Testosterone Levels Associated With Increased Risk Of Death In Men.

ScienceDaily (Aug. 17, 2006) — Men who have a low testosterone level after age 40 may have a higher risk of death over a four-year period than those with normal levels of the hormone, according to a report in the August 14/28 issue of Archives of Internal Medicine, one of the JAMA/Archives journals (Arch Intern Med. 2006;166:1660-1665.

(8) http://www.sciencedaily.com/releases/2008/01/080109111320.htm
Testosterone May Improve Mental Function. ScienceDaily (Jan. 14, 2008) — When we think about the powers of testosterone, we usually do not consider mental processes. However, research suggests that testosterone levels may affect men's cognitive performance, reports the January 2008 issue of Harvard Men's Health Watch.

(9) http://www.worldhealth.net/pdf/bookstore/thera6_ch7.pdf
Chapter 7 Testosterone, The Male Hormone Connection: Treating Diabetes and Heart Disease Michael Klentze, M.D., Ph.D. Medical Director, Klentze Institute of Anti-Aging, Munich,

(10) *http://www.hotzehwc.com/attachments/wysiwyg/2/Testosterone101.pdf*
Testosterone for Men and Women By Steven F. Hotze, M.D., e-book.

(11) *https://secure.pharmacytimes.com/lessons/200410-03.asp*
State-of-the-Art Update on Testosterone Replacement: A Clinical and Pharmacological Approach Narinder Duggal Pharmacy Times

(12) *http://www.drmirkin.com/men/M227.html*
TESTOSTERONE REPLACEMENT FOR OLDER MEN? Gabe Mirkin, M.D.

(13) *http://www.endo-society.org/publications/OldContent/testosterone-Feb2004.cfm*
Treating With Testosterone: Endocrine Society Audioconference Spotlights IOM Report, Practical Approach to Testosterone Therapy of Elderly Men Endocrine News Volume 29, Number 1 - February 2004

(14) *http://www.hormone.org/Resources/Patient_Guides/upload/patients_guide_low_testosterone.pdf*
PATIENT'S GUIDE to Low Testosterone *(*2003 Edition*)*. Editors:Glenn R. Cunningham, MD, Alvin M. Matsumoto, MD, Ronald Swerdloff, MD.

(15) *http://www.healthline.com/sw/hr-nl-a-harvard-expert-shares-his-thoughts-on-testosterone-replacement-therapy*
An interview with Abraham Morgentaler, M.D.A Harvard expert shares his thoughts on testosterone-replacement

(16) *http://www.pubmedcentral.nih.gov/articlerender.fcgi?artid=1502320*
New Advances in the Treatment of Hypogonadism in the Aging Male Christopher P Steidle, MD. Rev Urol. 2003; 5*(*Suppl 1*)*: S34–S40.

(17) *http://www.ncbi.nlm.nih.gov/pubmed/15799128. Testosterone therapy--what, when*
and to whom? Jockenhövel F. Aging Male. 2004 Dec;7*(*4*)*:319-24

(18) *http://www.ncbi.nlm.nih.gov/pubmed/15329035*
Androgen replacement therapy: present and future.Gooren LJ, Bunck MC. Drugs. 2004;64*(*17*)*:1861-91.

(19) *http://www.ncbi.nlm.nih.gov/pubmed/16918944. Testosterone treatment comes of* age: new options for hypogonadal men. Nieschlag E. Clin Endocrinol *(*Oxf*)*. 2006 Sep;65*(*3*)*:275-81

(20) *http://www.med.unc.edu/~mcoward/urology/Harrison's*
Aging-Related Changes in Male Reproductive Function.pdf Harrison's Internal Medicine > Part 14. Endocrinology and Metabolism > Section 1. Endocrinology > Chapter 325.

Disorders of the Testes and Male Reproductive System > Aging-Related Changes in Male Reproductive Function

(21) *http://www.andrologyjournal.org/cgi/content/full/27/2/126*
Testosterone Replacement Therapy for Older Men. MOSHE WALD et al, Journal of Andrology, Vol. 27, No. 2, March/April 2006

Testosterone and the Heart

(22) *http://www.ncbi.nlm.nih.gov/pubmed/13678385*
An assessment of correlations between endogenous sex hormone levels and the extensiveness of coronary heart disease and the ejection fraction of the left ventricle in males. Dobrzycki S et al. J Med Invest. 2003 Aug;50*(*3-4*)*:162-9.

(23) *http://www.ncbi.nlm.nih.gov/pubmed/14609611*
Effect of testosterone therapy on QT dispersion in men with heart failure. Malkin CJ, Morris PD, Pugh PJ, English KM, Channer KS. Am J Cardiol. 2003 Nov 15;92*(*10*)*:1241-3.

(24) *http://www.ncbi.nlm.nih.gov/pubmed/16093267*
Testosterone therapy in men with moderate severity heart failure: a double-blind randomized placebo controlled trial. Malkin CJ, Pugh PJ, West JN, van Beek EJ, Jones TH, Channer KS. Eur Heart J. 2006 Jan;27*(*1*)*:57-64. Epub 2005 Aug 10. Testosterone replacement therapy improves functional capacity and symptoms in men with moderately severe heart failure.

(25) *http://www.drdach.com/wst_page15.html*
Testosterone Information Page Jeffrey Dach MD

(26) *http://drcranton.com/hrt/testosterone_replacement.htm*
Testosterone Replacement: The Male Andropause, Taken from a chapter in the book, Resetting the Clock, by Elmer M. Cranton, M.D. and William Fryer

(27) *http://archneur.ama-assn.org/cgi/content/abstract/59/11/1750*
Beneficial Effects of Testosterone Replacement for the Nonmotor Symptoms of Parkinson Disease. Michael S. Okun, MD et al. Arch Neurol. 2002;59:1750-1753.

Risks of Testosterone

(28) *http://www.ncbi.nlm.nih.gov/pubmed/16526980. Testosterone replacement therapy*
and prostate risks: where's the beef? Morgentaler A. Can J Urol. 2006 Feb;13 Suppl 1:40-3

(29) *http://www.ncbi.nlm.nih.gov/pubmed/16042371*
Monitoring androgen replacement therapy: testosterone and prostate safety. Morales A. No evidence exists that appropriate androgen administration with knowledgeable

monitoring carries significant or potentially serious adverse effects on the prostate gland. J Endocrinol Invest. 2005;28(3 Suppl):122-7.

(30) *http://www.drdach.com/uploads/testosterone_rhoden.pdf*
Risks of Testosterone-Replacement Therapy and Recommendations for Monitoring Ernani Luis Rhoden, M.D., and Abraham Morgentaler, M.D. N Engl J Med 2004;350:482-92.

(31) *http://www.ncbi.nlm.nih.gov/pubmed/10415627*
Androgens and dry eye in Sjögren's syndrome. Ann N Y Acad Sci. 1999 Jun 22;876:312-24. Sullivan DA et al. Our results demonstrate that androgens regulate both lacrimal and meibomian gland function, and suggest that topical androgen administration may serve as a safe and effective therapy for the treatment of dry eye in Sjögren's syndrome.

(32) *http://www.ncbi.nlm.nih.gov/pubmed/12114274*
Androgen deficiency, Meibomian gland dysfunction, and evaporative dry eye. Sullivan DA et al. Ann N Y Acad Sci. 2002 Jun;966:211-22. Overall, these results support our hypothesis that androgen deficiency may be an important etiologic factor in the pathogenesis of evaporative dry eye in women with Sjögren's syndrome.

(33) *http://www.aace.com/pub/pdf/guidelines/sexdysguid.pdf*
Male Sexual Dysfunction, Endocr Pract. 2003;9 (No. 1) January/February 2003 77 AMER ASSOC OF CLIN ENDOCRIN MEDICAL GUIDELINES FOR CLIN PRACTICE FOR THE EVAL AND TREATMENT OF MALE SEXUAL DYSFUNCTION: A COUPLE'S PROBLEM–2003 UPDATE AACE Male Sexual Dysfunction Task Force. Andre T. Guay, MD et al.

(34) *http://www.fda.gov/medwatch/SAFETY/2003/03SEP_PI/AndroGel_PI.pdf*
Androgel FDA approved topical version of testosterone.

(35) *http://www.cardiosource.com/cjrpicks/CJRPick.asp?cjrID=3849*
Endogenous Testosterone and Mortality due to All Causes, Cardiovascular Disease, and Cancer in Men: European Prospective Investigation Into Cancer in Norfolk (EPIC-Norfolk) Prospective Population Study 2/6/2008 Khaw KT, Dowsett M, Folkerd E, et al. Circulation. 2007;116:2694-2701.

(36) *http://www.nih.gov/news/pr/jan2004/nia-26.htm*
Low Free Testosterone Levels Linked to Alzheimer's Disease in Older Men

(37) *http://jcem.endojournals.org/cgi/content/full/87/11/5001*
The Journal of Clinical Endocrinology & Metabolism Vol. 87, No. 11 5001-5007 Longitudinal Assessment of Serum Free Testosterone Concentration Predicts Memory Performance and Cognitive Status in Elderly Men Scott D. Moffat et al.

(38) *http://www.mbschachter.com/male_andropause.htm*
The Male Andropause, by Michael B. Schachter M.D., F.A.C.A.M.

(39) *http://www.usdoctor.com/Chapter13.html*
NATIONAL FEATURED ARTICLE TESTOSTERONE for MEN with DIABETES

(40) *http://www.touchbriefings.com/pdf/2782/jones.pdf*
Testosterone – Clinical Associations with the Metabolic Syndrome and Type 2 Diabetes Mellitus. T Hugh Jones at al.

(41) *http://www.svedyn.com/web/revistas/deficit%20androgenos%20adultos.pdf*
Androgen Deficiency in Men. Daniel S. Tung, MD, and Glenn R. Cunningham, MD The Endocrinologist Volume 17, Number 2, April 2007

(42) *http://care.diabetesjournals.org/cgi/content/full/30/4/911*
Diabetes Care 30:911-917, 2007 Clinical and Biochemical Assessment of Hypogonadism in Men With Type 2 Diabetes, Correlations with bioavailable testosterone and visceral adiposity. Dheeraj Kapoor, MD, et al.

(43) *http://jcem.endojournals.org/cgi/content/full/89/12/5920#R4*
The Journal of Clinical Endocrinology & Metabolism Vol. 89, No. 12 5920-5926 Prevalence and Incidence of Androgen Deficiency in Middle-Aged and Older Men: Estimates from the Massachusetts Male Aging Study. Andre B. Araujo et al.

(44) *http://www.ncbi.nlm.nih.gov/pubmed/11016912*
Metabolism. 2000 Sep;49*(9)*:1239-42.Validation of a screening questionnaire for androgen deficiency in aging males. *(*ADAM*)* Morley JE, Charlton E et al.

Chapter 17

Hypothyroidism, the Thyroflex and Reflex Time

On February 8, 2007, Ann Nicole Smith apparently overdosed and died 5 minutes away from my office at the Seminole Indian Hard Rock Hotel, a gambling casino on a nearby Indian reservation. Anna Nicole's death was officially attributed to drug overdose. However, the autopsy report described a low thyroid condition called Hashimoto's thyroid disease, a common condition causing low thyroid.*(1)* Anna Nicole Smith was also said to be taking human growth hormone *(*HGH*).(7)* Of course, this information wasn't mentioned in the autopsy report. The obvious question is why was Ann Nicole taking Growth Hormone when she really needed thyroid medication?

Although mainstream medicine is staunchly opposed to *HGH use by Aging Baby Boomers*, the practice has caught the attention of some *seniors groups*, and seems to be growing in spite of opposition by the Institute of Medicine and *JAMA .(2)(3)(4)(5)(6)* As in the case of Anna Nicole, I propose that it's usually thyroid deficiency rather than growth hormone deficiency that is the more urgent problem.

Human Growth Hormone at Cenegenics

A few years ago in 2005, I spent a week doing a clinical fellowship at the *Cenegenics Clinic in Las Vegas* with Alan Mintz MD.*(8)* My opinion after visiting the clinic is the Las Vegas Cenegenics clinic is excellent with good doctors and support staff devoted to Age Management Medicine. You may have seen Dr. Alan Mintz when he appeared on *CBS Television 60 Minutes* to describe his clinic program and talk about the Age Management Medicine Protocols offered there.*(9)*

In his CBS 60 minutes television interview, Alan Mintz disclosed that about 800 of the Cenegenics patients were using human growth hormone *(*HGH*)* based on a *protocol* for Adult Growth Hormone Deficiency.*(11)* The online community is indebted to Dr. Mintz for creating a useful online medical library containing many articles relating to aging and hormones.*(12)* Dr. Alan Mintz passed away June 3, 2007, a little less than a year after his interview on the 60 minutes CBS television show.*(10)* Dr. Mintz started his career as a radiologist, and later founded the Cenegenics clinic. He was a visionary and a pioneer in his field, and he inspired many other doctors, including myself, to enter the field of natural medicine and bio-identical hormones.

Thyroid Hormone, The Missing Piece of the Puzzle

Various vitamin and hormone treatments such as HGH *(*human growth hormone*)*, testosterone, DHEA, estrogen and progesterone are considered by aging baby boomers to have anti-aging properties. However I would suggest that one need look no further than thyroid hormone, which is perhaps the quintessential anti-aging medication, since it changes the body composition, skin and hair quality, and produces a more youthful appearance after a few months of treatment. In my experience these observed youthful changes are much more profound with thyroid hormone than any other treatment in patients with low thyroid.

Yet, many the large clinics involved in Age Management or so-called anti-aging medicine tend to be conservative when it comes to offering thyroid treatment. They usually hesitate to give thyroid medication if the labs are normal, or if they do give thyroid hormone, it is usually Synthroid. We prefer to use natural desiccated thyroid hormone such as *Nature-Throid from Western Research*, or Armour because clinical results are better.*(13)(32)*

Synthroid is a thyroid pill which contains only T4 *(*thyroxine*)*, while the natural thyroid medication contains both T3 and T4, accounting for the better clinical results of the natural thyroid.*(32)* Mainstream medical practice relies on the TSH test to determine when to treat with thyroid hormone *(*lab range 0.5 – 5.5*)* , so most people with low thyroid are missed by the medical system, and are not given thyroid hormone medication.

Mark Starr and Type Two Hypothyroidism

A few months after meeting with Alan Mintz, M.D. at the Cenegenics clinic, I attended a medical meeting of the ICIM *(*Integrative and Complementary Medicine*)* in Grand Rapids Michigan. At this meeting, I spoke with Mark Starr, M.D. who presented his approach to diagnosis and treatment of the low thyroid condition, which he calls Type Two Hypothyroidism.*(14)* Mark Starr's lecture and his book on the same topic were a real eye opener for me because he claimed that while 30% of the population are low thyroid, they are ignored and go untreated by mainstream medicine. These unfortunate souls drag themselves from doctor to doctor with labels such as chronic fibromyalgia, and chronic fatigue, and suffer from hair loss, constipation, depression and a host of other symptoms described by Dr. Jacob Teitelbaum.*(15)* Dr. Starr explained why thyroid blood tests such as the TSH are unreliable. Dr. Starr instead relies on old fashioned clinical judgment to decide when to treat with thyroid hormone and how much thyroid medication to give. *(16)(17)(18)*

Enter The Thyroflex Machine

One of the tried and true clinical parameters of thyroid function is the delayed Achilles reflex time which the old time docs used routinely for practical management of low thyroid before the blood tests were devised. Checking the Achilles reflex is still accepted and used by mainstream medicine today as an indicator of thyroid function.*(19)(20)(21)(22)(23)(24)*.

I was therefore really excited to meet Drs. Konrad Kail and Daryl Turner at their booth at the *American Academy of Anti-Aging Medicine Meeting* in 2005.*(25)(26)(27)(28)* Drs. Kail and Turner developed the Thyroflex instrument, a reflex hammer connected to a laptop computer which measures reflex time in milliseconds.*(27)*

They do not routinely use the Achilles Tendon reflex though. Instead, they decided to use the Brachio-Radialis muscle of the forearm, a more convenient way to illicit the reflex while the patient is seated in a comfortable chair. A delayed reflex time is the finding which indicates low thyroid.

They found excellent correlation between reflex time and thyroid function as measured by basal metabolic rate in patients before and after treatment with natural thyroid. Their study found a predictive Value of a Positive Test = 0.95 and a Predictive Value of a Negative Test= 0.017, which I thought was quite good.*(29)(30)*

Our Thyroflex Experience

We are proud to be the first medical clinic in Florida to offer this noninvasive Thyroflex test which really represents the best modern medicine has to offer, while at the same time validating the original knowledge of early thyroid clinical practice. After using the Thyroflex machine for about one year, we have found it to be especially useful in those cases in which the TSH is paradoxically low even though the patient is low thyroid. Note: a low TSH indicates high thyroid function, while a high TSH indicates low thyroid function. Many people are confused by this.

This paradoxically low TSH is called *hypothalamic dysfunction*, and Jacob Teitelbaum MD sees this frequently in his chronic fatigue patients.*(31)* Since in these cases the TSH is usually below 3, no mainstream doctor would be willing to give thyroid hormone treatment to these unfortunate souls. With the confidence of a delayed reflex time on a Thyroflex test, we can feel comfortable giving these people the badly needed thyroid, and the results have been astounding.

Our approach to diagnosis of low thyroid uses a lengthy questionnaire which goes over 70 symptoms of low thyroid *(listed below)*, a complete thyroid blood panel including TSH, free T3 and free T4, and a physical examination which includes measurement of reflex time with the Thyroflex. Also included is a basal body temperature chart filled out by the patient at home.

A Trial of Low Dose Thyroid is Very Safe

Once it has been determined that thyroid hormone is likely to be beneficial, a trial of low dose Nature-Throid from RLC labs *(Western Research)* is given with a small half grain tablet every other day, while a log book is kept by the patient describing any changes in energy or other symptoms. Any symptoms of thyroid excess such as palpitations, feeling of warmth, anxiety or insomnia are noted in the log book. After 8 days, the log book is reviewed to determine if the thyroid was of benefit. In addition, Iodine supplementation with Iodoral is routinely given as described in a previous article on Iodine and Breast Cancer Prevention.*(45)*

We have found that monitoring symptoms by recording any changes in a log book, as well as small half grain gradual increments in thyroid dosage makes this program very safe. In the event the patient experiences palpitations, they are instructed to hold any further thyroid medication and inform the physician. For more information, visit my web site *thyroid page.*

Checklist of Common Symptoms of Low Thyroid:

____Weight gain
____Puffy face
____Loss or thinning of eyebrows
____Cold intolerance
____Low sex drive
____Depression
____Abdominal bloating
____Cold hands or feet
____Dry or thinning hair
____Joint or muscle pain
____Thickening of the skin
____Thin, brittle fingernails

Longer List of Commonly Reported Symptoms of Hypothyroidism

1. Dry skin
2. Thick, scaling skin
3. Coarse skin
4. Fineness of hair
5. Dry, coarse, brittle hair
6. Sparse eyebrows, especially outer ends
7. Hair loss
8. Brittle nails
9. Dry ridges down nails
10. Cold skin
11. Swelling of face (edema)
12. Swelling around the eyes (edema)
13. Swelling of eyelids (edema)
14. Nonpitting edema of ankles
15. Fluid accumulation in abdomen (ascites)
16. Thick tongue
17. Swelling of ankles
18. Paleness of skin
19. Paleness of lips
20. Bluish or purplish coloration of skin, nail beds, lips
21. Weight gain unexplainably
22. Hoarseness
23. Low basal & activity level temperature
25. Slow speech
26. Slow pulse rate despite low physical fitness
27. Slow thinking
28. Sluggish movement
29. Slow relaxation phase of the knee or ankle reflex
30. Listless, dull look to eyes
31. Wasting of tongue
32. Nervousness
33. Slow heart rate despite low aerobic fitness

References

(1) *http://www.thesmokinggun.com/archive/years/2007/0326071anna1.html*
Anna Nicole Smith Autopsy Released, Coroner: Ex-Playmate died from accidental sedative overdose.

(2) *http://www.sfgate.com/cgi-bin/article.cgi?file=/chronicle/archive/2003/11/17/MNGEV33KQD1.DTL*
Aging Baby Boomers turn to hormone, Some doctors concerned about growing 'off-label' use of drug. Sabin Russell, November 17, 2003. San Francisco Chronicle.

(3) *http://www.seniormag.com/caregiverresources/articles/hgh.htm*
HGH (Human Growth Hormone) HGH and effects on aging - An exciting discovery made about 15 years ago has linked the aging process to declining levels of certain hormones. SeniorMag.com

(4) *http://www.natap.org/2005/HIV/102705_01.htm*
Provision or Distribution of Growth Hormone for "Antiaging", COMMENTARY Clinical and Legal Issues. Thomas T. Perls, MD, MPH; Neal R. Reisman, MD, JD; S. Jay Olshansky, PhD. JAMA. Oct 26 2005;294:2086-2090. Full Text PDF.

(5) *http://jama.ama-assn.org/cgi/content/extract/294/16/2086*
Provision or Distribution of Growth Hormone for "Antiaging", COMMENTARY Clinical and Legal Issues. Thomas T. Perls, MD, MPH; Neal R. Reisman, MD, JD; S. Jay Olshansky, PhD. JAMA. Oct 26 2005;294:2086-2090. Abstract.

(6) *http://www.iom.edu/ Institute of Medicine web site*

(7) *http://www.newsweek.com/id/35905*
What Anna Nicole Smith Was Shooting? The dead starlet's autopsy revealed that she was injecting human growth hormone to counter the effects of aging and promote weight loss. Does that work? Inside the HGH boom—and the backlash. By Lynn Waddell and Arian Campo-Flores, Newsweek Web Exclusive Mar 28, 2007

(8) *http://www.cenegenics.com/*
Cenegenics Medical Institute, 851 S Rampart Blvd Ste 210, Las Vegas, NV 89145-4886, Phone: (702) 240-4200, Toll Free 866.953.1510

(9) *http://www.cbsnews.com/stories/2006/04/19/60minutes/main1512855.shtml*
60 Minutes. Aging In The 21st Century, Steve Kroft Reports On The New Field Of Anti-Aging Medicine, Aug. 20. 2006

(10) *http://www.reviewjournal.com/obituaries/individual_display.jsp?obitID=2211636*
ALAN MINTZ M.D. Alan P. Mintz, M.D., cofounder and CEO of Cenegenics Medical Institute, passed away June 3, 2007, as a result of a brain hemorrhage. He was 69 years old. Born in Chicago, Alan was a graduate of the University of Chicago and earned a doctor of medicine degree from the University of Illinois - School of Medicine. He served as a physician in the U.S. Navy, prior to postgraduate training in radiology.

(11) *http://www.cenegenicsfoundation.org/library/Guidelines_hGH_Rx_on_LH.pdf*
Guidelines for the Diagnosis and Treatment of Adult Growth Hormone Deficiency Background. Cenegenics Foundation.

(12) *http://www.cenegenicsfoundation.org/library/*
Online Cenegenics Medical Library offered via nonprofit Cenegenics Education and Research Foundation.

(13) *http://www.nature-throid.com/*
Nature-Throid from RLC labs Western Research, Western Research Laboratories 2404 West 12th Street, suite #4 - Tempe, Arizona - 85281, Toll-Free: 1-877-797-7997

(14) *http://www.type2hypothyroidism.com/*
Type Two Hypothyroidism Book by Mark Starr.

(15) *http://www.healthy.net/scr/column.asp?ColumnId=28&Id=648*
Hypothyroidism, The Tragic and Invisible Epidemic of Thyroid Disease. Dr Jacob Teitelbaum MD

(16) *http://www.vitality101.com/*
Jacob Teitelbaum MD Chronic Fatigue Web Site

(17) *http://www.mercola.com/article/hypothyroid/diagnosis_comp.htm*
Optimum Diagnosis and Treatment of Hypothyroidism With Free T3 and Free T4 Levels Mercola.com

(18) *http://articles.mercola.com/sites/articles/archive/2003/03/01/hypothyroidism-part-two.aspx*
Major Revision of Hypothyroid Diagnosis Guidelines, Mercola.com

Achilles Tendon Reflex Time

(19) *http://www.ncbi.nlm.nih.gov/pubmed/5520306*
Med Klin. 1970 Nov 6;65*(*45*)*:1973-82. [Validity of Achilles tendon reflex measurement during thyroid gland function disorders][Article in German] Gillich KH, Krüskemper HL, Stendel A.

(20) *http://www.ncbi.nlm.nih.gov/pubmed/6895943*
Probl Endokrinol *(*Mosk*)*. 1982 Jan-Feb;28*(*1*)*:34-8. [Reflexometry as a supplementary study method in thyroid hypofunction][Article in Russian] Gaïdina GA, Matveeva LS, Lazareva SP.

(21) *http://www.ncbi.nlm.nih.gov/pubmed/2391297*
J Assoc Physicians India. 1990 Mar;38*(*3*)*:201-3. Ankle reflex photomotogram in thyroid dysfunctions.Khurana AK, Sinha RS, Ghorai BK, Bihari N.

(22) *http://www.ncbi.nlm.nih.gov/pubmed/952638*
A screening test for thyroid function.Goodman E. Aust Fam Physician. 1976 May; 5*(*4*)*:550-9, 561.

(23) *http://www.ncbi.nlm.nih.gov/pubmed/995289*
Achilles reflexogram and hemodynamic parameters in the evaluation of thyroid function. Franco G, Malamani T. Minerva Med. 1976 Oct 27;67*(*51*)*:3325-34

(24) *http://www.ncbi.nlm.nih.gov/pubmed/3658939*
Changes in the duration of the Achilles reflex in euthyroid goiter in children . Probl Endokrinol (Mosk). 1987 May-Jun;33(3):6-9.

(25) *http://www.googlesyndicatedsearch.com/u/scnm?q=kail*
Konrad Kail, P.A., N.D. Director. Southwest College Research Institute. Tempe, AZ (602) 363-9237 Associate Professor of Naturopathic Medicine; Special Consultant for External Research Affairs; BS, University of Houston, 1974; BS, Baylor College of Medicine, 1976; ND, National College of Naturopathic Medicine, 1983.

(26) *http://www.azadvancedmed.com/CV_Kail.html*
Curriculum Vitae for Dr. Konrad Kail

(27) *http://www.thyroflex.com/*
Thyroflex, Nitek Web Site, Daryl Turner

(28) *http://www.worldhealth.net/*
A4M, American Academy of Anti-Aging Medicine

(29) *http://www.thyroflex.com/docs/Predictability%20of%20Brachioradialis%20Reflexometry.doc*
Predictability of Brachioradialis Reflexometry, Thyroflex, Nitek

(30) *http://www.thyroflex.com/docs/Subclinical%20Hypothroidism.doc*
Managing Subclinical Hypothyroid Using Resting Metabolic Rate and Brachioradialis Reflexometry Konrad Kail, N.D.1, Robert F. Waters, Ph.D., Thyroflex, Nitek

(31) *http://www.townsendletter.com/Oct_2002/fibromyalgia1002.htm*
From the Townsend Letter for Doctors & Patients, October 2002. Highly Effective Treatment of Fibromyalgia and Chronic Fatigue Syndrome: Results of a Placebo Controlled Study and How to Apply the Protocol, by Jacob Teitelbaum, MD

(32) *http://www.armourthyroid.com/default.aspx*
Armour Thyroid Web Site

(33) *http://www.armourthyroid.com/hypothyroidism/symptoms.html#summary*
Summary List of Symptoms of Hypothyroidism , Armour web site

(34) *http://thyroid.about.com/cs/basics_starthere/a/hypochecklist.htm*
Hypothyroidism Risk/Symptoms Checklist, Help in Diagnosis and Finetuning Your Treatment By Mary Shomon, About.com, December 22, 2003

(35) *http://www.drlowe.com/geninfo/hyposigns.htm*
Do You Have Signs of Hypothyroidism or Thyroid Hormone Resistance? Dr. John C. Lowe

(36) *http://www.drlowe.com/articles/blinded.htm#process%20of%20change*
Lowe, J.C., Reichman, A., & Yellin, J.: The process of change with T3 therapy for euthyroid fibromyalgia: a double-blind placebo-controlled crossover study. Clin. Bull. Myofascial Ther., 2*(2/3)*:91-124, 1997.

(37) *http://www.drdach.com/wst_page10.html*
Thyroid Page on Jeffrey Dach MD web site

(38) *http://www.stopthethyroidmadness.com/*
Stop the Thyroid Madness, devoted to natural thyroid medication rather than synthroid

(39) *http://www.brodabarnes.org/*
Broda Barnes Institute

(40) *http://www.starrpainclinic.com/*
Mark Starr MD Pain Clinic

(41) *http://www.thyroidpower.com/linksfr.html*
Richard L. Shames, M.D.THYROID POWER

(42) *http://www.cfsfibromyalgia.com/links/index.htm*
Living Well With Chronic Fatigue Syndrome & Fibromyalgia, Mary Shomon, patient advocate.

(43) *http://thyroid.about.com/*
By Mary Shomon Thyroid Disease Guide About.com Thyroid

(44) *http://members.aol.com/jefferiesw/*
William McK. Jefferies, M.D. *(*Retired*)* Web Page, Dr. Jefferies has retired from active medical practice. *(*Honorary*)* Professor, Division of Endocrinology and Metabolism University of Virginia School of Medicine Charlottesville, Virginia

(45) *http://jeffreydach.com/2007/05/05/jeffreydachdrdachiodine.aspx*
Breast Cancer Prevention and Iodine Supplementation by Jeffrey Dach MD

(46) *http://www.reviewjournal.com/lvrj_home/2006/Jan-22-Sun-2006/news/5425933.html*
Jan. 22, 2006 Las Vegas Review-Journal IN DEPTH: Hormone therapy: CENEGENICS: Photo of Alan Mintz

(47) *http://en.wikipedia.org/wiki/Anna_Nicole_Smith*
Ann Nicole Smith Wikipedia Photo. American actress Anna Nicole Smith in the red carpet for 2005 MTV Video Music Awards

(48) *http://www.flickr.com/photos/foraggio/213328404/*
Anna Nicole Smith, Luna Park, Sydney. Toby Forage Anna died on February 8, 2007.

Section Five

Medical Conditions, Hypertension, Diabetes

Chapter 18

Fifty Million Americans have High Blood Pressure

Fifty Million Americans have High Blood Pressure and if you are one of them, then your doctor has you on pressure pills costing 3 billion dollars a year nationwide. Despite over 100 antihypertensive medications that have been approved, sadly, we have been unsuccessful in controlling hypertension. A survey reported in the July 9 issue of The Journal of the American Medical Association *(*JAMA*)* found that "Almost 30 percent of people with high blood pressure are unaware of their illness and 42 percent are not being treated".*(1)(2)*

The reason high blood pressure is bad for you is that it can damage the arteries causing heart disease, kidney damage, and stroke. There are two major types of hypertension with pills that work best for each type. Natural alternatives like Co-Enzyme Q-10 and Nattokinase can reduce reliance on blood medications.

Dr. John H. Laragh is the Expert on Hypertension:

My pick for best expert on hypertension is *John H. Laragh, M.D.,* who founded the American Society of Hypertension in 1986. He is chief editor of the American Journal of Hypertension, and has written over 900 articles and several textbooks dealing with hypertension. He was featured on the *cover* of Time magazine in 1975 for discovering the role of the renin-angiotensin-aldosterone system in regulating blood pressure.*(3)(4)(5)*

Hypertension is Caused by Elevated Renin Levels:

Dr. Laragh says that common hypertension is caused by excess renin in sixty percent of cases and can be permanently controlled with one drug by measuring blood renin activity, a procedure that Dr. Laragh pioneered and perfected over thirty years at his lab. This test is called the PRA test *(*plasma renin activity*)*. As a hospital based interventional radiologist for over 25 years, I sometimes did renin measurements by placing small catheters into each renal vein and collecting blood samples from the kidneys.*(6)* This is unnecessary for most people, because a routine blood sample from an arm vein is all that is needed to run the PRA test. We also used captopril renography to identify patients with renal artery stenosis who would benefit from renal artery angioplasty.*(7)*

Two types of Essential Hypertension:

Low Renin Hypertension

Dr Laragh says that essential hypertension exists in two forms. The first form is low renin hypertension, occurring in about a third of hypertensives. This is called Volume *(V)* hypertension. The plasma rennin activity PRA test shows low renin *(*less than 0.65 ng/m/hr*)* and the "water pills" such as the thiazides and calcium channel blockers work best for this type of low renin hypertension.

High Renin Hypertension

The second type is high renin hypertension, occurring in the other two thirds of hypertensives, is labeled *(*R*)* for Renin Hypertension, and the PRA levels are greater than 0.65 ng/m/hr. This hypertension is due to the renin-angiotensin system, and the newer drugs such as the ACE Inhibitors *(*angiotensin converting enzyme inhibitors*)* and Beta Blockers work best for this type.

Measuring renin allows your doctor to identify which type of antihypertensive medication is most likely to be effective and possibly safer for you. If the "water pills" have been tried and don't work for you, then you are probably have high renin hypertension and need one of the newer drugs such as an Ace Inhibitor. The advantage here is that once this is established, it is possible for you have your blood pressure controlled with one drug permanently. Single drug therapy for life is the major goal of treatment.

Problems with older "water pills":

What is really worrisome is the harm that can result from traditional diuretic "water pills". The thiazide diuretic, hygroton, produced an 11 percent incidence of permanent diabetes over five years in the ALLHAT drug study.*(*8*)(*9*)* Diabetes is a super high risk factor for heart disease. In other studies, thiazide "water pills" have been shown to regularly produce potassium and magnesium depletion that leads to cardiac arrhythmias, muscle weakness, EKG changes and fatal heart problems. All of these thiazide "water pill complications can be avoided by using a spirolactone type water pill instead *(*called aldactone*)*. Spironolactone is off-patent and therefore inexpensive costing 22 cents per tablet. The aldactone corrects the sodium-volume related hypertension without ever causing diabetes or depletion of potassium and magnesium. An incidental side effect of spironolactone is that this drug has an anti-testosterone effect. This may be useful in young females with PCOS and high testosterone levels, however, this may contribute to gynecomastia *(*breast enlargement*)* in aging males.

It hard to understand why Dr. Laragh's information has been overlooked *(*if not deliberately omitted*)* in official recommendations for the treatment of hypertension.

And as a result, your doctor may not do the renin test for high blood pressure unless you bring it up.

Alternatives to Drug treatment: Coenzyme Q-10 and Nattokinase:

Co-Enzyme Q-10 is a vitamin like nutritional supplement that has been useful in eliminating the need for blood pressure medications in about half the people who try it.*(*10*)(*11*)* One such program is advocated by Stephen Sinatra, M.D. in his books, "The Sinatra Solution, Metabolic Cardiology" and "Lower Your Blood Pressure in 8 weeks".*(*12*)* Co-Enzyme Q-10 has also been credited with saving many people from death from congestive heart failure when other drugs have failed. In addition, since the statin anti-cholesterol drugs cause depletion of Co-Enzyme Q-10 in the body, all patients on a statin drug should be supplementing with Co-Enzyme Q-10. Since Co-Q10 is not a drug, your doctor may not be aware of it.

The Benefits of Nattokinase on Blood Pressure

In 1980, while studying physiological chemistry at the University of Chicago Medical School, Japanese researcher Hiroyuki Sumi accidentally discovered that a traditional Japanese soy cheese which had been consumed for centuries, called "natto", had the ability to dissolve clots. His research group published a paper on the discovery in 1987.*(*13*)*

Traditionally, Natto has been consumed not only for cardiovascular support, but also to lower blood pressure. This was confirmed by several clinical trials in 1995, at Miyazaki Medical College and Kurashiki University in Japan where the effects of nattokinase on blood pressure in both animal and human subjects was studied. The researchers found that natto inhibits angiotensin converting enzyme *(*ACE*)*, which has a lowering effect on blood pressure. In one human study, Nattokinase ingestion was associated with a 10 percent drop in blood pressure. Natto is a nutritional supplement which is considered safe, However, people with bleeding disorders or on blood thinners should use nattokinase only under medical supervision. *(*14*)(*15*)(*16*)*

Check your own blood pressure:

If you are not sure what you blood pressure number is, you can have your doctor check it, or you can check it yourself with your own inexpensive machine obtainable from most drug stores. The normal blood pressure is commonly stated as 120 over 80 mm Hg. What is the desirable healthy blood pressure range? In the next chapter we will discuss this question.

References:

(1) http://pubs.ama-assn.org/media/2003j/0708.dtl#hypertension
JULY 8, 2003 PREVALENCE OF HYPERTENSION INCREASING IN THE U.S.— Nearly one-third of the U.S. adult population, an estimated 58 million people, have hypertension, an increase from previous reports, and reversing a three decade decline in the prevalence rate, according to a study in the July 9 issue of The Journal of the American Medical Association (JAMA). Hypertension was defined as a measured blood pressure (BP) of 140/90 mm Hg or greater or reported use of antihypertensive medications.

(2) http://jama.ama-assn.org/cgi/content/abstract/290/2/199
Trends in Prevalence, Awareness, Treatment, and Control of Hypertension in the United States, 1988-2000 Ihab Hajjar et al. JAMA. 2003;290:199-206.

(3) http://hcr3.isiknowledge.com/author.cgi?id=2331&cb=2453
John Laragh MD, CV and publication list. Cornell University

(4) http://www.time.com/time/covers/0,16641,1101750113,00.html
John Laragh MD Cover of Time Magazine credited to Bill Pierce Jan 13, 1975

(5) http://www.time.com/time/magazine/article/0,9171,917084-1,00.html
Time Magazine article on John Laragh and Hypertension, CONQUERING THE QUIET KILLER Monday, Jan. 13, 1975

(6) http://www.nature.com/jhh/journal/v16/n4/full/1001365a.html
Hypertension and renovascular disease: follow-up on 100 renal vein renin samplings. P Hasbak et al. Journal of Human Hypertension, April 2002, V16, N4, P275-280

(7) http://jnm.snmjournals.org/cgi/reprint/39/7/1297
Procedure Guideline for Diagnosis of Renovascular Hypertension, Andrew T. Taylor, Jr. et al. J Nucl Med. 1998 Jul;39(7):1297-302.

(8) http://www.medicinenet.com/script/main/art.asp?articlekey=51967
Water Pills Help All With Hypertension By Sid Kirchheimer WebMD Feature Reviewed By Charlotte Grayson

(9) http://www.diabetesincontrol.com/modules.php?name=News&file=article&sid=1189
Water Pills Increase Diabetes Risk in Major Study. Diuretics More Likely To Cause Diabetes Then ACE Inhibitors Or Calcium Channel Blockers. Patients randomized to diuretics in the landmark ALLHAT were more likely to develop new onset diabetes than patients randomized to either a calcium channel blocker or an angiotensin-converting enzyme (ACE) inhibitor to control high blood pressure.

(10) *http://lpi.oregonstate.edu/infocenter/othernuts/coq10/*
Coenzyme Q-10 Page at the Linus Pauling Inst.

(11) *http://www.ncbi.nlm.nih.gov/sites/entrez?db=pubmed&cmd=Retrieve&dopt=AbstractPlus&list_uids=10204818&query_hl=71&itool=pubmed_docsum*
Effect of hydrosoluble coenzyme Q10 on blood pressures and insulin resistance in hypertensive patients with coronary artery disease.Singh RB, Niaz MA, Rastogi SS, Shukla PK, Thakur AS. J Hum Hypertens. 1999 Mar;13*(3)*:203-8.

(12) *http://www.drsinatra.com/index.asp*
Dr. Steven Sinatra Web Site:

(13) *http://www.vrp.com/art/1227.asp?c=1177727946671&k=/det/6251.asp&m=/&p=no&s=0*
Nattokinase and Serrapeptase: Nature's Clot-Busters James South, M.A.

(14) *http://www.wellnesstrader.com/herbal-remedies/natto-nattokinase/nattokinase-research*
Nattokinase Research

(15) *http://www.mercola.com/forms/cardioessentials_scientific_research.htm*
Nattokinase research at Mercola.com

(16) *http://www.smart-publications.com/heart_attacks/nattokinase.php*
Nattokinase at Smart Punlications

Chapter 19

Blood Pressure Pills for Hypertension, When to Treat?

A good friend, age 60, has a mild hypertension, 147 mm Hg systolic, and accordingly takes blood pressure pills. The current guideline recommends treatment for blood pressure above 140 mm Hg systolic, regardless of age, usually with a "water pill" called a thiazide diuretic.*(1)* My friend asks me, does he need to take these blood pressure pills forever?

Blood Pressure 101, the Real Story

As we age, we all develop "hardening of the arteries", also called atherosclerotic vascular disease. This involves the gradual loss of flexibility and increased stiffness of the arterial walls from loss of elastin fibers as we age. This process also involves a more serious caking up of plaque inside the arteries which can block blood flow and cause a heart attack or stroke.

Mechanical Stress from Pulsations Produces Damage

Our hearts beat about 80 times per minutes at rest, and each heart beat produces a pulsatile wave of pressure which expands the arterial wall. These pulsatile waves produce mechanical stress which cause small cracks at weak points where the arteries divide. The body must repair these cracks, and the repair mechanism involves deposition of cholesterol plaque to seal these small cracks and prevent leakage. The final result of the repair process is the plaque buildup which blocks blood flow causing heart attacks and strokes. Sometimes the repair process involves inflammation which causes more damage to the lining of the artery.

A Lower Blood Pressure Reduces Mechanical Stress on the Arteries

Reducing the blood pressure obviously reduces the mechanical stress on the arteries, and thereby reduces the risk of heart attack and stroke. The real question is, "what blood pressure level requires treatment?", and "what is the optimal target area for the lowered blood pressure?" A blood pressure brought too low with pills leads to dizziness and fainting, so too low is not good either.

Blood Pressure Normally Rises with Age

The blood pressure increases gradually with age, a normal consequence of aging, but the guidelines ignore this, and use the same number, 140 mm Hg as a treatment threshold for all ages, and genders.*(22)* Why is this?

The Famous Framingham Study, the Basis for the BP Guideline

The blood pressure treatment guideline is based on the famous Framingham Study which showed the benefits of blood pressure reduction. The 18 year Framingham Blood Pressure study found increased risk of heart disease and death in people with blood pressure 140 to 160 mm Hg, and even more risk above 160 mm Hg. *(NEJM, Levy)(2)(4)(5)(6)(7)(8).*

Discrepancy Between Raw Data and Computer Smoothed Data:

The Framingham Study Data is usually presented in journals with computer smoothing with a smooth gradual line of increasing mortality as blood pressure goes up between 140 and 160 mm Hg. This is called the Linear Model. A mathematician, Dr. Port, has examined the Framingham raw data and Dr. Port concluded that the raw data is actually non-linear.*(17)(18)(28)* Dr. Port point out that the mortality rate is fairly constant at 15 deaths per 1000 until a blood pressure of 160 mm Hg is exceeded. This suggests a threshold of 160 mm Hg blood pressure above which treatment is desirable and beneficial.

Doctor Port then introduces a new model which takes into account age and gender. The mortality risk increases steadily with blood pressures that exceed a threshold based on sex and age. The threshold blood pressure formula is 110 + *(2/3)* *(*age*)* for a man aged 45-74, and 104 +*(5/6)* age for a woman aged 45-74. Here is the Dr. Port's chart in Lancet for the blood pressure thresholds, showing treatment thresholds based on age and gender.*(17)(18)(28)*

Blood Pressure Thresholds Based on Age *(*Port, Lancet*)*

Age.	Male BP Threshold	Female BP Threshold 70th percentile
45	139	142 mm Hg
50	143	146 mm Hg
55	147	150 mm Ng
60	150	154 mm Hg
65	153	158 mm Hg
70	157	162mm Hg

According to Dr. Port's chart *(*above*)*, a blood pressure of 147 mm Hg in a 60 year old man does not require treatment with "water pills". Blood pressure goes up with age, and this is normal.

Before you run to your doctor with a copy of this book, please be aware of the response by Dr. Lenfant, Director National Heart, Lung, and Blood Institute *(*NHLBI*)*, the agency which funded Dr. Port's report. Dr. Lenfant has outright rejected Dr. Port's non-linear model, and he restates his belief in the linear relationship between mortality and blood pressure.*(9)*

Here is what Dr. Lenfant says,

> "A study funded by the National Heart, Lung, and Blood Institute *(*NHLBI*)* and published in the January 15 issue of the Lancet *(*by Port*)* challenges [us] by asserting that the relationship between systolic blood pressure and mortality is not "continuous and graded." After careful review of this study, the NHLBI finds that it does not offer a basis for changing the current hypertension guidelines....We attach great value to new scientific findings and our careful review of Dr. Port's paper finds his analysis thought provoking. However, we would not recommend a change in the guidelines based on one epidemiological analysis....The totality of evidence found a clear linear relationship between systolic blood pressure, diastolic blood pressure and deaths."

Perhaps Dr. Lenfant didn't actually look at Dr. Port's raw data chart which clearly shows the data to be non-linear.

Dr. Lewiston published a rebuttal in Lancet 2002 which says, "Throughout middle and old age, usual blood pressure is strongly and directly related to vascular *(*and overall*)* mortality, without any evidence of a threshold down to at least 115/75 mm Hg" *(*12*)*. Dr. Lewiston didn't look at Dr. Port's raw data, either.

Jan Basile, MD, Walter A. Brzezinski, MD published a rebuttal in the Journal of Clinical Hypertension J Clin Hypertens 2*(4)*:290-294, 2000. which says that the Port paper did not evaluate morbidity, *(*i.e. non-fatal strokes and heart attacks*)*, which the SHEP study did examine, and the SHEP study showed considerable reduction in morbidity by reducing systolic pressure.*(29)(*15*)* Basile argues that the reduction in stroke morbidity in the SHEP study justifies treatment with blood pressure pills for the 140-160 range. This discussion can be found on the internet at the AngryDoc Blog.*(14)*

The problem with this reasoning is the SHEP study patients all started with blood pressures above 160, and does not address the below 160 question asked by Dr. Port. The SHEP study data showed a reduction of 5 years stroke rate from 8.2 to 5.2 per cent. However the average blood pressure was 170, with all patients above 160 at the start. There is no question that BP's above 160 require treatment, our question pertains to the 140 to 160 range which showed no increased mortality in the Framingham raw data. **"No randomized trial has ever demonstrated any reduction in risk of either overall or cardiovascular death by reducing systolic blood pressure from the thresholds in the above chart by Dr. Port to below 140 mm HG".** *(*17*)(*18*)(28)*

Multiple Factors at Work on Blood Vessels

What is the risk of stroke and heart attack at any particular blood pressure? Is a lower blood pressure better, and if so, how low is better? Perhaps the use of blood pressure to assess cardiovascular disease risk is too simplistic. The cause of damaged and diseased arteries is more complicated than a simple blood pressure measurement. There are multiple factors at work to produce damaged blood vessels which lead to heart attack and stroke.

First Factor is Mechanical Stress

The first factor is the mechanical stress on the artery wall represented by the blood pressure. This pressure wave is pulsatile, and has a waveform which is more complex than a simple blood pressure number. The second factor is the intrinsic strength of the arterial wall which is made of collagen. The third factor is the vigor of the reparative mechanism mounted as a defense against the small cracks in the wall from mechanical stress which may cause an inflammatory response inside the arterial wall. The fourth factor is the extent of underlying arterial disease. If the arteries are already severely damaged with extensive plaque formation, then even small increases in blood pressure could be potentially damaging. In patients with severe underlying arterial disease with known claudication, angina, or history of stroke and heart attack, controlling the blood pressure is a more urgent issue.

Arterial Stiffness

Arterial stiffness increases with age, requiring more pressure to perfuse the arterial system than the younger, more elastic arterial tree. This "arterial stiffness" can be studied with various techniques such as ultrasound of carotid artery thickness, the pulse pressure and the pulse wave form, and these techniques are all excellent indicators of cardiovascular disease risk and strong predictors of stroke, and actually may be more representative of mechanical stress on the arterial wall than simple blood pressure measurement.*(21) (22) (24) (25)*

Second Factor is Arterial Strength

The second factor is the intrinsic strength of the arterial wall which is made of the protein called collagen. For example, vitamin C deficiency is associated with poor collagen formation and increased risk of stroke as discussed in a previous chapter.*(27)* Blood pressure pills do nothing to improve the strength of the arterial system, on the other hand, supplemental vitamin C increases collagen formation and strengthens artery walls.

The trace mineral Copper is required as a cofactor for elastin production which allows the arteries to be flexible and elastic. Copper deficiency is associated with weakening in the wall and bubble formation in the arteries, called aneurysms, caused by lack of elastin.*(26)* The third factor, which is inflammation inside the artery as a repair mechanism, can be addressed with options discussed on my web site Heart Disease *page.(30)*

Complete Evaluation is More than a Simple Blood Pressure

A more complete vascular evaluation includes an ultrasound of the carotid arteries to measure wall thickness, an aortic ultrasound to screen for aneurysm, and measurement of the pulse pressure *(*this is the difference between systolic and diastolic pressures*)*. Knowledge of the medical history and pre-existing risk factors such as smoking, diabetes and presence of underlying arterial disease is important. After reviewing all this information, an informed decision can be made to treat or not to treat patients with blood pressures below 160.

Linear or Nonlinear Model is a Personal Choice

In a healthy adult with no other risk factors, and a blood pressure below 160, the Framingham Study raw data clearly shows no mortality risk. Therefore, following the guidelines published in Lancet by Port is a valid personal choice. The current blood pressure treatment guidelines are based on deceptive data smoothing on the Framingham data set, resulting in lower treatment thresholds which translate into extra billions of dollars for the drug companies. Should you accept the "Linear Model" or the Nonlinear model? That is an individual decision that is up to you depending on your knowledge of your own risk factors. After all, it's your body and your blood pressure.

Patients with normal arteries have the luxury to explore all options. However, in patients with known vascular disease with history of angina, claudication, previous stroke or heart attack, controlling the blood pressure becomes more urgent. In this severely diseased group, even small elevations of blood pressure may be harmful.

More information on lowering your blood pressure naturally without drugs can be found at my web site at this *page.(31)* Thanks to Joel Kauffman PhD for chapter 4 in his book, Malignant Medical Myths which brought this information to my attention.*(10)*

References:

(1) *http://www.guideline.gov/summary/summary.aspx?ss=15&doc_id=4771&nbr=003 450&string=blood+AND+pressure*
Seventh Report of the Joint National Committee on Prevention, Detection, Evaluation, and Treatment of High Blood Pressure. Chobanian AV et al. Seventh report of the Joint National Committee on Prevention, Detection, Evaluation, and Treatment of High Blood Pressure. Hypertension 2003 Dec;42*(6)*:1206-52.

(2) *http://www.framingham.com/heart/*
Framingham Heart Study

(3) *http://www.framinghamheartstudy.org/*
Framingham Study

(4) *http://www.framinghamheartstudy.org/biblio/index.html*
list of publications from the Framingham heart study

(5) *http://www.nhlbi.nih.gov/about/framingham/index.html*
NIH Framingham study web site

(6) *http://www.nhlbi.nih.gov/about/framingham/biblio.htm*
1288 publications from the Framingham data

(7) *http://www.hypertensiononline.org/slides2/cme_notes.cfm?tk=13*
hypertension online, PowerPoint Slides of all the major studies

(8) *http://content.nejm.org/cgi/content/full/329/26/1912*
The Natural History of Borderline Isolated Systolic Hypertension. Alex Sagie, Martin G. Larson, and Daniel Levy. NEJM Volume 329:1912-1917 December 23, 1993 Number 26

(9) *http://www.nhlbi.nih.gov/new/press/nhlbijan13.htm*
Statement from Claude Lenfant, M.D., NHLBI Director, on Systolic Blood Pressure, Deaths, and Treatment Guidelines, NIH

(10) *http://ourworld.compuserve.com/homepages/dp5/kauffman.htm*
"Malignant Medical Myths" by Joel Kaufman, PhD, page 105 to 129, Myth 4.

(11) *http://www.rxlist.com/script/main/srchcont_rxlist.asp?src=thiazide*
listing of 151 different thiazide blood pressure medications on RxList.com

(12) *http://www.ncbi.nlm.nih.gov/pubmed/12493255*
Prospective Studies Collaboration. Age-specific relevance of usual blood pressure to vascular mortality: a meta-analysis of individual data for one million adults in 61 prospective studies. Lewington S, et al. Lancet. 2002 Dec 14;360*(9349)*:1903-13. This

Confirms Linear Model **"INTERPRETATION: Throughout middle and old age, usual blood pressure is strongly and directly related to vascular (and overall) mortality, without any evidence of a threshold down to at least 115/75 mm Hg."**

(13) *http://www.ncbi.nlm.nih.gov/pubmed/12748199*
The Seventh Report of the Joint National Committee on Prevention, Detection, Evaluation, and Treatment of High Blood Pressure: the JNC 7 report. JAMA. 2003 May 21;289(19):2560-72. This article confirms the Linear Model.

(14) *http://www.ncbi.nlm.nih.gov/pubmed/12748199*
The Seventh Report of the Joint National Committee on Prevention, Detection, Evaluation, and Treatment of High Blood Pressure: the JNC 7 report. Vol. 265 No. 24, June 26, 1991 JAMA. Chobanian AV et al. Advocates the Linear Model for Hypertension.

(15) *http://jama.ama-assn.org/cgi/content/abstract/265/24/3255*
SHEP Cooperative Research Group. Prevention of stroke by antihypertensive drug treatment in older persons with isolated systolic hypertension: final results of the Systolic Hypertension in the Elderly Program (SHEP). JAMA. 1991;65:3255–3264. **CONCLUSION. In persons aged 60 years and over with isolated systolic hypertension, antihypertensive stepped-care drug treatment ...reduced the incidence of total stroke by 36%, with 5-year absolute benefit of 30 events per 1000 participants. Major cardiovascular events were reduced, with 5-year absolute benefit of 55 events per 1000.**

(16) *http://content.nejm.org/cgi/content/full/329/26/1912*
FRAMINGHAM HEART STUDY. NEJM Volume 329:1912-1917 December 23, 1993 Number 26. The Natural History of Borderline Isolated Systolic Hypertension Alex Sagie, Martin G. Larson, and Daniel Levy

(17) *http://www.math.ucla.edu/~scp/publications/mortality.PDF*
Lancet. 2000 Jan 15;355(9199):175-80. Systolic blood pressure and mortality. Port S, Demer L, Jennrich R, Walter D, Garfinkel A. (**Port article #1**)

(18) *http://www.ncbi.nlm.nih.gov/pubmed/10675116*
Abstract, Lancet. 2000 Jan 15;355(9199):175-80. Systolic blood pressure and mortality. Port S, Demer L, Jennrich R, Walter D, Garfinkel A. INTERPRETATION: The Framingham data contradict the concept that lower pressures imply lower risk and the idea that 140 mm Hg is a useful cut-off value for hypertension for all adults. There is an age-dependent and sex-dependent threshold for hypertension. A substantial proportion of the population who would currently be thought to be at increased risk are, therefore, at no increased risk.

(19) *http://angrydr.blogspot.com/2007/03/numb3rs.html*
Angry Doc blog discusses Hypertension Treatment Guidleines and Port Lancet Article.

(20) *http://www.hypertensiononline.org/index.cfm*
Hypertension Online PowerPoint Slides, Baylor College of Medicine

(21) *http://qjmed.oxfordjournals.org/cgi/content/full/95/2/67*
Assessment of arterial stiffness in clinical practice. I.S. Mackenzie, I.B. Wilkinson and J.R. Cockcroft. Q J Med 2002; 95: 67-74. Over 100 years ago, arterial stiffness was recognized as important in predicting cardiovascular disease.

(22) *http://circ.ahajournals.org/cgi/content/full/96/1/308*
Hemodynamic Patterns of Age-Related Changes in Blood Pressure The Framingham Heart Study Stanley S. Franklin, MD; William Gustin, IV, BS; Nathan D. Wong, PhD; Martin G. Larson, ScD; Michael A. Weber, MD; William B. Kannel, MD; ; Daniel Levy, MD. Framingham study which shows BP increases with age. Circulation. 1997;96:308-315.

(24) *http://circ.ahajournals.org/cgi/content/full/100/9/951*
Common Carotid Intima-Media Thickness and Arterial Stiffness, Indicators of Cardiovascular Risk in High-Risk Patients The SMART Study (Second Manifestations of Arterial disease) Petra C. G. Simons, MD, PhD; Ale Algra, MD, PhD; Michiel L. Bots, MD, PhD; Diederick E. Grobbee, MD, PhD; Yolanda van der Graaf, MD, PhD; for the SMART Study Group. Circulation. 1999;100:951-957.

(25) *http://hyper.ahajournals.org/cgi/content/full/34/3/375*
Isolated Systolic Hypertension Prognostic Information Provided by Pulse Pressure Michael J. Domanski et al. (Hypertension. 1999;34:375-380.)

(26) *http://www.ncbi.nlm.nih.gov/pubmed/7202350*
Decreased hepatic copper levels. A possible chemical marker for the pathogenesis of aortic aneurysms in man. Arch Surg. 1982 Sep;117(9):1212-3. Tilson MD. Copper is a cofactor for elastin production. Copper is needed for the proper function of the enzyme lysyl oxidase, which is required in the crosslinking of collagen and elastin.

(27) *http://jeffreydach.com/2007/05/05/jeffreydachdrdachvitaminc.aspx*
Vitamin C and StrPrevention by Jeffrey Dach MD.

(28) *http://eurheartj.oxfordjournals.org/cgi/reprint/21/20/1635.pdf*
European Heart Journal (2000) 21, 1635–1638, EUHJ.2000.2227, There is a non-linear relationship between mortality and blood pressure. S. PORT A. GARFINKEL N. BOYLE

(29) *http://www.blackwell-synergy.com/doi/abs/10.1111/j.1524-6175.2007.06287.x*
Analysis of Recent Papers in Hypertension, Jan Basile, MD, Senior Editor
Michael J. Bloch, MD. The Journal of Clinical Hypertension, Volume 9 Issue 7 Page 576-581, July 2007

(30) *http://www.drdach.com/wst_page7.html*
Reversing Heart Disease by Jeffrey Dach

(31) *http://www.drdach.com/wst_page13.html*
Hypertension by Jeffrey Dach MD

Chapter 20

How To Improve Insulin Resistance in Type Two Diabetes

Mrs. Duvalier is an insulin dependent diabetic on daily insulin injections. She uses a home glucometer to measure her fasting blood sugar which ranges from 200 to 300. She explained to me that she is interested in natural treatments to reduce her need for insulin. She wants to be able to get off insulin entirely. I replied the best we could hope to achieve would be a partial improvement. Getting off insulin altogether with a normal blood sugar would be a tall order, I told her. This article discusses our approach to improving insulin sensitivity and reducing the insulin requirement with diet, exercise, and nutritional supplements.

Natural Approach with Diet, Exercise and Nutritional Supplements

A logical and natural approach to treatment for diabetes involves modifying the diet to a low glycemic diet, exercise program, and weight loss.

The Atkins Diabetes Revolution, The Low Glycemic Diet *(6)(7)*

The Atkins type diet which is low carbohydrates diet, and high in fat and protein has been known to improve insulin resistance and reduce fasting blood sugar values. It is also helpful for weight loss. Eliminate refined sugar and refined carbohydrates for maximal benefit. Also recommended is Protein Power by Drs. Michael and Mary Dan Eades.*(46)*

An excellent resource is Jenny Ruhl's book, *Blood Sugar 101*, which explains how to improve insulin sensitivity by using a glucometer to measure blood sugar after a meal. Knowing how high your blood sugar goes after a carbohydrate loaded meal gives you information about what types of carbohydrates to avoid and keeps your blood sugar under control with diet. By keeping blood sugar under control, the insulin resistance improves automatically.*(45)*

Exercise and Weight Loss

Weight Loss associated with a vigorous exercise program will improve insulin sensitivity and reduce fasting blood sugar values.

Nutritional Supplements for Improving Insulin Resistance

Chromium Iodinate *(***chromium polynicotinate***)* 500-1000 mcg daily. This is the first FDA approval of a qualified health claim for a supplement. **Biotin** 9-16 mg daily. **R-Alpha-lipoic acid** has been shown to improve insulin sensitivity and resistance in individuals with existing type 2 diabetes. 100-600 milligrams 1-3 times daily of

R-Lipoic Acid.*(7)* **Vitamin D**, check vitamin D level and supplement if found to be low. Recheck every six months to keep in target area. **Vitamin B-1 thiamine. Coenzyme Q10** 30 to 60 milligrams of coenzyme Q10 daily. **Acetyl L Carnitine** shuttles fatty acids across mitochondrial membrane. Useful for fat metabolism. Works together with Coenzyme Q 10 and D Ribose to increase mitochondrial function. **Cinnamon** has been recommended by some, considered ineffective by others. It is cheap and available as a spice at the grocery store.

Iodine Supplementation to Reverse Insulin Resistant Diabetes

It is not widely known that iodine supplementation is beneficial in reversing diabetes. The following is a link to a case report of an individual treated by Dr George Flechas. This patient had thyroid cancer treated with surgery and radioactive iodine, and was later treated with 75 mg of Iodine per day with improvement in insulin resistant adult onset diabetes. Apparently the iodine was beneficial in reversing the diabetes.

Case Report Mr. Mack - Thyroid Cancer, Hypothyroidism

> "Mack is a 58 year old social worker living in North Carolina. Mack went to Dr. Flechas to see if he had Fibromyalgia as he was experiencing constant pain. Dr. Flechas did a thorough physical on Mack and discovered a thyroid nodule on the first visit. He also discovered that Mack had diabetes and high blood pressure. Mack had already been diagnosed with sleep apnea and restless leg syndrome.
>
> Dr. Flechas' first course of action was to begin a series of tests to diagnose the thyroid nodule. He was also started on medicines to control his diabetes and high blood pressure. A ultrasound of his thyroid was performed in the office and revealed that the nodule was solid. He then sent him for a thyroid uptake nuclear scan. The test revealed that the nodule was "cold". A "cold" nodule is an indicator that the nodule could be malignant. The next was a fine needle biopsy of the nodule. The biopsy was inconclusive saying that the nodule could neither be defined as malignant or benign. After much discussion between three doctors including Dr. Flechas, an endocrinologist, and a ENT, it was decided that Mack would have surgery to remove the nodule. During the surgery the nodule was sent directly to pathology and it was discovered to be Papillary Thyroid Cancer and the decision was made to go ahead and remove all of Mack's thyroid.
>
> After Mack had recovered from the surgery, he was then sent back into the hospital for a radioactive iodine treatment to kill any remaining thyroid tissue that may be in his body.
>
> When the course of treatment for his thyroid cancer was completed, Dr. Flechas started Mack on Iodoral - 3 tablets in the morning and 3

tablets at night. Since starting the Iodoral, Mack's diabetes had almost completely disappeared. He is no longer on diabetes medicines and his blood sugars have been in the normal range for over a year.

Update April, 2005: Mack is now down to 240 lbs after starting at a weight of about 320 lbs when first starting treatment with Dr. Flechas. His overall general health is wonderful. He is sleeping well for the first time in years and very active." Quoted directly from Dr Flechas' Web Site.*(16)*

Iodine Supplements Found to be Beneficial in Diabetics

"It was while treating a large 320-pound woman with insulin dependent diabetes that we learned a valuable lesson regarding the role of iodine in hormone receptor function. This woman had come in via the emergency room with a very high random blood sugar of 1,380 mg/dl. She was then started on insulin during her hospitalization and was instructed on the use of a home glucometer. She was to use her glucometer two times per day. Two weeks later on her return office visit for a checkup of her insulin dependent diabetes she was informed that during her hospital physical examination she was noted to have FBD.

She was recommended to start on 50 mg of iodine *(4 tablets)* at that time. One week later she called us requesting to lower the level of insulin due to having problems with hypoglycemia. She was told to continue to drop her insulin levels as long as she was experiencing hypoglycemia and to monitor her blood sugars carefully with her glucometer. Four weeks later during an office visit her glucometer was downloaded to my office computer, which showed her to have an average random blood sugar of 98.

I praised the patient for her diligent efforts to control her diet and her good work at keeping her sugars under control with the insulin. She then informed me that she had come off her insulin three weeks earlier and had not been taking any medications to lower her blood sugar. When asked what she felt the big change was, she felt that her diabetes was under better control due to the use of iodine. Two years later and 70 pounds lighter this patient continues to have excellent glucose control on iodine 50 mg per day.

We since have done a study of twelve diabetics and in six cases we were able to wean all of these patients off of medications for their diabetes and were able to maintain a hemoglobin A1C of less than 5.8 with the average random blood sugar of less than 100.

To this date these patients continue to have excellent control of their Type II diabetes. The range of daily iodine intake was from 50 mg to 100 mg per day. All diabetic patients were able to lower the total amount of medications necessary to control their diabetes. Two of the twelve patients were controlled with the use of iodine plus one medication. Two patients have control of diabetes with iodine plus two medications. One patient had control of her diabetes with three medications plus iodine 50 mg. The one insulin dependent diabetic was able to reduce the intake of Lantus insulin from 98 units to 44 units per day within a period of a few weeks." quoted from George Flechas MD web site.*(17)*

Diabetes Drugs: More is not always better.

The large NIH Diabetes study *(***ACCORD***)* was halted recently because of higher mortality in the intensive treatment group, according to a New York Times article by Gina Kolata.*(30)* The patients with the tighter control of blood sugar had the higher mortality. This shocked and stunned the medical community because it has always been believed that the closely or "tightly controlled" blood sugar had the best results for diabetes. One possible explanation for these shocking results is that in order to control blood sugar, the intensive group was given large doses of insulin and other medications which created high insulin levels which are harmful to the heart as discussed by Ron Rosedale in his article posted on *Mercola.com*, "Insulin and Its Metabolic Effects" BoulderFest August 1999 Seminar. *(42)(32)(33)*

Diabetes Drugs

Drugs which increase Insulin Output by Pancreas: Chlorpropamide, Tolbutaminde, Glyburide, Glipizide, Glimepiride.

Drugs which decrease glucose from the liver: Metformin (Glucophage). Metformin does not alter concentrations of insulin in the blood and, therefore, rarely causes low blood glucose levels. Metformin is one of the most commonly used first line drugs.

Drugs which increase Insulin Sensitivity: Troglitazone (Rezulin) which was taken off the market in March 2000 due to liver toxicity, or rosiglitazone (Avandia) whose long-term safety profile is not known.

Drugs which decrease the absorption of carbohydrates from the intestine: Precose. Precose has significant gastrointestinal side effects. Abdominal pain, diarrhea, and gas are common and are seen in up to 75% of patients.

Drugs which increase the amount of Insulin: Insulin Injectable Humulin.

Much has been written about the limitations of diabetes drugs, and the superiority of diet and lifestyle changes to improve insulin resistance and blood sugar in type two diabetes.*(28)(29)* More intensive drug treatment with intensive lowering of blood sugar and HGB-A1C does not always translate into improvement in health in high risk diabetes, as the ACCORD study demonstrates. The ACCORD study was halted early because the more intensive treatment group had a **higher mortality**. *(30)-(41)*

We shall now return to our patient, Mrs. Duvalier, who followed the above diet, lifestyle and supplement program, and returned to the office for a follow up visit. She declared that her family members were pleased with her new appearance after losing 20 pounds, and her home glucometer readings showed better control of her blood sugar with fewer drugs. She still required insulin, but her insulin requirement had decreased consideraby.

References

Chromium, Biotin and Cinnamon

(1) http://jn.nutrition.org/cgi/reprint/123/4/626
Chromium in Human Nutrition: A Review WALTER MERTZ U.S. Department of Agriculture, Agricultural Research Service,Beltsuille Human Nutrition Research Center, Beltsville, MD 20705, American Institute of Nutrition. Received 21 July 1992.

(2) http://www.ncbi.nlm.nih.gov/pubmed/15208835
Diabetes Educ. 2004;Suppl:2-14.A scientific review: the role of **chromium** in insulin resistance.

(3) http://www.ncbi.nlm.nih.gov/pubmed/17952838
Horm Metab Res. 2007 Oct;39(10):743-51. **Chromium** in metabolic and cardiovascular disease.Hummel M, Standl E, Schnell O. Diabetes Research Institute & Academical Hospital Munich-Schwabing, Munich, Germany.

(4) http://www.ncbi.nlm.nih.gov/pubmed/17109595
Diabetes Technol Ther. 2006 Dec;8(6):636-43. The effect of **chromium picolinate and biotin** supplementation on glycemic control in poorly controlled patients with type 2 diabetes mellitus: a placebo-controlled, double-blinded, randomized trial.Singer GM, Geohas J. Section of Cardiovascular Medicine, Yale University School of Medicine, New Haven, Connecticut 06520-8017, USA. Biotin 2 mg 667% Chromium 6000 mcg 500%

(5) http://www.ncbi.nlm.nih.gov/pubmed/16117721
Dis Manag. 2005 Aug;8(4):265-75. Use of **chromium picolinate and biotin** in the management of type 2 diabetes: an economic analysis. Fuhr JP Jr, He H, Goldfarb N, Nash DB. Department of Economics, Widener University, Chester, Pennsylvania, USA.

Atkins Diet

(6) *http://www.atkins.com/products/atkins-diabetes-revolution*
Atkins Diet Revolution for Diabetes

(7) *http://www.nutritionandmetabolism.com/content/1/1/14*
Book review, Review on "Atkins Diabetes Revolution: The Groundbreaking Approach to Preventing and Controlling Type 2 Diabetes" by Mary C. Vernon and Jacqueline A. Eberstein
Surender Arora and Samy I McFarlane, Nutrition & Metabolism 2004, 1:14

Alpha Lipoic Acid

(8) *http://www.thorne.com/altmedrev/.fulltext/11/3/232.pdf*
Alha Lipoic Acid Review Article Thorne

(9) *http://www.phlaunt.com/diabetes/20144672.php*
Supplements that are thought to work for diabetes in the opinion of Jenny's Blood Sugar101 (ALA, Benfotiamine, Vit D etc.)

(10) *http://www.phlaunt.com/diabetes/15877514.php*
Supplements that are questionale or not thought to be effective in the opinion of Jenny's Blood Sugar 101 (Cinnamon, Chromium etc.)

Vitamin B1 Thiamine

(11) *http://www.purecaps.com/NewsResearch/newsletter/20050920/index.asp*
BenfoMax (Benfotiamine): Novel Support for Nerve, Retina and Kidney Function
Benfotiamine, S-benzoylthiamine-O-monophosphate, is a fat soluble vitamin B1 (thiamine) derivative that has enjoyed over a decade of popular use in Europe.

(12) *http://www.benfotiamine.org/index.htm*
Benfotiamine.org Lipid soluble form of thiamine B1

(13) *http://www.benfotiamine.org/Benfo600Study.pdf*
Benfotiamine Inhibits Intracellular Formation of Advanced Glycation End Products in vivo. JIHONG LIN, ALEX ALT, JUTTA LIERSCH, REINHARD G. BRETZEL, MICHAEL BROWNLEE*, HANS-PETER HAMMES Third Medical Department, Justus-Liebig-University Giessen, Germany *Albert-Einstein College, New York, NY,

Chromium and Cinnamon

(14) *http://www.ncbi.nlm.nih.gov/pubmed/18234131*
Proc Nutr Soc. 2008 Feb;67(1):48-53. Chromium and polyphenols from cinnamon improve insulin sensitivity. Anderson RA. Beltsville Human Nutrition Research Center, USDA, Beltsville, MD 20705, USA.

(15) *http://www.purecaps.com/NewsResearch/newsletter/20050920/article_three.asp*
FDA Concludes that Chromium Picolinate is Safe;Approves First Qualified Health Claim.
In August, the FDA recognized chromium picolinate as a safe nutritional supplement with credible evidence to support the first qualified health claim with regard to the role of chromium in healthy glucose metabolism.

Iodine References

(16) *http://www.helpmythyroid.com/mack.html*
Case Report on Mack - Thyroid Cancer, Hypothyroidism George Flechas MD HelpMyThyoid.com

(17) *http://www.iodine4health.com/disease/diabetes/flechas_diabetes.htm*
George FLECHAS MD Orthoiodosupplementation in a Primary Care Practice, Flechas JD. Role of Iodine in Diabetes

References Dealing with Nutritional Supplements for Diabetes:

(18) *http://www.phlaunt.com/diabetes/index.php*
Blood Sugar 101 by Jenny

(19) *http://www.raysahelian.com/diabetes.html*
Natural Supplements for Diabetes by Ray Sahelian MD

(20) *http://www.encyclopedia.com/doc/1G1-81138246.html*
A Natural Approach to Diabetes - Brief Article Townsend Letter for Doctors and Patients, Jan, 2002 by Farhang Khosh. Excellent Reveiw with References

(21) *http://www.drlam.com/A3R_brief_in_doc_format/Diabetes.cfm#Diabetes*
Dr Lam's Diabetes Protocol

(22) *http://www.westonaprice.org/moderndiseases/diabetes.html*
Treating Diabetes: Practical Advice for Combating a Modern Epidemic By Tom Cowan, MD
Weston Price Org

(23) *http://healthmoz.org/how-to-reverse-type-2-diabetes-and-insulin-resistance-in-5-simple-steps/#comment-2040*
How To Reverse Type 2 Diabetes And Insulin Resistance In 5 Simple Steps Mark Hyman, MD is a pioneer in functional medicine, practicing physician and best-selling author. A sneak preview of his book "The UltraSimple Diet" is available.

More on Chromium, First Health Claim Approved by the FDA

(24) *http://www.purecaps.com/itemdy00.asp?T1=CRG61*
chromium polynicotinate from pure encapsulations, preferred type of chromium

(25) http://www.cfsan.fda.gov/~dms/qhccr.html
There was one study *(Cefalu et al., 1999)* that showed a benefit for chromium picolinate and insulin resistance. FDA finds that there is very limited credible evidence for a qualified health claim specifically for chromium picolinate and a reduced risk of insulin resistance, and therefore possibly a reduced risk of type 2 diabetes. However, the reported findings of Cefalu et al., 1999 have not been replicated.

(26) http://www3.interscience.wiley.com/cgi-bin/abstract/61004819/ABSTRACT
Cefalu, W.T., A.D. Bell-farrow, J. Stegner, Z.Q. Wand, T. King, T. Morgan, J.G. Terry. Effect of chromium picolinate on insulin sensitivity in vivo. Journal of Trace Elements in Experimental Medicine. 1999;12:71-83.

(27) http://care.diabetesjournals.org/cgi/content/full/27/11/2741
Diabetes Care 27:2741-2751, 2004 by the American Diabetes Association, Inc. Review Article Role of Chromium in Human Health and in Diabetes, William T. Cefalu, MD and Frank B. Hu, MD, PHD

Diabetes Drugs

(28) http://doctorjames.wordpress.com/2008/02/28/the-truth-about-diabetes-and-why-drugs-dont-work/
The Truth About Diabetes and Why Drugs Don't Work Posted by doctorjames on February 28, 2008, Dr. James R. Haakenson

(29) http://sparkofreason.blogspot.com/2008/02/insulin-insanity.html
insulin Insanity from Spark of Reason, Dave Dixon Ph.D.in physics

Accord Study Halted Early

(30) http://www.nytimes.com/2008/02/07/health/07diabetes.html February 7, 2008
Diabetes Study Partially Halted After Deaths By GINA KOLATA New York Times

(31) http://www.pbs.org/newshour/bb/health/jan-june08/diabetes_02-07.html
Diabetes Study Partially Halted Due to Cardiac Risk. PBS.

(32) http://doctorrw.blogspot.com/2008/02/accord-study-what-does-it-mean.html
The ACCORD study: what does it mean?

(33) http://www.diabetesmine.com/2008/02/accord-study-a.html
ACCORD Study: Wrong and Wronger

(34) http://www.cbsnews.com/stories/2008/02/06/health/main3797887.shtml
Diabetes Patients' Deaths Stunt Study. Unexpected Number Of Fatalities Cuts Short Experimental Treatment For Type 2 Diabetics WASHINGTON, Feb. 7, 2008. CBS News.

(35) *http://hcrenewal.blogspot.com/2008/02/is-more-always-better-accord-study.html*
Thursday, February 07, 2008 Is More Always Better? - the ACCORD Study Results. Health Care Renewal

(36) *http://diabetesupdate.blogspot.com/2008/02/how-advance-differs-from-accord.html*
How ACCORD differed from Advance by Jenny Ruhl Blood Sugar 101. Accord added statins and fibrates to the program.

(37) *http://public.nhlbi.nih.gov/newsroom/home/GetPressRelease.aspx?id=2551*
For Safety, NHLBI Changes Intensive Blood Sugar Treatment Strategy in Clinical Trial of Diabetes and Cardiovascular Disease. NIH News Release.

(38) *http://www.medscape.com/viewarticle/480545_print*
Expert Interview. The Incretin Hormones in the Treatment of Type 2 Diabetes: An Expert Interview With John Buse, MD, PhD Medscape Diabetes & Endocrinology 6*(1)*, 2004. Medscape 06/14/2004.

(39) *http://www.sourcewatch.org/index.php?title=GlaxoSmithKline,_the_Diabetes_Drug_Avandia_and_The_Intimidation_of_Dr._John_Buse*
GlaxoSmithKline, the Diabetes Drug Avandia and The Intimidation of Dr. John Buse

Statin Drugs for Diabetics

(40) *http://clinical.diabetesjournals.org/cgi/content/full/21/4/168*
Clinical Diabetes 21:168-172, 2003© American Diabetes Association ®, Inc., 2003 Practical Pointer Statin Treatment in Diabetes Mellitus John Buse, MD, PhD, CDE Athough cardiac events are reduced in diabetics, **where is the HPS all-cause mortality data**?

(41) *http://www.vitamincfoundation.org/statinalert/hps.html*
Comments by Statistician Eddie Vos *(*Health-heart.org*)*. **The full HPS mortality data have never been properly published** and one of the HPS authors just asked me WHY I wanted to know, instead of coming up with the data.

Harmful Effects of High Insulin Levels

(42) *http://www.mercola.com/2001/jul/14/insulin.htm*
Insulin and Its Metabolic Effects By Ron Rosedale, M.D. Presented at Designs for Health Institute's BoulderFest August 1999 Seminar, mercola.com

(43) *http://nourishedmagazine.com.au/blog/articles/insulin-resistance-the-real-culprit*
Insulin Resistance: The Real Culprit By Ron Rosedale, M.D.

(44) *http://www.amldiet.com/*
Advanced Metabolic Laboratories *(*AML*)* by Dr. Ron Rosedale, MD, author of THE ROSEDALE DIET.

(45) *http://www.phlaunt.com/technionbooks/20645175.php*
Jenny Ruhl Blood Sugar 101

(46) *http://www.proteinpower.com/*
The Official Web Site of Drs. Michael and Mary Dan Eades. Protein Power Book.

Chapter 21

The Epidemic of Type Two Diabetes, How to Get Rid of the Spare Tire

Currently, we have an epidemic of Type II Diabetes in the United States which affects 6 per cent of the population *(16 million people)* and is projected to grow to 10 per cent within a few years. This is a problem which affects adults as well as school age kids. With the kids, the problem is so bad that the State of Connecticut has actually outlawed junk food and soda pop vending machines from local schools. Many other states are considering similar legislation. We will examine the cause of our epidemic of Type II diabetes and what choices we can make to avoid this disease.

Lets assume you have just eaten a nice piece of chocolate cake with vanilla ice cream. This meal contains a huge load of refined sugar which is absorbed quickly into the bloodstream, raising your blood sugar to a high level. The Pancreas responds by secreting Insulin into the bloodstream, which is the major hormone involved in moving sugar out of the blood and into the cells. Insulin is a messenger which circulates to all the cells of the body giving them the message to open trillions of tiny doors in the cells, saying "let the sugar in, please". Another message tells the cells of the body to convert the newly arrived sugar into fat, hence the "spare tire" of belly fat.

If you are eating refined sugar products in junk food throughout the day, then you are probably running high Insulin levels all day long. A funny thing about hormone messages is that if the message is sent too often, the receptors in the cells becomes unresponsive. This is called "Insulin Resistance" in which the Insulin Message is simply ignored by all cells of the body. The constant high insulin level does a few more things that you should know about. It causes the liver to manufacture more triglycerides and cholesterol and may trigger high blood pressure. Secondly, another switch is turned on that causes Chronic Inflammation throughout the body. Thirdly, Insulin is a storage hormone, so it tells the machinery of the cell to store the excess glucose as body fat, thus creating the "spare tire" effect in the belly. Losing this extra body fat is a matter of controlling insulin levels with a low glycemic *(sugar)* diet, not a low fat diet.

Our current war on dietary fat in America was led by dietitians and government bureaucrats who have no understanding of the hormonal impact of our food choices. This type of is incorrect thinking is based on politics rather than science. The average percentage fat in our diet is lower than it was 50 years ago, yet we have more obesity now than ever before. Experts are now realizing that the enemy is not dietary fat, the real enemy is excess insulin provoked by a high carbohydrate diet.

Risk factors for type II Diabetes include high sugar diet, inactivity, obesity, and family history of diabetes. The Glucose-Insulin Tolerance Test can provide predictive testing years in advance of actual full blown diabetes disease. If your doctor tells you that your fasting blood sugar is above 125, then by definition, you have Adult Onset Diabetes (also known as Type II) Diabetes. If your fasting blood sugar level is above 100, then you may be Pre-Diabetic.

Conventional medical treatments are designed to raise the already high insulin levels in order to lower blood sugar. As you might have guessed by now, this can actually worsen rather than remedy the problem.

How does one get rid of the spare tire, improve Insulin Resistance and prevent Diabetes with all of its horrendous complications of renal disease, heart attack, stroke, visual impairment, and peripheral neuropathy?

Number one, keep blood insulin levels low by eliminating refined sugars and carbohydrates from the diet. Examples are the Zone Diet (Dr. Barry Sears) and the South Beach Diet (Dr. Agatson) which emphasize vegetables, fruits, and lean protein. Protein Power by Dr. Michael Eades is also an excellent resource.

Both diets follow a Glycemic Index food chart which tells you how much blood sugar the food item produces. Try to avoid the high Glycemic foods such as candy bars, soda pop, junk food, cookies, cakes, chips, and ice cream. We love to eat these foods and we sometimes have "sugar cravings". Don't worry; it only takes about a week of abstaining from sugar for the cravings to go away. Be careful with refined carbohydrates such as pasta, and white bread. These are also "High Glycemic" because rapid absorption raises the blood sugar same as eating pure sugar.

Number two, reduce your weight with an exercise program. Get up and go out and become more active. This will burn off the belly fat and improve insulin resistance and this will also lower your blood pressure and cholesterol. If you haven't been exercising lately, first check with your doctor for a treadmill test to see how much exercise you can tolerate.

Number three, there are some nutritional supplements which can help. For example, DHEA is a nutritional supplement at the health food store which was studied by Dr. Villareal at Washington University in St. Louis.(1) He published his findings in the prestigious medical journal, JAMA on Nov 10, 2004. In the study, he gave 50 milligrams of DHEA to 56 elderly men and women and used MRI scans to measure the "spare tire" belly fat. After the DHEA treatment, he found a 7 to 10 percent reduction in belly fat and significant improvement in Insulin Sensitivity. In women, adverse side effects of excess DHEA include testosterone-like effects such as unwanted facial hair, and acne, so it is best to work with a knowledgeable physician who can test your DHEA level and recommend the proper dosage.

Number Four, 1 to 2 teaspoons per day of pharmaceutical grade Omega-three fish oil is recommended by Dr. Barry Sears who reports that it improves insulin sensitivity.

Number Five, an important mineral called Chromium which is included in most multivitamin preparations improves insulin sensitivity. Chromium picolinate is very safe and not to be confused with the toxic tetravalent chromium 6 which leaked into the groundwater near Hinkley, California in 1996 from the Electric Company's Power Station. This was highlighted in the movie "Erin Brockovich", starring Julia Roberts.

Recommended Reading:

1) The Anti-Inflammation Zone: Reversing the Silent Epidemic That's Destroying Our Health by *Barry Sears.*

2) The Omega Rx Zone: The Miracle of the New High-Dose Fish Oil by *Barry Sears.*

3) The South Beach Diet Good Fats/Good CarbsGuide *(*Revised*)* : The Complete and Easy Reference for All Your Favorite Foods by *Arthur Agatson* MD.

4) The RoseDale Diet by Ron Rosedale MD

5) Protein Power by Drs. Michael and Mary Dan Eades

References

(1) http://jama.ama-assn.org/cgi/content/abstract/292/18/2243
Effect of DHEA on Abdominal Fat and Insulin Action in Elderly Women and Men, A Randomized Controlled Trial. Dennis T. Villareal, MD; John O. Holloszy, MD. JAMA. 2004;292:2243-2248.

Section Six- This section contains a collection of book reviews

Chapter 22 Book Reviews by Jeffrey Dach MD

From Fatigued to Fantastic by Jacob Teitelbaum MD, Third Edition.

The Definitive Book on Chronic Fatigue and Fibromyalgia, December 27, 2007

Most doctors are familiar with Dr. Teitelbaum featured as an eloquent keynote speaker on the medical lecture circuit, dazzling the audience with his encyclopedic knowledge of both conventional and natural medicine. Trained in internal medicine, Jacob Teitelbaum, is a gifted and brilliant medical researcher and clinician. He is also a model for ethical business conduct, because unlike other crass, commercially oriented docs who hide their knowledge or charge for it, Teitelbaum openly shares his medical knowledge with the public and other doctors. All of Teitelbaum's treatment protocols are listed in Appendix G of the book, and are posted on his web site. In addition, all profits from books and nutritional supplements are donated to charity.

The 400 page book is lengthy, and is actually four books in one. Where previous authors have written entire books on each of the four main topics, with the acronym SHIN for Sleep, Hormones, Infections and Nutrition, Teitelbaum combines them all into one large volume which can be used as desk reference on chronic fatigue and fibromyalgia.

In addition, the book can serve as an introductory text for the open minded MD interested in integrating natural medicine into a conventional medical practice, since sleep disorders, hormonal imbalance, chronic or hidden infections, and nutritional deficiencies are some of the more common reasons to seek medical attention.

This is the third edition of his book, and Teitelbaum has managed to make a great book even better. Those familiar with the work of the Connecticut cardiologist, Steven Sinatra MD, will recognize the triad of D-Ribose, L-carnitine and Co-Enzyme Q-10 mentioned by Teitelbaum to jump start energy in the chronically fatigued.

Insomnia or poor quality sleep is a major issue for many chronic fatigue sufferers, creating a vicious cycle which perpetuates the disorder. Teitelbaum provides a long list of natural remedies such as L-theanine 5-HTP, L-Tryptophan, Melatonin, and Magnesium, as well as prescription drugs seen on television advertising.

The Hormonal Support chapter is the meat of the book, with Teitelbaum crediting the landmark work, the Safe Use of Cortisol, by William McK Jefferies, and Broda Barnes' work on natural thyroid. To these medical greats, Teitelbaum adds his own unique insights gleaned from years of clinical practice. For example, Teitelbaum finds that most patients need only 5 to 12.5 mg of cortisol, and recommends keeping cortisol dosage below 20 mg per day to avoid adrenal suppression.

Like many other natural medicine docs, Teitelbaum finds bio-identical hormone supplementation important for a successful outcome, and asserts that bio-identicals are safe, a conclusion based on his own clinical experience and medical literature reviews by Kent Holtorf, MD, posted on Teitelbaum's website.

Teitelbaum found that many of his patients had chronic infections of sinuses, urinary tract, prostate, and respiratory system, and had taken multiple courses of antibiotics leading to kill-off of the friendly bacteria in the colon, as well as fungal overgrowth, also called Candidiasis. Teitelbaum credits The Yeast Connection by William Crooks for much of this information which includes a lengthy discussion of anti-fungal drugs and natural remedies for Candidiasis.

The Nutrition chapter covers a detailed program with a complete vitamin, mineral program with recommended dosages, and discusses dietary avoidance of caffeine, alcohol, sugar, white flour and other practical considerations.

My hat is off in admiration and thanks to Jacob Teitelbaum MD, for this third edition of an important book, the definitive work on chronic fatigue and fibromyalgia. No doubt, many have benefitted and will continue to benefit from the medical insights in this book. We expect and look forward to a continuing stream of valuable insights in future works as his medical career continues.

Other books recommended are Pain Free 1,2,3 by Jacob Teitelbaum MD, The Safe Use of Cortisol by McK Jefferies, and Adrenal Fatigue by Wilson.

The Testosterone Syndrome: The Critical Factor for Energy, Health, and Sexuality–Reversing the Male Menopause by Eugene Shippen

A Book About Testosterone Supplementation for the Aging Male, December 25, 2007

The Testosterone Syndrome, Reversing the Male Menopause by Eugene Shippen, M.D. is a book about testosterone replacement for aging males. Dr. Shippen is a popular lecturer on the medical meeting circuit where he covers testosterone replacement. Not only is he an expert on testosterone medical research, he also draws on his experience of many years using testosterone in clinical practice.

It is well known that institutional medicine has been staunchly opposed to the idea of testosterone for aging males. In spite of this opposition, national sales of testosterone has been increasing yearly, suggesting that consumer demand is now the driving force. For the medical consumer, since this information isn't available from your doctor or in the media, Shippen's book is the first step to learn about signs and symptoms of low testosterone, and whether testosterone supplementation is right for you. Although some areas of the book contain language suitable for health care professionals, the book is actually written for the lay reader.

According to Shippen, age related decline in testosterone levels cause muscle weakness, memory loss, erectile dysfunction, and the onset of a host of degenerative diseases. However, merely replenishing testosterone is not the whole solution. The missing piece of the puzzle is the male estrogen level which can go up with testosterone treatment because of the aromatase conversion of testosterone to estradiol. Shippen found that this aromatase conversion of testosterone to estradiol. was aggravated if testosterone blood levels fluctuated between high and low extremes. Shippen advocates the gradual release of testosterone with subcutaneous pellets to avoid this problem. I found it puzzling that Shippen did not mention aromatase inhibitor medication which is the current solution. Also, many other experts suggest daily topical testosterone creams, since this provides more stable delivery.

During a more recent lecture I attended, Shippen spoke about giving a series of small mini-injections of testosterone, rather than the pellets. So I would caution the reader to keep in mind that the book was written 10 years ago, and a future new edition would be welcome, including information on aromatase inhibitors and other new developments. In spite of this, there is much excellent information in the book. While drugs change with the passage of time, human physiology does not.

A key chapter deals with low testosterone, erectile dysfunction and sexual dysfunction. Here Shippen shares his insights about the importance of exercise *(Kegel exercises)*, to strengthen the pelvic muscles, in addition to testosterone for the return of sexual function.

Other chapters deal with beneficial effects of testosterone on the circulation, the heart, and mental functioning. Another chapter deals with testosterone and the prostate. One myth is that testosterone causes prostate cancer, and Shippen finds no evidence of this in the medical literature or in his clinical practice.

In conclusion, Shippen's book is recommended for any male over the age of 50 who is interested in testosterone supplementation to maintain youthful vigor, and as a preventive health measure.

The Andropause Mystery: Unraveling Truths About the Male Menopause by Robert S. Tan

An Honest Appraisal of Male Hormonal Decline and Treatment, December 24, 2007

In this book, Robert Tan MD , an astute clinician and a board certified specialist in geriatric medicine, describes his professional experience, diagnosing and treating hormonal decline in aging males. Tan describes a turning point in his career when he stumbled upon a bedridden male with the typical signs and symptoms of low testosterone, namely muscle weakness, frailty, memory loss, and hair loss. Lab testing confirmed low testosterone levels. Testosterone for aging males was new in those days, so Tan had difficulty convincing the pharmacy to release the testosterone injections *(* 200 mg twice a month*)*. After three months of injections, the patient grew a beard, began walking again, and his memory and libido improved.

The experience motivated Tan to do a Medline search on the topic, and he found very little research in the area of Male Menopause, also called Andropause. This book was written to unravel the truths and dispel the myths about the Male Andropause and Testosterone replacement for the aging male.

Tan asks a few obvious questions. The medical system treats women for the hormonal decline of Menopause, so why aren't men treated for their similar hormonal decline of male Andropause? The medical system recognizes Menopause, but does not recognize Andropause.

Many physicians deny that Andropause really exists. Tan says sorry, but it does exist, and his patients are testimony to this truth. Andropause is a real syndrome, and he clearly explains that 30% of males over 65 have low testosterone levels with the associated muscle weakness, memory loss, and loss of libido. Tan also explains the reasons why the syndrome is ignored by conventional medicine. There is no curriculum in medical school or residency, and very little research in the library due to lack of funding, and lastly, unlike females who are more expressive and communicative about their night sweats and hot flashes, males tend to be stoic, and in denial of their Andropause symptoms.

Tan discusses the beneficial affects of testosterone on cognitive function, finding that many *(*but not all*)* demented nursing home males are restored to normal after testosterone treatments. He also discusses the effect of testosterone on mood, cardiac function, muscle strength, bone density, and lastly improvement in libido and erectile function. In one humorous story, Tan recounts a demented nursing home patient whose testosterone treatment had to be discontinued because of hypersexual effects. Apparently, the old fellow had approached several nurses with inappropriate requests.

Tan also discussed the incorrect belief that Testosterone treatment increases the risk of prostate cancer. Tan dispels this myth, stating that in his clinical experience, he has yet to see a case of prostate cancer induced by testosterone replacement. Nonetheless, Tan advocates routine prostate surveillance with serial PSA *(*prostate specific antigen*)* and DRE *(*digital rectal examination of the prostate*)*.

Chapter 7 discusses the nuts and bolts of testosterone replacement with diagnostic blood testing, available testosterone preparations and dosage schedules. Tan feels that testosterone replacement for males should become as routine as HRT for the female menopause.

In conclusion, in a field with scant information, Tan's book fills a void. The book is an honest, courageous, down to earth, and occasionally humorous look at testosterone replacement for the aging male. Also recommended is The Testosterone Syndrome by Eugene Shippen MD.

Could It Be B12?: An Epidemic of Misdiagnoses by Sally M. Pacholok and Jeffrey J Stuart D.O.

The Definitive Book on B12 Deficiency, Diagnosis and Treatment, December 23, 2007

A good friend of ours had a sudden unrelenting pain in her leg which baffled her doctors. After many months of suffering, and many failed treatments and medications, she tried inexpensive vitamin B12 injections which immediately worked, providing complete relief. Occasionally the pain returns and reminds her it's time for another B12 injection. The injections are easy with a small syringe and tiny needle, and the B12 is injected under the skin twice a week.

There are many more stories of B12 misdiagnosis in Pacholok's book. Nurse Pacholok first describes her own ordeal with pernicious anemia and B12 deficiency which motivated her to become an expert on the topic. Working within the health care system, she was appalled at the numbers of patients with obvious signs and symptoms of B12 deficiency who were misdiagnosed.

Finding the medical system apathetic and unresponsive to her advice about B12 deficiency, Pacholok wrote this book to empower medical consumers and to educate their physicians. Pacholok is on a crusade to change medical practice to routinely screen for B12 deficiency, and her book is one giant step in that direction.

Vitamin B12 deficiency is estimated to affect 10%-15% of individuals over the age of 60 years. 40% of elderly hospitalized patients have low or borderline serum B12 levels, and 50% of long term vegetarians have B12 deficiency.

B12 absorption depends on many cofactors, so it is possible to take adequate amounts of B12 in the diet, and still have a B12 deficiency. Absorption of B12 requires gastric acid, so anything which reduces gastric acid production such as gastric surgery, atrophic gastritis, or antacid drugs could produce B12 deficiency. The very popular antacid drug Prilosec *(omeprazole)* has been clearly shown to decrease B12 absorption. Other antacid pills such as Prevacid, Protonix, antac, Nexium, Aciphex,

Zantec, Tagamet, Pepcid, Maalox, mylanta, reduce gastric acid, inhibit B12 absorption and may produce B12 deficiency. Drugs such as Metformin and other diabetes drugs can cause B12 deficiency. The anesthetic agent, Nitrous Oxide, or "laughing gas", used in dental or surgical procedures causes B12 deficiency Pernicious anemia is the second most common cause of B12 deficiency. This is an autoimmune disease with loss of Intrinsic Factor, in which antibodies damage the stomach lining interrupting the B12 absorption mechanism.

Other people at risk for B12 deficiency include vegetarians, people with eating disorders such as bulimia and anorexia, inflammatory bowel disease with malabsorption (ie. crohn's).

Auto-immune diseases such as Hashimoto's thyroiditis may be associated with B12 deficiency(pernicious anemia).

Vitamin B12 deficiency can cause unusual neurological symptoms such as tremor, gait disturbance, severe pain, and can mimic MS (multiple sclerosis) or even Parkinson's Syndrome. The physical signs and symptoms can often mimic other diseases and the diagnosis is frequently missed.

B12 deficiency damages the myelin sheath around the nerve fibers, this is a soft fatty insulating material which is also damaged in demyelinating diseases such as multiple sclerosis.

B12 deficiency can cause mental changes such as irritability, apathy, sleepiness, paranoia, personality changes, depression (including post-partum depression), memory loss, dementia, cognitive dysfunction or deterioration, fuzzy thinking, psychosis, dementia, hallucinations, violent behavior, in children; autistic behavior, developmental delay.

B12 deficiency can cause neurological signs and symptoms of abnormal sensations (pain, tingling, and/or numbness of legs, arms trunk or anywhere),diminished sense of touch, pain or temperature (may mimic diabetic neuropathy Charcot foot), loss of position sense, weakness, clumsiness, tremor, any symptoms which may mimic Parkinson's or multiple sclerosis, spasticity of muscles, incontinence, paralysis, vision changes, damage to optic nerve (optic neuritis).

Atherosclerotic vascular disease is increased by B12 deficiency including; Coronary artery disease, TIAs, CVA, heart attack, heart failure, claudication, all associated with elevated homocysteine levels caused by B12 deficiency.

B12 deficiency causes Megaloblastic Anemia (enlarged red blood cells with anemia). In this type of anemia, the red blood cells are fewer in number, yet they are larger in diameter (this large size is called megaloblastic and is measured on the CBC with the mean corpuscular volume, MCV). The anemia can cause fatigue, and weakness.

Cervical Dysplasia and increased risk for other dysplasias and cancers are associated with B12 deficiency. B12 supplementation is cancer prevention.

Most doctors do not test for B12, and if they do a test it is the serum B12 which may be unreliable because of the wide normal range. A more accurate test, urinary methyl malonic acid was developed by Eric Norman MD, and is inexpensive and widely available (MMA). The Methyl Malonic Acid MMA is elevated in the urine and serum in patients with B12 deficiency. Pacholok makes the case that everyone presenting for medical care should be routinely screened for B12 deficiency with the MMA, serum B12 and Homocysteine tests.

Treatment is Curative:

Treatment with inexpensive B12 injections or sublingual tablets is curative. Recent work by Kuzminski showed that daily 2 mg. oral B12 serves as well as monthly 1 mg intramuscular B12 injections. Serum Homocysteine is elevated in B12 deficiency. It is important to discover B12 deficiency early, since nerve damage can be irreversible if not discovered right away.

In conclusion, this is the definitive book on B12 deficiency, diagnosis and treatment for the lay reader and for the interested physician. As a result of reading this book, I now routinely test serum B12 and Urinary MMA on ALL patients, and have been surprised to find many symptomatic B12 deficient patients completely missed by the medical system. Needles to say, it is very gratifying to see ill patients completely recover with B12 injections.

I applaud the authors on a job well done, bringing B12 deficiency to the attention of the public, and no doubt saving many lives in the process. This book will make a positive impact on the nation's health, and change medical for the better. The only thing I would change about the book is to give Sally a name that is easier to pronounce.

Adrenal Fatigue: The 21st Century Stress Syndrome by James L. Wilson

A Self-Help Book for Chronic Burn-Out called Adrenal Fatigue, December 21, 2007

Adrenal Fatigue by James L Wilson, ND, DC, PhD is unquestionably the definitive work on low cortisol adrenal fatigue, written by the top expert in the field after compiling 2400 medical references. Originally intending to educate physicians about adrenal fatigue, a syndrome currently ignored by mainstream medicine, Wilson changed his mind, and wrote a self-help guide for all of us chronically stressed out members of the "rat race" suffering from this new 21st century epidemic.

Chapter 5, the Signs and Symptoms of Adrenal Fatigue contains humorous illustrations which communicate very clearly in non-technical language the symptoms of fatigue, lethargy, craving of salty foods, hypoglycemic episodes, decreased libido, stress intolerance, light headed upon standing, depression, loss of memory and cognitive decline, and prolonged recovery time from flu-like illnesses, which characterize adrenal fatigue, the net result of years of chronic stress.

In Chapter 7, Wilson explains that adrenal fatigue is not recognized by mainstream medicine because there is no ICD-9 code, and health insurance companies will not pay for diagnosis and treatment without a code. This is perhaps a simplification because the ICD-9 code 255.4 for adrenocortical insufficiency can be used. Wilson goes on to explain that the only codes and lab tests are for Addison's disease which is complete adrenal failure, so even if testing is done, most people with mild adrenal insufficiency will be told the test results are normal. Thanks to Wilson's efforts to publicize the syndrome, hopefully this is changing.

Chapter 8 contains a lengthy questionnaire which will assist the reader in self-diagnosis.

I found Chapter 10 on physical signs of adrenal fatigue the most useful, describing findings on physical examination such as the unstable pupil, blood pressure reduction upon standing, and Sergent's white line test.

Chapter 11 provides complete coverage of laboratory testing for cortisol levels in saliva, blood, and urine samples, as well as ACTH stimulation. Wilson favors the 4 sample salivary cortisol test as the easiest and most convenient method, with the added advantage that salivary testing can be done at home without a prescription

The largest section of the book, Part Three, deals with treatment and recovery from adrenal fatigue discussing lifestyle, diet, food allergies, replacement hormones, and supplements, and a discussion of cortisol vs. adrenal cortical extracts.

Adrenal fatigue is the net result of years of continuous high cortisol output by the adrenals caused by chronic stress from job, family, illness, injury, and poor diet and lifestyle associated with high-tech modern living. After years of chronic stress, the two small triangular supra-renal glands poop out, and we become another casualty of adrenal fatigue, the 21st century epidemic. Since mainstream doctors can't seem to help, either ignoring the syndrome, or prescribing anti-depressants for it, this self-help book may be a life-saver. Thank you, Dr. Wilson.

Other books recommended are Safe Uses of Cortisol by McK Jefferies, Hypothyroidism the Unsuspected Illness by Broda Barnes, From Fatigued to Fantastic by Teitelbaum.

Avoiding Breast Cancer While Balancing Your Hormones by Joseph F. McWherter M.D.

Natural Hormone Program to Decrease Breast Cancer Risk, December 20, 2007

Any woman hesitant about hormone replacement because of fear of breast cancer should read this book.

Joseph McWherter MD, an OB/Gyne doctor in Texas with a large natural hormone practice, wrote this book in response to the Women's Health Initiative Study (WHI) published in JAMA in 2002. The WHI Study was halted early because of increased heart disease and breast cancer. As usual, the newspaper headlines were misleading and got the story wrong, failing to mention the important distinction between the unsafe synthetic hormones used in the WHI study, and the safe natural hormones used by Dr. McWherter and many others.

Chapter 2 discusses the causes of breast cancer, namely accumulated DNA damage related to junk food diets, stressful lifestyle, environmental toxins, radiation, hormonal imbalance, and genetic predispositions, etc.

Chapter 3, Estrogen Explained, goes over rather detailed and technical information about the three types of human estrogens (E1,E2,E3) and their metabolism. Also clarified are the differences between synthetic estrogen, natural estrogen, xeno-estrogen and phyto-estrogen.

Chapter 4 is devoted to explaining the WHI Women's Health Initiative Study, and a discussion of the importance of testing estrogen metabolites, namely the 2/16 hydroxy-estrogen ratio. Increasing this 2/16 ratio by consuming broccoli, or with supplements such as I3C and DIM reduces breast cancer risk.

Separate chapters are devoted to exercise, diet, and detoxification, all very detailed and complete. Before studying medicine, Dr. McWherter was a mathematician, and he covers these topics with mathematical precision. The exercise chapter contains actual photos showing how to do each exercise. The diet chapter contains menus and a glycemic index chart. The detoxification chapter includes a questionnaire and 21 day Detox diet.

The real crux of the book, of course, is the hormone chapter in which McWherter discusses natural hormones called Bi-Est and Tri-Est topical preparations. McWherter found that blood testing under treatment usually shows an estradiol level in the 20-50 pg/ml range. On page 140, McWherter reveals startling information about the low incidence of breast cancer in his treatment group. There was only one case of breast cancer in 2,300 women over 5 years on his clinic program. This single case is compared to the 60 cases expected based on the WHI placebo arm data. Needless to say, this is an excellent result.

Chapter 10, Breast Care Nutrients, covers McWherter's Nutritional supplement program to prevent breast cancer, and the first item mentioned is iodine supplementation. Mc Wherter is familiar with the work of Derry and Brownstein on Iodine as the key to breast cancer prevention, and he gives credit to their work. Other supplements such as I3C, DIM and Calcium-D-glucarate are also mentioned.

A final chapter is devoted to breast cancer surveillance and detection with self breast examination, mammography and thermography.

Missing from the book is a chapter discussing heart disease. Suffice it to say that the second arm of the WHI using premarin alone actually showed less heart disease in the premarin treated group, and a recent NEJM study showed less coronary calcification on CAT scan in the premarin treated group. These revelations indicate that estrogen is protective, not causative of heart disease.

In conclusion, McWherter's book serves as an educational tool for his own clinic patients, and provides a glimpse into his program for every one else. I have found the book a valuable resource, and have adopted the breast cancer prevention protocol for my own clinical practice.

McWherter's excellent book sets a very high standard for future authors of natural hormone replacement for women, and the book deserves a prominent place in every medical library. Also recommended is Natural Hormone Balance for Women by Uzzi Reiss MD, Iodine and Breast Cancer Prevention by Derry, and Iodine by Brownstein.

Natural Hormone Balance for Women: Look Younger, Feel Stronger, and Live Life with Exuberance by Uzzi Reiss MD

A Woman's Practical Guide to Natural Hormones, December 18, 2007

This is currently one of the best books for women who want to know about natural bio-identical hormones for the menopausal symptoms of night sweats, hot flashes, insomnia, weight gain, and foggy mind.

I met Uzzi Reiss at a medical meeting a few years ago, and he mentioned his new book during conversation. After returning from the meeting, I read Suzanne Somers' book in which she mentioned that Uzzi Reiss had been one of her doctors during her long odyssey to find bio-identical hormone replacement. As a gynecologist with a large clinical practice in Los Angeles, Dr. Uzzi Reiss has accumulated a considerable amount of knowledge and experience using natural hormones for women, and Dr. Reiss is one of the few physicians willing to share this knowledge.

Reiss's book provides a practical guide for the safe use of natural hormones, and answers the following questions:

1) When to use natural hormones, when to not use them

2) The difference between unsafe patented synthetic hormones, and the safe natural hormones.

3) Why natural hormones are safe.

4) What route of administration is best, pills, gels, creams, drops, etc.

5) What are your possible responses to each hormone in terms of how you will feel.

6) How to monitor our response and adjust your hormone dosage individually.

7) How to work with your doctor to adjust your hormone dosage for optimal effect avoiding hormone excess symptoms.

Regarding hormone testing:

Dr. Reiss uses blood testing for baseline hormone levels, however, he says:"The heavy reliance on normal-range readings is nothing less than a tragic, medical addiction"

Dr. Reiss's approach:

After a routine history and physical exam, baseline blood hormone levels and a pelvic sonogram, treatment is started at a relatively low hormone dosage, adjusting upward as needed. For the adjustment phase, Dr. Reiss empowers his patients with the knowledge to adjust their individual hormone levels. This is done based on symptoms of hormone deficiency or excess, clearly described in detail in his book, which serves as an educational tool for his patients.

Separate chapters are devoted to Estrogen, Progesterone and Testosterone with very detailed descriptions of symptoms of hormonal deficiency and hormonal excess. Dr. Reiss does not discuss thyroid, leaving that for other authors. Also, there are only limited comments about adrenal fatigue and the problems associated with low cortisol.

A major strength of the book is that Dr. Reiss provides exact hormone dosages and route of administration for his Los Angeles patient population. However, as a matter of practical experience, I have found his starting estrogen dosage somewhat on the high side of the scale for my area of the country, so I would caution the reader about that. Also, Dr. Reiss does not explain why he changed the standard formulation of Tri-Est (10/10/80) to a different unique formulation of Tri-Est gel (0.25E1/ 0.75E2/ 2.75E3). According to most large national compounding pharmacies, the most common formulation is Bi-Est in 0.625 mg to 1.25 mg dosage with (20 E2 / 80 E3) formulation.

In any event, these minor flaws are outweighed by the many strengths of the book which empowers women to learn about natural hormone balance. I applaud Dr. Reiss for providing a valuable public service with a book that should be in every woman's library on natural hormone replacement.

Curing the Incurable: Vitamin C, Infectious Disease, and Toxins by Thomas E. Levy MD JD

A Remarkable Medicine Has Been Overlooked, December 15, 2007

Written with an eloquent flowing style, this book makes the case for Vitamin C as a remarkable medicine that has been overlooked by the medical establishment. Although the crowning achievement of modern medical science is the invention of antibiotics which cures bacterial infections, we have no antibiotics effective for acute viral illness.

Dr. Levy says this is incorrect because Vitamin C is a curative "antibiotic" for viral diseases when used properly in high enough dosage by IM or IV route.

Dr. Levy's book makes a number of points:

1) Vitamin C is not really a vitamin needed in trace amounts, it is needed in large amounts as a co-factor in oxidation-reduction reactions in the cellular biochemistry.

2) All animals, with the exception of primates, have the enzymes to make their own vitamin C. They do not need to consume Vitamin C in their diet, they make their own.

3) All humans (and primates) lack this final enzyme for the manufacture of vitamin C, and therefore we must consume Vit C in our diet. We have a genetic deficiency in GLO gulano-lactone-oxidase, the final step for the manufacture of vitamin C.

4) Because of this genetic defect, we all have a subclinical Vitamin C deficiency making us more susceptible to infectious diseases.

5) The 60 mg dosage RDA for vitamin C is adequate to prevent scurvy but is insufficient for optimal health.

6) Adequate human "Opti-Doses" of vitamin C based on animal studies is in the range of 3-5 grams per day, and this requirement increases during periods of stress or infection.

7) IV or IM Vitamin C in the appropriate dosage ranges has been clinically proven to cure acute viral diseases such as polio, acute hepatitis, measles, mumps, chickenpox, shingles, and viral encephalitis.

The most amazing evidence presented in the book is the work of Frederick R Klenner, a doctor in North Carolina who cured 60 of 60 acute polio cases with IM or IV vitamin C and published his findings in Southern Medicine & Surgery, Volume 103, Number 4, April, 1951, pp. 101-107. Klenner wrote more than 20 other publications. Polio vaccine was introduced shortly afterwards, and Klenner's work with Vitamin C was simply ignored.

Because of the unconstitutional FDA ruling which prohibits Vitamin C manufacturers from informing the public, very few people are aware of this research showing the incredible benefits of vitamin C.

I have had numerous conversations about vitamin C with other doctor friends, and colleagues I have known for 25 years, and invariably any comment about Vitamin C is met with ridicule, laughter, and disbelief. Sadly, that is the current state of the medical establishment. Perhaps Dr. Thomas Levy's book will serve to change this, and one day soon, mainstream medicine will embrace a remarkable medicine that has been overlooked.

Breast Cancer and Iodine : How to Prevent and How to Survive Breast Cancer by Dr. David Derry M.D., Ph.D.

Proposes Iodine as Prevention and Treatment for Breast Cancer, December 14, 2007

Breast Cancer and Iodine by David Derry MD PhD, is a unique 100 page volume which presents the academic case for iodine as prevention and treatment of breast cancer. The book should be handed out freely during October Breast Cancer Awareness Month. Although written for the lay reader, it should be required reading for all medical students, breast surgeons, mammographers, breast cancer oncologists and any doctor who orders mammograms.

With ten pages of medical references including the work of B A Eskin and W R Ghent, Dr. Derry discloses the remarkable connection between iodine deficiency, fibrocystic breast disease and breast cancer. Iodine's anti-cancer activity lies in its control of apoptosis, or programmed cell death.

Derry presents case studies complete with surgical pathology confirmation showing regression of both fibrocystic breast disease and carcinoma-in-situ breast cancer with iodine treatment. He also presents a case report case of infiltrating breast cancer involving the skin which regressed after prolonged application of topical Lugol's iodine solution.

I can report from the experience of my own family members that iodine supplementation causes regression of fibrocystic breast disease.

Derry's ideas in the book could be easily revised into an NIH grant proposal to research and confirm the role of iodine. To do so would advance the nation's health and be a great public service. Iodine is safe, inexpensive and readily available without a prescription. A US policy of iodine supplementation matching the Japanese dietary intake of iodine could very well be our best preventive measure against breast cancer.

Iodine, Why You Need It and Why You Can't Live Without It by David Brownstein MD

This Book Invokes a Renaissance in the Use of Iodine , December 12, 2007

Iodine, Why You Need It and Why You Can't Live Without It by David Brownstein MD is written for the lay reader, however, all health care professionals should find the information useful in clinical practice.

Brownstein says we are in the "Medical Dark Ages" concerning iodine supplementation, and his book attempts to invoke a Renaissance. David Bronstein MD has a clinical practice in the goiter belt of Michigan, and is involved with an ongoing iodine research project with Guy Abraham MD and George Flechas MD.

According to Brownstein, iodine is safe and beneficial, preventing not only goiter, but also preventing the many thyroid cysts, nodules and auto-immune thyroid disease rampant in the population. Iodine is anti-microbial, anti-parasitic, anti-cancer, important for hormone production, reverses fibrocystic breast disease, and shrinks ovarian and thyroid cysts. It may be our most important preventive measure against breast cancer.

The book dispels a number of myths about Iodine supplementation.

Myth number one: There is no iodine deficiency because of Iodized Salt.

The iodine in Iodized salt is not very bio-available, and government surveys show decreasing Iodine levels in the population. Brownstein found that 90% of his patients were iodine deficient based on a 24 urine test for excreted iodine after a 50 mg loading dose.

Myth Number two: Too much Iodine above the RDA of 150 mcg is not safe.

In reality Iodine supplementation is very safe. The average Japanese diet contains 12 mg per day which is 100 times the RDA in the US. In the event of a nuclear power plant accident, the government gives everyone 50 mg. of Iodine to prevent thyroid cancer.

A chapter is devoted to iodine deficiency and fibrocystic breast disease and breast cancer. Brownstein presents case reports of women with fibrocystic disease as well as breast cancer who benefit from iodine supplementation. Another chapter devoted to the thyroid describes patients with Graves' disease and Hashimoto's disease who benefit from iodine supplementation.

Iodine tablets are inexpensive and widely available as a nutritional supplement called Iodoral without a prescription. Another book, Breast Cancer and Iodine, by David Derry MD PhD, is also recommended.

Hypothyroidism Type 2: The Epidemic by M.D., Mark Starr MD

A Sequel to Broda Barnes and a Tribute to Thyroid Medical Pioneers , December 12, 2007

Hypothyroidism, Type Two by Mark Starr MD is a tribute to many of the great pioneers of thyroid medicine, Broda Barnes MD, Eugene Hertoge, and Lawrence Sonkin MD. The book is a sequel to the Broda Barnes classic on low thyroid and a compilation of evidence that modern lab testing is unreliable for the diagnosis of low thyroid, and the current treatment equally lacking.

Partly to seek treatment for his own musculoskeletal pain, Starr went to New York to study pain medicine with Hans Krauss at Cornell Medical Center. Starr later opened his own pain clinic and quickly realized that the majority of his patients responded to thyroid medication with pain relief.

If you have read the Broda Barnes book, Hypothyroidism, the Unsuspected Illness, you will find many of the same ideas explained and elaborated by Mark Starr's tribute to the earlier work. For example, the definition of Type Two Hypothyroidism is defined as cellular resistance to the action of thyroid hormone.

While thyroid hormone's main action is to increase the size and number of mitochondria, the mitochondrial DNA is highly susceptible to genetic mutations because of maternal transmission.

An unforeseen outcome of the medical victory over infectious diseases with modern antibiotics is the creation of new generations of low thyroid children who in earlier times would have succumbed to childhood infectious diseases. They now survive to adulthood thanks to antibiotics, and according to both Starr and Barnes, later develop heart disease as undiagnosed low thyroid adults.

The book contains fascinating reprints of old medical book photos of patients with low thyroid before and after treatment, and adds a valuable chapter on clinical signs and symptoms of low thyroid. Another chapter covers Starr's area of expertise which is musculoskeletal pain syndromes and their relation to the low thyroid condition. Another useful chapter explains in detail why desiccated thyroid is more effective than the synthetic T4 commonly used by the medical system.

Unlike the Broda Barnes book which was written at the end of a long medical career, Starr's book appears at the relative beginning of his, and one can only wonder what future additional insights he will share after 30 years of medical practice.

Your Thyroid and How to Keep It Healthy by Barry Durrant-Peatfield

Excellent Thyroid Book Follows Tradition of Broda Barnes MD, December 10, 2007

I recommend to you the book by Barry Durrant Peatfield, "Your Thyroid and How to Keep It Healthy". Peatfield was a general practitioner in the British National Health service who came to America and trained at the Broda Barnes Institute. He returned to England and started a thyroid private practice. His book summarizes over 25 years of clinical diagnosing and treating thyroid illness. One section of the book is devoted to the question, "Why thyroid blood tests can be unreliable".

Here is what Dr. Peatfield says:

"Anxiety in the medical establishment about rules and dogma has led to a slavish reliance on blood tests, which are often unreliable and can actually produce a false picture of the true situation"

"I have sadly come across very few doctors who can accept the fact that a normal, or low TSH, may still occur with a low thyroid."

"as a result of this test *(*TSH*)*, thousands are denied treatment"

Peatfield lists several reasons why thyroid blood tests are flawed:

1*)* They measure hormone levels in the blood. What we really want to know is tissue levels, not blood levels.

2*)* The blood tests do not measure cellular receptor hormone resistance.

3*)* The blood tests do not measure conversion block. Some patients cannot convert their inactive T4 to active T3.

4*)* The thyroid tests do not account for adrenal insufficiency.

5*)* Paradoxical low TSH may occur with a low thyroid function.

These sentiments are shared by the teachings of Broda Barnes MD, and the Broda Barnes Foundation. However, Peatfield's book elaborates beyond the classic teachings of Broda Barnes by including chapters on the adrenal as well as a chapter on iodine supplementation. I found this book excellent, and it belongs in every medical library dealing with thyroid disease.

Hypothyroidism: The Unsuspected Illness by Broda Barnes

A Medical Classic from a Medical Giant which Still Rings True, December 9, 2007

Hypothyroidism the Unsuspected Illness, by Broda Barnes MD, is a medical classic and should be required reading for every medical student and doctor. I have read the book many times. The book contains the condensed wisdom of a lifetime of research and clinical experience with the thyroid, and it rings true today as it did in 1976. Thyroid blood tests come and go, yet human physiology remains the same.

Broda Barnes estimated that up to 40% of the population suffers from a low thyroid condition and would benefit from thyroid medication. Of course, Barnes' opinion differed with that of mainstream medicine of his time which relied dogmatically on thyroid blood tests to make the diagnosis of low thyroid. Barnes felt the blood tests were unreliable and instead used the basal temperature, history and physical examination. This medical debate regarding unreliability of thyroid blood testing continues today.

Being an astute clinician, Dr. Barnes makes a number of observations about the low thyroid condition. Firstly, low thyroid is associated with a reduced immunity to infectious diseases such as TB. Before the advent of modern antibiotics in the 1940's, most low thyroid children succumbed to infectious diseases before reaching adulthood. Secondly, low thyroid is associated with a peculiar form of skin thickening called myxedema which causes a characteristic appearance of the face, puffiness around the eyes, fullness under the chin, loss of outer eyebrows, and hair thinning or hair loss.

A third observation by Dr. Barnes is that low thyroid is associated with menstrual irregularities, miscarriages and infertility. Barnes treated thousands of young women with thyroid which restored cycle regularity and fertility. In his day, the medical system resorted to the drastic measure of hysterectomy for uncontrolled menstrual bleeding. Although today's use of birth control pills to regulate the cycles is admittedly a far better alternative, Barnes found that the simple administration of desiccated thyroid served quite well. Again, Barnes noted that blood testing was usually normal in these cases which respond to thyroid medication.

A lengthy chapter is devoted to heart attacks and the low thyroid condition. Based on autopsy data from Graz Austria, Barnes concluded that low thyroid patients who previously would have succumbed to infectious diseases in childhood go on years later to develop heart disease. Barnes also found that thyroid treatment was protective in preventing heart attacks, based on his own clinical experience. Likewise for diabetes, Dr. Barnes found that adding thyroid medication was beneficial at preventing the onset of vascular disease in diabetics. Again, blood tests are usually normal.

Dr. Barnes devotes separate chapters in the book to discussion of chronic fatigue, migraine headaches and emotional/behavioral disorders all of which respond to treatment with thyroid medication.

The final chapter describes Dr. Barnes work on obesity when he resided over a hospital ward of volunteer obese patients, and monitored everything they ate. He found that the obese patients invariably ate a high carbohydrate diet, and avoided fat. Barnes added fat back into the menu and reduced the refined carbohydrates and found that his obese patients lost 10 pounds a month with no hunger pangs.

Missing from the book are discussions of Iodine supplementation and the role of the Adrenal, both of which are covered in later updated versions of Barnes thyroid book by other authors. See Hypothyroidism Type Two by Mark Starr, and Your Thyroid by Barry Durrant Peatfield. Iodine supplementation is covered by both Derry and Brownstein. The Safe Uses of Cortisol by William McK Jefferies is the companion medical classic devoted to the adrenals and cortisol.

Safe Uses of Cortisol by William McK Jefferies MD

Safe Use of Cortisol is a Unique Medical Classic, December 7, 2007

The Safe Use of Cortisol by William McK Jefferies MD is a medical classic, and along with its companion classic by Broda Barnes, Hypothyroidism, the Unsuspected Illness, both books should be required reading by every medical student and MD and deserve a prominent place in every medical library. I have read both numerous times, and plan to re-read both again.

This book contains a condensation of clinical knowledge from the career of a medical giant, and a wealth of knowledge not found anywhere else, and is complete with references to the medical literature, case histories, laboratory studies and dosages.

In this slim volume, Safe Use of Cortisol, Dr. McK Jefferies points out an important distinction which is not widely known by mainstream doctors or the public. This is the distinction between the lower and completely safe, physiologic doses of cortisol, and the dangerous higher pharmacologic dosage levels commonly used by mainstream doctors to treat rheumatoid arthritis and other auto-immune diseases.

While the lower cortisol doses below 40 mg per day are safe, above this dosage level, one finds increased risk of adrenal suppression, and increased risk of adverse side effects including moon face, osteoporosis with spontaneous fractures, thinning of skin with easy bruising, striae, subcutaneous hemorrhages, fluid retention with edema, and cataracts.

Cortisol is widely available as inexpensive Cortef from the corner drug store, and is the bio-identical hormone secreted by the adrenal gland. Since it is a natural hormone, it cannot be patented, explaining the lack of funding for research by the pharmaceutical companies.

Chapter 4 of the book discusses generally accepted uses of Cortisol, starting with the most logical use which is adrenal insufficiency, also called Addison's disease. However, McK Jefferies also discusses mild adrenal insufficiency, which is not usually recognized by mainstream doctors, and should be. Other uses of low dose cortisol include ovarian dysfunction with infertility, chronic fatigue, allergies and auto-immune diseases.

McK Jefferies relies on the Cortrosyn ACTH stimulation test to evaluate adrenal function, as well as urinary cortisol metabolites and serum cortisol tests. He also addresses thyroid function as part of the overall clinical picture; hence the connection with Broda Barnes and the continued advocacy of McK Jefferies' work by the Broda Barnes Institute.

I found Chapter 5, Gonadal Dysfunction and Infertility, to be the most fascinating and clinically useful chapter. McK Jefferies used low dose cortisol to successfully treat thousands of young women suffering from irregular menstrual cycles, ovarian dysfunction, hirsutism *(*facial hair, and acne, both signs of elevated testosterone*)*.

Nowadays, teenagers with irregular menstrual bleeding are routinely given birth control pills with synthetic hormones to regulate their cycles. The synthetic hormones in BCPs are associated with adverse side effects and do not address the underlying fertility issues.

Unknown to the mainstream medical system, the real treatment for irregular menstrual bleeding is found in this medical classic book, namely low dose cortisol and thyroid which successfully normalizes menstrual cycles and restores fertility. Dr. McK Jefferies suggests that the cause of the infertility and irregular periods in these patients is usually excess adrenal production of either androgen *(*PCOS*)* or estrogen, and the low dose cortisol serves to suppress this excess hormone production by the adrenals and allow normal ovarian function.

Now recognized as the most common genetic disorder in the population, *(*CYP21A2*)* non-classical 21-hydroxylase deficiency is associated with menstrual irregularities, hirsutism and acne from elevated testosterone. Rather than low dose cortisol *(cortef)*, current treatment practice is to use a similar low dose dexamethasone *(See the 2006 review in J Clin Endo & Metab Vol. 91, No. 11 4205-4214, by Maria I New)*. Perhaps non-classical 21-OH should be renamed McJefferies Syndrome to give proper credit to this great clinician, since many of his cases were in retrospect probably 21 hydroxylase deficiency.

McJefferies stresses that normalization of thyroid function is also required for menstrual regularity and fertility. Broda Barnes agrees with McK Jefferies on the importance of thyroid for normalizing menstrual cycles, and both treat with thyroid medication even though the thyroid blood tests may be completely normal. They have found the blood tests to be unreliable. This is at variance with mainstream medical practice which clings dogmatically to the thyroid blood tests. Most mainstream doctors would refuse to offer thyroid medication unless there is a documented "out of range" lab value.

Chapter 9 deals with using low dose cortisol for viral infections such as influenza. Although there was some initial concern that low dose cortisol would reduce immunity in some way, Dr. Mc Jefferies was surprised to find in clinical practice that his patients maintained on low dose cortisol typically reported fewer common colds and other viral illnesses than their family members, suggesting an enhancement of immunity. Another practice he used was to increase the cortisol dosage when patients felt a common cold or viral influenza coming on. He found that this enabled the patient to ward off or recover from the illness more quickly. Of course, he also points out that excess doses of cortisol would have the opposite effect and impair resistance to infection.

The final chapters of the book discuss the use of low dose physiologic cortisol for rheumatoid arthritis, allergies, auto-immune disease, chronic fatigue.

In addition to the ACTH stimulation tests still in use today, we now have the newer, salivary cortisol testing which I am sure Mc Jefferies would have found useful in his day. What he would have written about the use of salivary cortisol testing ? Unfortunately we will never know. Perhaps a future medical author will build on McK Jefferies work and incorporate salivary testing and other new developments in a future book.

I reviewed the third edition which was published in 2004. The first edition was published in 1983. Other books recommended along side this one are, Adrenal Fatigue by James Wilson, Hypothyroidism, the Unsuspected Illness by Broda Barnes, From Fatigued to Fantastic: by Jacob Teitelbaum, Your Thyroid and How to Keep it Healthy by Barry Durrant Peatfield.

Section Seven Infertility PCOS CAH

Chapter 23

Understanding PCOS, the Hidden Epidemic

PCOS Polycystic Ovary Syndrome - Anovulatory Androgen Excess

Seventeen year old Alice has PCOS *(*Polycystic Ovary Syndrome*)*. Alice came with her Mom into the office and told me her story. Alice has been overweight, borderline diabetic, and has facial hair and acne caused by elevated testosterone. At age 12, Alice started normal menstrual cycles, but her cycles began fluctuating and periods stopped at age 15. Her gynecologist diagnosed PCOS *(*Polycystic Ovary Syndrome*)*, and put her on birth control pills to regulate her cycles. The birth control pills caused adverse side effects of weight gain weight and elevated blood pressure *(*hypertension*)*, so she stopped them.

Progesterone is the Most Logical Form of Treatment and Actually Works

Two months ago, Alice was switched over from the birth control pills to natural progesterone, taking a 100 mg capsule twice a day for 14 days on, 14 days off. The progesterone was successful, restoring a normal menstrual period, and a return to regular cycles.

BCP's *(*birth control pills*)* are usually prescribed by the OB-Gyne doctor to regulate cycles in the PCOS patient. This standard treatment is not the best one. There is a more logical alternative that actually works called natural progesterone. Both John R Lee MD, and JeriLynn Prior MD advocate the use of natural progesterone as a far better alternative to birth control pills. After all, birth control pills *(*BCP's*)* are a chemical form of castration, and work by inhibiting ovulation.

This chapter will explain the cause of PCOS, and will describe the signs and symptoms of PCOS, including the clinical features of PCOS, and give you a simple questionnaire to determine if you have PCOS. This article will also explain why natural progesterone is the best treatment, and a much better choice compared to birth control pills.

PCOS was Rare When First Described in 1935, Now Quite Common.

When PCOS *(*polycystic ovary syndrome*)* was first described in 1935 by Stein and Leventhal, it was fairly rare.*(55)* Nowadays, it is quite common, involving 6 to 10 per cent of the female population, affecting 3.5 to 5 million women.*(24)* Why the increased incidence? Some believe that endocrine disruptor chemicals in the environment are to blame.*(60A)*

List of Clinical Signs and Symptoms Of PCOS

Oligomenorrhea or amenorrhea (no periods) Anovulation (no ovulation) Weight gain, obesity Hirsutism (excessive hair growth, male pattern) Insulin resistance (pre-diabetes) Acne Male-pattern baldness Multiple small ovarian cysts on sonogram Acanthosis nigrans *(*darkening of the skin at the nape of the neck and under arms*)*-indicator of hyperinsulinemia

Definition of Ovulation:

Ovulation describes the event when an egg is released from a follicle in the ovary, and starts the long trip down the fallopian tube to the uterine cavity, where the egg can be fertilized and start growing into an embryo. This same ovulation event causes high progesterone production by the corpus luteum in the ovary. When ovulation occurs normally every month, menstrual cycles are regular.

Definition of Anovulation:

If no egg is released from the ovary, there is no subsequent progesterone production. This is called anovulation which causes irregular menstrual cycles. Long periods of anovulation lead to increased testosterone production and eventually, the periods may stop altogether.

How Do You Know If You Have PCOS?

PCOS Questionnaire.(63)(64)

Length of Menstrual Cycle, Variable Length

1) Between the ages of 16 and 40, was length of your menstrual cycle (on average) greater than 35 days and/or totally variable ?

Hair Growth (Male Pattern)

2) During your menstruating years (not including during pregnancy), did you have dark, coarse hair on your three or more of these sites? Upper lip? chin? breasts? chest between the breasts? back? belly? upper arms? upper thighs?

Obesity

3) Were you ever obese or overweight between the ages of 16 and 40?

If you answer **Yes, to 2 out of 3** of the following questions, this indicates high likelihood (80%) of PCOS.

What Causes PCOS ?

The world's greatest authority, Leon Speroff MD, says in his book page 493: "A question which has puzzled gynecologists and endocrinologists for many years is what causes polycystic ovaries. There is an answer which is appealing in its logic and clinical applicability. The characteristic polycystic ovary emerges when a state of anovulation persists for any length of time" *(1)*

PCOS is the end result of not ovulating, *(*no progesterone production*)* for a long time *(*a few years*)*, resulting in a vicious cycle which self perpetuates anovulation, causing increased testosterone production by the ovary. Insulin resistant diabetes and obesity aggravate the problem. As you might expect, PCOS is a major cause of infertility.

About 10% of patients thought to have PCOS actually have an underlying genetic enzyme defect in adrenal steroid synthesis called Non-Classical CAH. This can be diagnosed with a Cortrosyn stimulation test measuring 17 hydroxy-progesterone, and a 21-OH genetic test called CAHDtex from Esoterix. If present, treatment is successful with low dose adrenal steroid tablets *(*cortef, dexamethasone, prednisone*)* which restores fertility and reverses the acne. *(*see below discussion on non-classical CAH*)*.

Oral Contraceptives for PCOS *(*BCP's*)* Aggravate Insulin Resistance

Birth control pills are a chemical form of castration, which prevent ovulation. Lack of ovulation is the primary defect in PCOS, so birth control pills merely perpetuate the primary defect. Birth control pills can restore regular bleeding periods, however, this is artificial, and aggravate the underlying PCOS problem rather than solve it. In addition, birth control pills are known to worsen insulin resistance and diabetes.*(2)*

"PCOS may affect between 3.5 and 5.0 million young women in the United States, it arguably may be the most important general health issue affecting young women. BCP's *(OCPs)* are the traditional therapy for the chronic treatment of PCOS...... limited evidence raises the issue that BCP's *(OCPs)* may aggravate insulin resistance and exert other untoward metabolic actions that possibly enhance the long-term risk for diabetes and heart disease." *(2)*

JeriLynn Prior MD Says:

> "The fundamental problem with PCOS is not making progesterone for two weeks every cycle. This lack of progesterone leads to an imbalance in the ovary, causes the stimulation of higher male hormones and leads to the irregular periods and trouble getting pregnant. Progesterone is usually missing—replacing it therefore makes sense. " *(5)*

John R Lee MD says:

> "I recommend supplementation of normal physiologic doses of progesterone to treat PCOS. If progesterone levels rise each month during the luteal phase of the cycle, as they are supposed to do, this maintains the normal synchronal pattern each month, and PCOS rarely, if ever, occurs. Natural progesterone should be the basis of PCOS treatment, along with attention to stress, exercise, and nutrition.
>
> If you have PCOS, you can use 15 to 20 mg of progesterone cream daily from day 14 to day 28 of your cycle. If you have a longer or a shorter cycle, adjust accordingly. The disappearance of facial hair and acne are usually obvious signs that hormones are becoming balanced, but to see these results, you'll need to give the treatment at least six months, in conjunction with proper diet and exercise." This is quoted from the *John R Lee Medical Letter 1999.(10)*

Can PCOS be Treated with Natural Progesterone?

Dr. JeriLynn Prior says yes it can.*(3)*

> "Progesterone talks back to the hypothalamic and pituitary *(brain)* hormones that control the ovaries and stops them from stimulating

the ovaries to make too much testosterone." Dr Prior recognizes that the *(*BCP*)* pill, with its synthetic type of progesterone, does help women with PCOS to a certain degree. But her goal for PCOS patients is, "to return the brain/ovary system to a normal balance. The goal of the BCP Pill is the **opposite** - it must suppress the brain-ovary system to prevent pregnancy." JeriLynn Prior MD Web Site.*(3)*

To help her PCOS patients achieve a normal hormonal balance, Dr. Prior prescribes oral micronized **progesterone** *(*trade name Prometrium*)* which is a bio-identical hormone. Patients who take this natural progesterone for two weeks every month *(*called cyclic progesterone therapy) note improvement in menstrual cycle regularity, and this may help the brain to develop the normal cyclic rhythm that is missing in PCOS. Dr. Prior thinks another benefit of cyclic progesterone therapy is that progesterone inhibits the 5-alpha reductase enzyme that converts testosterone into DHT causing excess facial hair and oily skin and acne.

Help for PCOS - Cyclic Progesterone Therapy
JeriLynn C. Prior MD Says:
"I use ***cyclic progesterone therapy*** as the heart of treatment for PCOS-anovulatory androgen excess.*(6)* Progesterone is the hormone made by the ovary after an egg is released.

The fundamental problem with PCOS is not making progesterone for two weeks every cycle. This lack of progesterone leads to an imbalance in the ovary, causes the stimulation of higher male hormones and leads to the irregular periods and trouble getting pregnant. Progesterone is usually missing—replacing it therefore makes sense. Progesterone talks back to the hypothalamic and pituitary *(*brain*)* hormones that control the ovary, and stops them from stimulating the ovary to make too much testosterone.

Taking progesterone for two weeks every month *(*called cyclic progesterone*)* may help the brain to develop the normal cyclic rhythm that is missing in PCOS. Progesterone also counterbalances the steadily high estrogen levels that the PCOS ovary produces even if you have no periods. Progesterone will prevent estrogen over-stimulation of the uterine lining *(*endometrial hyperplasia*)* and heavy flow. It may also interfere with the action of high estrogen on the breasts, therefore preventing tenderness and "lumpiness" and perhaps even the risk for breast cancer.

Finally, and most doctors don't realize this, progesterone antagonizes and inhibits the enzyme *(*called 5-alpha reductase*)* that is needed to make testosterone into dihydrotestosterone. Dihydrotestosterone is the powerful male hormone that talks hair follicles into making coarse hair and too much oil that causes acne." Quote by Dr. JeriLynn C. Prior and Celeste Wincapaw *(5)*

Useful Tools for Patients from Dr. Prior

A ***Cyclic Progesterone Therapy*** patient handout sheet can be found at Dr. Prior's web site.*(6)* A useful menstrual cycle diary log sheet can also be found there.

Guidelines for Progesterone Cream Dosage for PCOS *(8)*

32mg to 64 mg of progesterone cream applied topically in divided doses from day 12-26 of the menstrual cycle depending on severity.*(8)*

Dr. Lam Progesterone Guidelines for Polycystic Ovary Syndrome *(9)*

Dr. Lam follows Dr John R Lee pioneering use of progesterone. He recommends topical application of 20 mg of progesterone cream during day 14 to 28 of the menstrual cycle. He will adjust accordingly if for longer or shorter cycles are noted. He reports facial hair and acne, two commonly associated symptoms, will disappear as the hormonal balance is restored.*(9)*

Other treatable causes of anovulation

1*)* Low thyroid function *(*hypothyroid*)* causes menstrual irregularity, anovulation and infertility. Ovulation and fertility is restored by thyroid medication. Ovarian cysts also resolve.

2*)* Vitamin D deficiency is associated with anovulation and resolves with Vitamin D supplementation.

3*)* Iodine deficiency causes ovarian cysts and anovulation, and resolves with iodine supplementation.

Other Useful Drug Treatments for PCOS:

Issue	***Drug Treatment***
infertility, anovulation	Clomid clomephine, induces ovulation.
Insulin Resistance:	Metformin improves insulin sensitivity.*(39)(39A)*
Acne, Facial Hair:	Spironlactone, Aldactone inhibits testosterone.

REFERENCES

(1) *http://www.amazon.com/Clinical-Gynecologic-Endocrinology-Infertility-Editorial/dp/0781747953*
The Clinical Gynecologic Endocrinology and Infertility: Leon Speroff MD

(2) *http://jcem.endojournals.org/cgi/content/full/88/5/1927*
A Modern Medical Quandary: Polycystic Ovary Syndrome, Insulin Resistance, and Oral Contraceptive Pills, The Journal of Clinical Endocrinology & Metabolism Vol. 88, No. 5 1927-1932

(3) *http://www.pcosupport.org/newsletter/articles/article122707-3.php*
Can PCOS be Treated with Natural Progesterone? Jerilynn Prior, PCOSA Today Newsletter

(4) *http://www.virginiahopkinstestkits.com/priorovaries.html*
WHAT MAKES YOUR OVARIES TICK, Insights about ovulation, fertility, PCOS and more.An Interview with Jerilynn C. Prior, M.D. FRCPC

(5) *http://www.cemcor.ubc.ca/help_yourself/articles/challenge_pcos*
Help for Anovulatory Androgen Excess (AAE)—Challenge PCOS! by Dr. Jerilynn C. Prior and Celeste Wincapaw

(6) *http://www.cemcor.ubc.ca/files/uploads/Cyclic_Progesterone_Therapy.pdf*
INFORMATION FOR WOMEN: CYCLIC PROGESTERONE THERAPY Protocol for treatment.

(7) *http://www.cemcor.ubc.ca/files/uploads/Menstrual_Cycle_Diary_with_treatments.pdf*
Menstrual Cycle Diary / Log Book / Calendar

(8) *http://www.natural-progesterone-advisory-network.com/what-is-the-guidelines-to-progesterone-dosage/*
What is the guidelines to progesterone dosage for PCOS ? National Progesterone Advisory Network

(9) *http://www.drlam.com/A3R_brief_in_doc_format/progesterone.cfm*
Dr. Lam Progesterone Page

(10) *http://www.virginiahopkinstestkits.com/pcos.html*
What Your Dr. May Not Tell You about PCOS, Polycystic Ovary Syndrome (PCOS), A New Epidemic that Causes Infertility, Excess Hair, Acne and More By John R. Lee, M.D. and Virginia Hopkins

(11) *http://www.townsendletter.com/Nov2004/phyto1104.htm*
Townsend Letter, Phytotherapy for Polycystic Ovarian Syndrome (PCOS) by Angela Hywood N.D. & Kerry Bone, Townsend Letter message Boards

(12) *http://pcos.meetup.com/217/*
PCOS GROUPS and Message Boards, The Arizona Polycystic Ovarian Syndrome Meetup Group,

(13) *http://search.yahoo.com/search?p=pcos+message+board&fr=yfp-t-501-s&toggle=1&cop=mss&ei=UTF-8*
Hundreds of PCOS Message Boards

(14) *http://www.early-pregnancy-tests.com/vitex.html*
Home Ovulation Tests, Pregnancy Test Kits, Basal Thermometers

Birth Control Pills

(15) *http://www.sensible-alternative.com.au/polycystic_ovarian_syndrome.html*
The Birth Control Pill is NOT the Answer. The birth control pill does absolutely nothing to improve insulin resistance, and can actually worsen it

(16) *http://jcem.endojournals.org/cgi/content/full/82/9/3074*
The Journal of Clinical Endocrinology & Metabolism Vol. 82, No. 9 3074-3077. The Effect of a Desogestrel-Containing Oral Contraceptive on Glucose Tolerance and Leptin Concentrations in Hyperandrogenic Women Shahla Nader, Maggy G. Riad-Gabriel and Mohammed F. Saad

(17) *http://jcem.endojournals.org/cgi/content/full/88/5/1927*
Diamanti-Kandarakis, E et al. A modern medical quandary: Polycystic Ovary Syndrome, Insulin Resistance, and Oral Contraceptive Pills. J Clin End Met 2003.88(5): 1927-1932 CONTROVERSIES IN ENDOCRINOLOGY Evanthia Diamanti-Kandarakis, Jean-Patrice Baillargeon, Maria J. Iuorno, Daniela J. Jakubowicz and John E. Nestler

(18) *http://www.ncbi.nlm.nih.gov/pubmed/16409223*
Panzer et al. Impact of Oral Contraceptives on Sex Hormone-Binding Globulin and Androgen Levels: A Retrospective Study in Women with Sexual Dysfunction. The Journal of Sexual Medicine. 2006. 3:p.104-113

(19) *http://www.eurekalert.org/pub_releases/2006-01/bpl-ocp121305.php*
Birth Control Pill Side effects. Oral contraceptive pill may prevent more than pregnancy

New research indicates birth control pill could cause long-term problems with testosterone

(20) http://ditchthepill.org/
Ditch the Pill . org, very negative about BCPs

Jones, M.D. Medical Director, Women's Health Institute

THYROID References

(21) http://www.ncbi.nlm.nih.gov/pubmed/16208308
Abstract Minerva Endocrinol. 2005 Sep;30*(3)*:193-7. Relationship between insulin secretion, and thyroid and ovary function in patients suffering from polycystic ovary. CONCLUSIONS: The data obtained in our study enable us to support the close connection between ovary function, thyroid function and insulin-resistance. In all patients, in fact, albeit at different times, an improvement was obtained in all 3 pathologies.

(22) http://www.ncbi.nlm.nih.gov/pubmed/17302862
Thyroid disease and female reproduction. Poppe K, Velkeniers B, Glinoer D. Clin Endocrinol *(Oxf)*. 2007 Mar;66*(3)*:309-21

(23) http://www.ncbi.nlm.nih.gov/pubmed/15012623
High prevalence of autoimmune thyroiditis in patients with polycystic ovary syndrome. Janssen OE. Eur J Endocrinol. 2004 Mar;150*(3)*:363-9. CONCLUSION: This prospective study demonstrates a threefold higher prevalence of Autoimmune Thyroid disorders in patients with PCOS

Prevalence of PCOS in Population

(24) http://jcem.endojournals.org/cgi/content/full/85/7/2434
A Prospective Study of the Prevalence of the Polycystic Ovary Syndrome in Unselected Caucasian Women from Spain. Our results demonstrate a 6.5% prevalence of PCOS, as defined, in a minimally biased population of Caucasian women from Spain. The polycystic ovary syndrome, hirsutism, and acne are common endocrine disorders in women. The Journal of Clinical Endocrinology & Metabolism Vol. 85, No. 7 2434-2438

Thyroid References

(25) http://www.ncbi.nlm.nih.gov/pubmed/8053991
Hypothyroidism presenting with polycystic ovary syndrome.Sridhar GR. J Assoc Physicians India. 1993 Feb;41*(2)*:88-90.

(26) http://www.ncbi.nlm.nih.gov/pubmed/17954423
Precocious puberty and large multicystic ovaries in young girls with primary hypothyroidism.Sanjeevaiah AR et al. Endocr Pract. 2007 Oct;13*(6)*:652-5.

(27) http://www.ncbi.nlm.nih.gov/pubmed/17917634.
Vaginal bleeding with multicystic ovaries and a pituitary mass in a child with severe hypothyroidism. Mohsin F, Nahar et al. Mymensingh Med J. 2007 Jul;16*(2 Suppl)*:S60-62

(28) *http://www.ncbi.nlm.nih.gov/pubmed/2729396*
Spontaneous ovarian hyperstimulation syndrome associated with hypothyroidism. Rotmensch S et al. Am J Obstet Gynecol. 1989 May;160*(5 Pt 1)*:1220-2.

(29) *http://www.ncbi.nlm.nih.gov/pubmed/17954423?*
Precocious puberty and large multicystic ovaries in young girls with primary hypothyroidism.Sanjeevaiah AR et al. Endocr Pract. 2007 Oct;13*(6)*:652-5.

(30) *http://www.ncbi.nlm.nih.gov/pubmed/16864150*
Primary hypothyroidism presenting as ovarian tumor and precocious puberty in a prepubertal girl. Campaner AB et al. Gynecol Endocrinol. 2006 Jul;22*(7)*:395-8.

(31) *http://www.ncbi.nlm.nih.gov/pubmed/16995569*
Ovarian cysts in young girls with hypothyroidism: follow-up and effect of treatment. Sharma Y et al. J Pediatr Endocrinol Metab. 2006 Jul;19*(7)*:895-900.

(32) *http://www.jacemedical.com/articles/Sub-laboratory%20Hypothyroidism%20.pdf*
"Sub-laboratory" Hypothyroidism and the Empirical use of Armour Thyroid Alan R. Gaby, MD . Excellent review on subclinical hypothyroidism.

Iodine and PCOS

(33) *http://www.optimox.com/pics/Iodine/pdfs/IOD02.pdf*
Orthoiodosupplementation: Iodine sufficiency of the whole human Guy. E. Abraham M.D.1, Jorge D. Flechas M.D.2 and John C. Hakala R.Ph. Our preliminary experience with I supplementation at 12.5 mg/day.

(34) *http://optimox.com/pics/Iodine/opt_Research_I.shtml*
Listing of Iodine publications at the Optimox Web Site.

(35) *http://optimox.com/pics/Iodine/IOD-10/IOD_10.htm*
Orthoiodosupplementation in a Primary Care Practice Jorge D. Flechas, M.D.

(36) *http://cypress.he.net/~bigmacnc/drflechas/index.htm*
HelpMyThyroid, George Flechas MD web site

Vitamin D and PCOS

(37) *http://www.ncbi.nlm.nih.gov/pubmed/17177140*
Low serum 25-hydroxyvitamin D concentrations are associated with insulin resistance and obesity in women with polycystic ovary syndrome. Exp Clin Endocrinol Diabetes. 2006 Nov;114*(10)*:577-83. Hahn S et al.

(38) *http://www.ncbi.nlm.nih.gov/pubmed/10433180*
Vitamin D and calcium dysregulation in the polycystic ovarian syndrome.Thys-Jacobs S et al. Steroids. 1999 Jun;64*(6)*:430-5.

METFORMIN

(39) *http://content.nejm.org/cgi/content/extract/358/1/47*
Metformin for the Treatment of the Polycystic Ovary Syndrome John E. Nestler, M.D. N. Engl. J. Med., January 3, 2008; 358(1): 47 - 54.

(39A) *http://www.ovarian-cysts-pcos.com/glucophage-metformin-pcos.html*
PCOS and Metformin (Glucophage)

Diet and Weight Loss

(40) *http://www.ovarian-cysts-pcos.com/pcos-book-res.html*
The Natural Diet Solution for PCOS and Infertility Nancy Dunne, ND Bill Slater, MBA

(41) *http://www.ovarian-cysts-pcos.com/PCOS-success.html#sec1*
PCOS success stories by Nancy Dunne

Conventional Medical Diagnosis and Treatment of PCOS

(42) *http://www.amazon.com/Clinical-Gynecologic-Endocrinology-Infertility-Editorial/dp/0781747953*
Speroff on PCOS: Clinical Gynecologic Endocrinology and Infertility by Leon Speroff MD p.493

(43) *http://assets.cambridge.org/97805218/48497/excerpt/9780521848497_excerpt.pdf*
Exerpt from Book: Introduction: Polycystic ovary syndrome is an intergenerational problem. Gabor T. Kovacs and Robert Norman Cambridge University Press 978-0-521-84849-7 - Polycystic Ovary Syndrome, Second Edition

(44) *http://findarticles.com/p/articles/mi_qa3890/is_200407/ai_n9457295/pg_1*
Hoyt, Karri Lynn "Polycystic Ovary (Stein-Leventhal) Syndrome: Etiology, Complications, and Treatment". Clinical Laboratory Science. Summer 2004.

(45) *http://health.nytimes.com/health/guides/disease/polycystic-ovary-disease/overview.html*
Polycystic Ovary Disease article in the New York Times

(46) *http://www.ebmonline.org/cgi/content/full/229/5/369*
MINIREVIEW, Screening for and Treatment of Polycystic Ovary Syndrome in Teenagers.

Experimental Biology and Medicine 229:369-377 (2004) Darren J. Salmi et al.

(47) *http://www.drgalen.com/pcos.html*
Dr. Galen, Reproductive Science Center[a] of the San Francisco Bay Area, POLYCYSTIC OVARY SYNDROME (PCOS) Treatment of PCOS:

(48) *http://www.clinmedres.org/cgi/content/full/2/1/13*
Clinical Medicine & Research Volume 2, Number 1 : 13 -27, 2004, Polycystic Ovarian Syndrome: Diagnosis and Management Michael T. Sheehan, MD. Marshfield Clinic. Excellent review of conventional diagnosis and treatment for PCOS.

(49) *http://www.inciid.org/printpage.php?cat=pcos&id=505*
Understanding and managing Polycystic Ovarian Syndrome *(*PCOS*)* by Sam Thatcher, M.D., Ph.D. director of the Center for Applied Reproductive Science in Johnson City, TN,. Conventional Approach.

(50) *http://www.perspectivespress.com/0-944934-25-0.html*
PCOS: The Hidden Epidemic. a Book by Sam Thatcher MD PhD, Conventional Approach to PCOS.

(51) *http://www.emedicine.com/ped/topic2155.htm*
Polycystic Ovarian Syndrome Last Updated: September 15, 2006, on E-Medicine.

(52) *http://www.endotext.org/female/female6/female6.htm*
ENDOTEXT.COM, HYPERANDROGENISM, HIRSUTISM AND POLYCYSTIC OVARY SYNDROMEChapter 6 - Randall B. Barnes, M.D., Adrienne B. Neithardt, M.D. and Suleena K. Kalra, M.D.November 19, 2003 on Endotext.com

(53) *http://jcem.endojournals.org/cgi/content/full/89/2/453*
EXTENSIVE PERSONAL EXPERIENCE Androgen Excess in Women: Experience with Over 1000 Consecutive Patients R. AZZIZ et al. The Journal of Clinical Endocrinology & Metabolism 89*(*2*)*:453–462.

(54) *http://www.joplink.net/prev/200201/ref/01-02.html*
Stein IF, Leventhal ML. Amenorrhoea associated with bilateral polycystic ovaries. Am J Obstet Gynecol 1935;29:181–91. Original article 1935.

The Environment, Endocrine Disruptor Chemicals and PCOS

(55) *http://www.ourstolenfuture.org/Consensus/2005/2005-1030vallombrosa.htm*
Vallombrosa Consensus Statement on Environmental contaminants and human fertility compromise. October 2005.

(56) *http://www.ourstolenfuture.org/index.htm*
Our Stolen Future, endocrine disruptors in the environment

(57) *http://www.ovarian-cysts-pcos.com/news13-pcos-pesticides.html#sec1*
Pesticides and PCOS

(58) *http://humupd.oxfordjournals.org/cgi/reprint/7/3/323.pdf*
Endocrine Disruptors as environmental cause of PCOSThe impact of Endocrine Disruptors on the Female Reproductive System, Stamati and pitsos et al.

Testosterone for Women

(59) *http://www.asrm.org/Literature/Menopausal_Medicine/menomedsummer01.pdf*
Testosterone Treatment: Psychological and Physical Effects in Postmenopausal Women. Susan R. Davis, Ph.D. Menopausal Volume 9, Number 2, Summer 2001

Diet for PCOS

(61) *http://pcos.is/files/pcosbook1.pdf*
A complete online book on Diet and Nutrition for PCOS by Nancy Dunn

(62) *http://www.topfitonline.com/chartglycemic.htm*
Glycemic Index Chart - handy and useful.

Questionnaire for PCOS

(63) *http://www.cfp.ca/cgi/content/full/53/6/1041/T50531041*
Table 5 Clinical tool for diagnosis of polycystic ovary syndrome. Can Fam Physician Vol. 53, No. 6, June 2007, pp.1041 - 1047 , Polycystic ovary syndrome. Validated questionnaire for use in diagnosis, Sue D. Pedersen, et al.

(64) *http://www.pubmedcentral.nih.gov/articlerender.fcgi?tool=pmcentrez&artid=194 9220*
Can Fam Physician. 2007 June; 53*(6)*: 1041–1047. Polycystic ovary syndrome. Validated questionnaire for use in diagnosis, Sue D. Pedersen, et al.

(65) *http://www.acamnet.org/site/c.ltJWJ4MPIwE/b.2242497/k.2C78/Integrative_Medicine_Physicians/apps/kb/cs/contactsearch.asp*
ACAM doctor's directory to find a physician.

(66) *http://www.worldhealth.net/pages/directory*
A4M doctor's directory to find a physician.

(67) *http://jeffreydach.com/2008/02/27/a-commonly-missed-cause-of-infertility-non-classical-cah-by-jeffrey-dach-md.aspx*
A Commonly Missed Cause of Infertility, NonClassical CAH by Jeffrey Dach MD

Chapter 24

NonClassical CAH, Congenital Adrenal Hyperplasia

Irregular Menstrual Cycles, Acne, and Hirsutism

Our nation spends millions of dollars on laser hair removal treatments, and acne skin treatments.*(1)* Infertile women spend small fortunes on sophisticated in-vitro fertilization techniques. Many of these women actually have a common genetic disorder called **Non-Classical CAH** which occurs in 3% of certain ethnic groups, and the diagnosis may be missed by the medical system. Curative treatment is an inexpensive tablet costing pennies a day, called Dexamethasone, given at bedtime which restores fertility and cycle regularity, and eliminates the hirsutism *(*facial hair*)* and acne.

An estimated ten percent of Poly Cystic Ovary Syndrome *(*PCOS*)* patients may have underlying Non-Classical CAH causing irregular menstrual periods, acne, hirsutism *(*unwanted facial hair*)* and infertility. A previous chapter discussed PCOS, *Understanding PCOS, the Hidden Epidemic.(2)*

What is NonClassical CAH? NonClassical Congenital Adrenal Hyperplasia, Non-Classical 21 Hydroxylase Deficiency *(*NC21OHD*)*

Non Classical CAH- A Common Genetic Disorder

Non-Classical CAH or 21-Hydroxylase Deficiency is the most common genetic disease known, occurring in 1% of New Yorkers, and up to 3% in ethnic groups such as Ashkenazi Jews, Hispanics, Italians, and Yugoslavs.*(3)*

Adrenal Gland Enzyme Deficiency, and Reduced Ability to Make Cortisol

The underlying genetic disorder causes an enzyme deficiency in the adrenal gland which reduces the ability of the adrenal to make cortisol. Instead of making cortisol, the adrenal steroid pathways are shunted towards testosterone causing elevated testosterone and the typical symptoms of hair growth *(*hirsutism*)*, and acne and there may also be menstrual irregularities, anovulation, and infertility.*(3)(4)*

What is the 21 Hydroxylase Enzyme?

This is a key enzyme in the adrenal gland involved in the conversion of cholesterol into cortisol. In the Classical form of CAH, the 21 hydroxylase enzyme *(*21-OH*)* is severely deficient with resulting low cortisol levels, and high testosterone levels. In the Non-Classical form however, the 21 hydroxylase *(*21-OH*)* enzyme is still working fairy well with only a slight reduction in activity, and cortisol levels are usually normal, while testosterone levels may be elevated to a variable degree. The Adrenal Steroid synthesis pathways are displayed as a chart, which can be found on Quest web site.*(5)*

How to Make the Diagnosis of Non-Classical CAH? Use Cortrosyn Stimulation.

The most definitive diagnosis is done with a Cortrosyn Stimulation test *(*0.25 mg*)* which measures 17-hydroxyprogesterone *(*17-OHP*)* at 0 and 60 minutes after SQ injection of the Cortrosyn *(*ACTH*)*. This is a description of how this test is performed: First a preliminary *(*baseline *)* blood test is done for various hormones including 17-OHP, this is followed by a subcutaneous injection of 0.25 mg of a drug called Cortrosyn which is a form of ACTH which stimulates the adrenal glands to make more hormones. An hour *(*60 minutes*)* after the Cortrosyn injection, a post stimulation blood sample is drawn for lab testing for 17-OHP and other hormones. Classification of CAH depends on 17-OH-Progesterone *(*17-OHP*)* values on stimulated test. Patients with Non Classic 21-OH Deficiency typically show 60-min stimulated 17-OHP values between 1,500 and 10,000 ng/dl. The 17-OHP values cluster at three areas. Normal is below 1,500, Non-Classical CAH clusters from 1500 to 10,000 and, and Classical CAH is above 10,000.*(6)(7)*

Genetic Testing for 21-OH Deficiency

Genetic testing for non-classical CAH is now available and very useful. The genetic test shows whether or not there is a mutation in the CYP21A2 gene coding for the 21-Hydroxylase Enzyme.*(8)* This test is available at both Quest and LabCorp. The **CAHDtex** test by Esoterix is useful in showing the exact mutation in the CYP21A2 gene.*(9)* Once the exact mutation in the CYP21A2 gene is known, one can refer to a *chart* to determine the severity of the enzyme defect.*(10)* Genetic testing of other family members is usually recommended once a sibling is found with the mutation. Dr. Maria New has her own in-house lab in New York which does genetic testing for CAH.*(11)*

Clinical Presentation in Children

In children, the signs of non-classical CAH include premature onset of puberty, cystic acne, accelerated growth, and advanced bone age. Premature development of pubic hair may occur as early as 6 months of age *(*due to elevated testosterone*)*. The severe cystic acne may be unresponsive to oral antibiotics and retinoic acid *(*Accutane*)*. Although the child may be taller than the other kids in early childhood, this early growth spurt finishes early *(*because of epiphyseal fusion*)*, and final height ends up shorter than usual. Thus, these kids are tall children but short adults. Another feature may be male pattern baldness in a female involving the top of the head and sparing the sides.

Teenagers and Young Adults - Major Cause of Infertility

Teenage girls may present with features of elevated testosterone such as facial hair *(*hirsutism*)*, acne and menstrual irregularities or anovulation. Young adult females may present with the chief complaint of infertility. It has been generally recognized that infertility of undetermined cause in women may be reversed with glucocorticoid *(*cortef or prednisone*)* therapy, which most likely treats an occult Non-Classical CAH Syndrome. William Mc Jefferies MD successfully treated thousands of such cases described in his 1983 medical classic, The Safe Uses of Cortisol.*(12)* Dr. McJefferies speculated correctly that an abnormality in adrenal steroid synthesis was present in many young girls with infertility, and only years later was the exact molecular and genetic basis elucidated as non-classical CAH. In retrospect, non-classical CAH should be re-named McJefferies Syndrome, thus giving appropriate credit to this great clinician who successfully treated many of these cases from 1950 to 1990.

Treatment of Non Classical CAH with Cortisol Restores Fertility

Oral tablets containing low dose cortisol successfully treat Non-Classical CAH and reverse the symptoms restoring fertility. The cortisol suppresses ACTH and reduces the testosterone production by the adrenal. **Dr. Maria I New** is a national expert on non-classical CAH, and she has followed a large group of 400 patients with Non-Classical CAH. Dr. New treats them with 0.25 mg. dexamethasone taken before bedtime. Dr. New reports that it takes about 3 months for reversal of acne and infertility. Hirsutism takes longer to respond, about 30 months.*(3)(13)*

The cost for a dexamethasone tablet is $0.50, and the 3-month treatment cost is estimated to be $45. Compare this $45 dollars to the infertility treatment cost of $30,000 for one cycle of in vitro fertilization. Dr. Maria New says that many patients presenting with infertility actually have NonClassical CAH, and fertility could be restored easily with treatment with oral cortisol tablets such as Dexamethasone, Prednisone or even the Cortef recommended by McJefferies.*(3)* Before spending a fortune on in-vitro fertilization for infertility, it would be prudent to rule out Non-Classical CAH with a simple genetic test.

Safety of Low Dose Cortisol

Low dose Cortef, Prednisone or Dexamethasone treatment is safe without the adverse side effects associated with high dose treatment. However, there is a chance of mild adrenal suppression which could require additional or extra doses of medication under periods of higher stress or illness such as the flu or when undergoing a surgical operation. Therefore McJefferies routinely gave instructions to increase the cortisol dosage when a flu illness is noted coming on or under similar stresses. He also advised his patients to wear a warning bracelet containing the information that the patient has non classical CAH, with cortisol dosage and timing.*(12)*

REFERENCES

(1) http://jcem.endojournals.org/cgi/content/full/91/11/4205/T7
TABLE 7. National health care burden for treatment of hyperandrogenic signs associated with NC21OHD. EXTENSIVE CLINICAL EXPERIENCE Nonclassical 21-Hydroxylase Deficiency Maria I. New The Journal of Clinical Endocrinology & Metabolism Vol. 91, No. 11 4205-4214

(2) http://jeffreydach.com/2008/02/13/understanding-pcos-the-hidden-epidemic-by-jeffrey-dach-md.aspx
Understanding PCOS, the Hidden Epidemic by Jeffrey Dach, M.D.

(3) http://jcem.endojournals.org/cgi/content/full/91/11/4205
EXTENSIVE CLINICAL EXPERIENCE. Nonclassical 21-Hydroxylase Deficiency by Maria I. New MD. The Journal of Clinical Endocrinology & Metabolism Vol. 91, No. 11 4205-4214.

(4) http://www.mcg.edu/pediatrics/pedsendo/21.pdf
Consensus Statement on Treatment of 21-Hydroxylase Deficiency. JCEM 87*(9)*:4048-4053, 2002.

(5) http://www.questdiagnostics.com/hcp/intguide/EndoMetab/Gen_Misc/TG_CAH/TG_CAH_Fig1.pdf
Adrenal Steroid Pathways chart Quest Labs

(6) http://jcem.endojournals.org/cgi/content/full/91/11/4205/F5
FIG. 5. Nomogram relating baseline to ACTH-stimulated serum concentrations of 17-OHP. From Maria New article.

(7) http://www.questdiagnostics.com/hcp/intguide/jsp/showintguidepage.jsp?fn=EndoMetab/Gen_Misc/TG_CAH/TG_CAH.htm
Congenital Adrenal Hyperplasia Test Guide Quest Labs

(8) http://www.questdiagnostics.com/hcp/intguide/EndoMetab/EndoManual_AtoZ_PDFs/CAH_Common.pdf
Quest Lab Test Code 14755X - a genetic test for the common mutations for CAH 21 hydroxylase deficiency

(9) http://www.esoterix.com/files/ss_cah.pdf
DNA TESTING FOR 21-HYDROXYLASE DEFICIENCY. Esoterix introduces a new DNA test to identify deficiency in the 21-hydroxylase gene, the most common cause of congenital adrenal hyperplasia *(CAH)*. **CAHDetx** evaluates the CYP21 gene, detecting mutations

and gene deletion/conversions that account for approximately 90% to 95% of all CAH cases.

(10) *http://jcem.endojournals.org/cgi/content-nw/full/91/11/4205/T1*
TABLE 1. Common gene mutations of the 21-hydroxylase gene CYP21A2 from Maria New

(11) *http://www.marianew.com/Laboratory.html*
CONGENITAL ADRENAL HYPERPLASIA DNA TESTING FOR 21-HYDROXYLASE DEFICIENCY FACT SHEET. Maria New MD Laboratory

(12) *http://www.amazon.com/review/R2IPB7XGMO20NE/ref=cm_cr_rdp_perm*
Safe Use of Cortisol is a Unique Medical Classic, December 7, 2007 By Jeffrey Dach MD

(13) *http://www.marianew.com/index.html*
Dr. Maria I. New is one of the world's leading pediatric endocrinologists and children's advocates. Professor of Pediatrics, Director, Adrenal Steroid Disorders Program, Mount Sinai School of Medicine1 Gustave L. Levy Place, Box 1198, New York, NY 10029-6574

Section Eight

Heart Disease, Clogged Arteries

Chapter 25

CAT Coronary Calcium Scoring, Reversing Heart Disease

How to Reverse Heart Disease with the Coronary Calcium Score

Finally Accepted by the AHA

The AHA *(*American Heart Association*)* has steadfastly denied for many years that Coronary Calcium Scoring was a valid marker of heart disease. Well guess what? They have recanted, and admitted that the amount of calcium in the coronary arteries reliably predicts heart attack risk. This is called the calcium score.*(1)* UCLA cardiologist, Dr. Matt Budoff, a long-time champion of the Coronary Calcium Scan, and author of the AHA paper says, "The total amount of coronary calcium *(*Agatson score*)* predicts coronary disease events beyond standard risk factors."*(1)*

Dr. Detrano, in an article in the New England of Medicine, wrote that "**The coronary calcium score is a strong predictor of incident coronary heart disease and provides predictive information beyond that provided by standard risk factors".***(31)* The Coronary Calcium Score is a precise quantitative tool for measuring and tracking heart disease risk, and is more valuable and accurate than other traditional markers *(*such as total cholesterol which is practically worthless as a heart disease risk marker*)*.

What is Coronary Artery Disease? It's Plaque Formation.

In youth, there is minimal plaque formation. However, as we age with passage of time, the plaque grows larger. About 20% of this plaque volume contains calcium which is measurable on CAT scan, providing a marker for the total plaque burden. Calcium score and by inference, plaque volume, typically increases every year in untreated patients. Eventually, as we age, the enlarging plaque eventually obstructs blood flow causing a heart attack. Another common scenario is plaque rupture which exposes the inflammatory debris of the plaque to the circulating blood. This quickly results in clot formation *(*thrombosis*)* resulting in a heart attack and possibly sudden death. To summarize, the calcified portion of the plaque is consistently 20% of the total plaque volume, allowing use of the calcium score as a marker for total plaque volume.

Arterial Calcification - Why Does it Happen?

Calcification in the soft tissues *(*connective tissue, ligaments, muscles, arteries*)* is found in many disease states, and commonly identified on pathology slides of human tissues. Whenever there is cell death or tissue necrosis *(*death of cells*)*, the body invokes a process of calcification which can be regarded as part of the healing process. Arterial calcification is actually a form of bone formation in the wall of the artery triggered by an inflammatory process. Pathology studies have shown that coronary artery calcium forms in areas of **healed plaque ruptures.** *(21)* Calcification and plaque formation increases with age, with calcium score typically increasing every year in untreated patients according to William Davis MD.

What is a Heart Attack?

A heart attack is cell death of heart muscle caused by lack of blood flow with oxygen deprivation. As previously mentioned, this is caused by arterial blockage by enlarging plaque formation which occludes the lumen, or plaque rupture which causes clot formation which occludes blood flow. If a small area of heart muscle is involved, the heart attack may be silent with no symptoms. If a large area is involved, there may be severe chest pain radiating to the left arm or jaw, or other symptoms such as shortness of breath. If the conduction system is involved, there may be irregular heart rhythm called ventricular tachycardia which can cause sudden death. Some people have chronic chest pain from diseased arteries and this is called angina pectoris, treated with medicines to dilate the coronary arteries, such as nitroglycerine.

Common Sites of Plaque Formation -Bifurcations and Mechanical Stress

Ask any interventional radiologist or invasive cardiologist where they find the most plaque formation and obstructions in the arterial tree, and they will say its the same few places over and over again. These places are the carotid bifurcation, the distal aorta at the bifurcation, the femoral bifurcation, the exit from the adductor canal. And of course, another common site is in the coronary arteries near their take off from the aorta, and bifurcations of the coronary arteries. A bifurcation is where the vessel branches into two vessels, making a Y pattern.

The bifurcations have maximal turbulence and mechanical stress on the vessel wall. Remember the blood is flowing under pulsatile pressure, and this mechanical pressure and turbulence, over time, causes little stress cracks in the vessel. The cracks appear at sites of maximal stress. The coronary arteries are a special case because of the extra motion of the cardiac muscle which moves and stretches the coronary arteries every heart beat, especially as the arteries branch off from the aorta which is relatively stationary, while lower down over the surface of the heart, the vessels move vigorously with each heart beat. Atherosclerosis is the net result of the healing process for these little cracks in the arterial wall resulting from mechanical stress.

William Davis MD, Advocate of the Coronary Calcium Score

William Davis MD recommends obtaining a calcium score with a CAT heart scan in males over 40 and females over 50. This allows visualization and measurement of the amount of calcium in the coronary arteries. Dr. Davis recommends calcium score screening starting at younger ages for these high-risk patients: with a strong family history of early heart disease, cigarette smoker, diabetes mellitus, or severe lipid or lipoprotein genetic disorders.*(2)(3)* The Coronary Calcium Score test is currently covered by Medicare and many health insurances.*(32)* Credit and thanks is given to William Davis MD at the Track Your Plaque Web site for much of the information presented here. I have added a few items, though.

All About Coronary Calcium Scoring

1) Calcium scoring may be superior to angiography as a means to track plaque. That's because the vast majority of heart attacks are due to plaque rupture and thrombosis at areas of thickened plaque with minimal lumen narrowing. Over time, the body's healing process automatically remodels the areas of thickened plaque, and increases lumen size to compensate for the reduced blood flow.

2) Calcium scoring gives a precise number which correlates with the amount of plaque volume. Although only the hard plaque, or calcium in the artery is actually measured, this is useful because it consistently occupies 20% of total plaque volume, *(*i.e. total hard and soft plaque*)*.

3) The new 64-slice CAT scanners provide reliable calcium scoring just like any other scanner, both multi-slice and EBT*(*Electron Beam Cat*)*.

The Track Your Plaque Program, advocated by William Davis MD.*(2)(3)*

1) Quantify plaque with Coronary Calcium Score with CAT scan *(*or with Electron Beam CT*)*. Obtain your CAT Scan serially, every 12 months to assess response to treatment and lifestyle modification *(*track your plaque*)*.

2) Use Sophisticated Lipoprotein Panel *(*Quest-VAP , LabCorp-NMR*) (7)(8)* to uncover hidden causes of plaque progression. LDL particle size and number, Lipoprotein *(*a*)*. Repeat every 6 months.

3) The Main Treatment Goal is the reduction in Coronary Artery Calcium Score, and by inference, reduction in plaque volume and reduction in cardiovascular mortality. The cardiology community still awaits the hard data on these results *(*CHD mortality and CHD events, treatment arm vs. no treatment arm*)*. These numbers have not been published as far as I know.

How to Measure Success in Halting or Reversing Heart Disease Plaque

According to Dr. Davis, calcium score typically increases at an astonishing rate of 30-35% per year without treatment. Therefore, Dr. Davis considers treatment success to be reduction in this rate from 30 to perhaps only a 5-10 per cent increase in calcium score per year. An absolute reduction in calcium score on follow up scanning is the optimal outcome, which is difficult to achieve even with strict adherence to the Track Your Plaque program, in Dr Davis's experience.

Track Your Plaque Program Details - Attain the Following Targets:

a*)* Reduction of LDL to 60 mg/dl *(*LDL should be measured directly, not calculated*)*.

b*)* Reduction of triglycerides to 60 mg/dl.

c*)* Raising HDL to 60 mg/dl.

d*)* Correction of hidden causes of plaque on Lipoprotein profile such as total number of small LDL particles, IDL, and Lp*(*a*)*.

e*)* Achieving normal blood pressure *(*<130/80*)* Even a small elevation of blood pressure in diseased arteries can cause increased mortality. Diseased arteries are fragile and plaque rupture can occur easily.

f*)* Achieving normal blood sugar *(*≤100 mg/dl*)*. Diabetes is a high risk factor for heart disease.

g*)* Reduction of C-reactive protein to <1 mg/l

Dietary Modification and Supplements to Attain Above Targets:

Niacin

a*)* Niacin vitamin B3 *(*Slo-Niacin Upsher-Smith *(44)* or Niaspan Kos Pharmaceuticals preferred*)* 500-1500mg. per day *(*avoid the no-flush niacin which contains inositol*).(6)(44)*

Omega 3 Fish Oil

b*)* Fish oil *(*Omega 3 oils*)* 4000 mg per day *(*providing 1200 mg omega-3 fatty acids*)*. *(*molecular distilled pharmaceutical grade*).(36)*

Vitamin D

c) Vitamin D level restored to above 50 ng/ml *(*Vitamin D3 2000-5,000 u/day*)*, Vitamin K2 also used. Low vitamin D is associated with increasing arterial calcification and increased heart disease risk.*(26)* Consumption of calcium tablets by women increases arterial calcification and heart attack risk.*(5)* A previous chapter dealt with vitamin D.*(60)*

d) Low Glycemic Diet (avoid Fructose Corn Syrup, avoid wheat products), and eliminate wheat products like Shredded Wheat cereal, Raisin Bran, and whole wheat bagels.

e) Consume foods such as raw almonds, walnuts, pecans; olive oil and canola oil. Beneficial for lipoprotein profile.

f) Increasing protein intake, our major building block for body tissues. Added benefit of protein intake is that it doesn't increase blood sugar. This is low glycemic nutrition.

g) Wine—Red wines contain resveratrol, (don't exceed two glasses/ day). Bioflavonoids and anti-oxidants have a strong anti-inflammatory effect.

h) Fiber - Ground flaxseed (2 tbsp/day)-Extra fiber aids in detoxifying liver and the entire body by interrupting the enterohepatic circulation. Psyllium (metamucil). Regulates bowel movements and has favorable effect on lipoprotein profile.

Vitamin C

Vitamin C (1000–3000 mg/day), is a key player, as it is the vitamin for strong collagen formation, strengthening the arterial wall. See Linus Pauling's patented protocol which includes Vitamin C and amino acids Proline and Lysine, the two amino acids that act as receptors for Lp(a). By consuming additional Lysine and Proline, the receptor sites on the Lp(a) and other lipoproteins are covered up and made less sticky, resulting in less deposition in the artery wall. The vitamin C is important not only for strong collagen formation, a major component of the arterial wall, but also for all other structural elements of the body, for that matter. *(37)(52)(53)(54)(55)(56)(57)*

Humans have a genetic deficiency in Gulano-Lactone-Oxidase (GLO), the final enzyme step in the manufacture of Vitamin C, and therefore unlike all the other animals who make their own Vitamin C, we cannot make this necessary vitamin. We share with all other primates this genetic disease, the inability to manufacture vitamin C, producing a vitamin C deficiency state in all humans.*(58)* For more on this topic, I strongly recommend Thomas Levy's two books on Vitamin C. *(49)(50)(51)*

j) Exercise and weight loss- improves insulin sensitivity, reduces inflammatory markers, reduces blood pressure, improves lipoprotein profile.

Magnesium

k) Magnesium supplementation is inexpensive and safe. Magnesium deficiency due to dietary deficiency or thiazide diuretics for hypertension is common, and is associated with increased heart disease risk. Magnesium reduces blood pressure, relaxes smooth muscle in arteries, and is needed for normal endothelial function.*(41)(42)(43)*

L-Arginine

L-arginine is converted to nitric oxide, an important substance for arterial health. Research by Furchgott and other showed that nitric oxide (NO) relaxes arterial smooth muscle, dilating coronary arteries by up to 50%.*(35)* However, Nitric Oxide (NO) is gone after a few seconds, so nitric oxide must be replenished at a constant rate to keep the arteries relaxed and open. Lack of NO is associated with constricted arteries, damage to the arterial lining, and accelerated plaque growth. L-arginine shrinks coronary plaque, corrects "endothelial dysfunction", improves insulin sensitivity, is anti-inflammatory and shrinks plaque.

Reverse Cholesterol Transport and Essential Phospholipid - Phosphatidyl Choline (PC) *(38)(39)*

James C. Roberts MD FACC, a practicing invasive cardiologist in Toledo Ohio, reports clinical success with Phosphatidylcholine (IV or in Liposomal oral form with EDTA). He gives a talk entitled, "Reverse Cholesterol Transport and Metal Detoxification". A DVD of his lectures is available which describes considerable clinical success with oral EDTA and phosphytidylcholine. His lecture material, complete with clinical case histories is posted on his web site.*(61)*

Essential Phospholipid is available under trade name Phoschol which increases Lecithin Cholesterol Acyl Transferase activity (LCAT) (Dobiasova M 1988).*(40)*(40b) Activating LCAT is beneficial because LCAT is the crucial substance which transports cholesterol from the arterial plaque back to the liver for metabolic breakdown into bile. This process reverses atherosclerotic plaque formation.*(38)(39)*

Thyroid Function

Normalize thyroid function. Broda Barnes MD showed that low thyroid function was a significant risk factor for heart disease. This conclusion was based on autopsy data from Graz Austria and detailed in his book, Hypothyroidism the Unsuspected Illness, and his other book, Solved the Riddle of Heart Attacks. Barnes felt that the thyroid lab tests were frequently unreliable, and he used clinical judgment instead of lab tests to determine when to treat with thyroid hormone. *(59)*

All About Reducing Lipoprotein (a)(2)(3)

Lipoprotein little A, also written as Lp(a) is a genetic variant lipoprotein which is associated with a high risk of heart disease, and therefore identification and reduction is essential for preventing heart attacks. The problem is that the conventional lipid test panels done in your doctor's office do not include Lp(a). Only the more sophisticated lipoprotein panels such as the VAP (Atherotech) or NMR (Liposcience) panels provide Lp(a) data.

Lp(a) and Lipoproteins:

1) Lp(a) is best to measured in (nmol/l), and target below 75 nmol/l .

2) Lp(a) measured in mg/dl (weight may not be accurate), then target below 30 mg/dl.

3) Measured (not calculated) LDL target 50–60 mg/dl.

4) Target the LDL particle number (by NMR) of 600–700 nmol/l or Apoprotein B of 50–60 mg/dl. Reduce small LDL to <10% of total LDL.

Treating Lp(a) with Niacin

The forms of Niacin recommended by Dr. Davis are Niaspan (prescription from Kos Pharmaceuticals) or over-the-counter Slo-Niacin(Upsher-Smith). Both are better tolerated than OTC plain niacin, with less side effects of the well known hot flushes from the niacin. The niacin induced hot flushes are aggravated by dehydration or alcohol consumption. Certain types of wine can magnify the hot flushing from niacin. The flushing can be reduced or avoided by drinking a full glass of water with each niacin gelcap. Some find that taking an aspirin tablet with the niacin helps to reduce the hot flushing.

Lp(a) and BioIdentical Hormones

Bio-Identical hormones are beneficial for reducing heart disease. In menopausal females, estrogen preparations such as Bi-Est are used. Estrogens have been shown to reduce coronary artery calcium score.(46) In males over 50, bio-identical testosterone cream may lowers Lp(a) by as much as 25% (William Davis MD). Medical studies show that optimizing Testosterone levels in aging males can reduce risk of coronary artery disease by 60%. (47)(48) DHEA can promote weight loss, and improve insulin sensitivity.(45)

Lp*(a)* and L-Carnitine

The supplement L-carnitine can be a useful adjunct; 2000–4000 mg per day *(*1000 mg twice a day*)* can reduce Lp*(a)* 7–8%, and occasionally will reduce it up to 20%.

Remember, reduction in calcium score on follow up calcium scan is the goal.

What about Statin-Cholesterol Lowering drugs, and Calcium ?

Dr. Davis admits that the total cholesterol and the LDL cholesterol numbers are of little value in predicting heart disease risk. And he says that the statin drug side effects, ie. muscle pain and weakness, are more common in actual practice than the drug advertising would suggest, making statin drugs difficult to take for the long term. In my opinion, statin drugs are not recommended for women as explained in my previous chapter on Statin Drugs for Women, Just Say No.*(33)* Also look at my other chapter on Statins, Lipitor and the Dracula of Medical Technology.*(34)* Dr. Davis points out that women who take calcium tablets have double the risk of heart attacks than those on placebo.*(5)*

A heartfelt thanks and credit goes to William Davis MD for putting together the best heart disease prevention program on the web at the Track Your Plaque Web Site and Blog. Much of the above information came from Dr. Davis.*(2)(3)*

References:

(1) http://circ.ahajournals.org/cgi/content/full/114/16/1761
*(*Circulation. 2006;114:1761-1791.*)* AHA Scientific Statement
Assessment of Coronary Artery Disease by Cardiac Computed Tomography
A Scientific Statement From the American Heart Association. Matthew J. Budoff, MD et al.

(2) http://www.trackyourplaque.com/index.asp
William R. Davis, MD, FACC, Track Your Plaque 2600 N. Mayfair Road, Suite 950 Wauwatosa, WI 53226 414-456-1123 414-456-1766

(3) http://heartscanblog.blogspot.com/
William Davis Track Your Plaque Blog

(4) http://atvb.ahajournals.org/cgi/content/full/19/5/1250
Fish Intake, Independent of Apo*(a)* Size, Accounts for Lower Plasma Lipoprotein*(a)* Levels in Bantu Fishermen of Tanzania The Lugalawa Study. Santica M. Marcovina et al. Arteriosclerosis, Thrombosis, and Vascular Biology. 1999;19:1250-1256.

(5) http://www.bmj.com/cgi/content/full/bmj.39440.525752.BEv1
Vascular events in healthy older women receiving calcium supplementation: randomised controlled trial. Bolland MJ, Barber PA, Doughty RN et al. BMJ, published 15 January 2008.

(6) http://www.upsher-smith.com/legacy/products/sloniacin/sloniacinintro.html
Slo Niacin Upsher Smith

(7) http://www.liposcience.com/
LipoScience NMR Lipiprotein Analysis through LabCorp

(8) http://www.thevaptest.com/
Atherotec VAP Lipid analysis through Quest

(9) http://www.scct.org/news/clinical_consensus_coronary_artery_calcium_scoring.pdf
ACCF/AHA 2007 Clinical Expert Consensus Document on Coronary Artery Calcium Scoring By Computed Tomography in Global Cardiovascular Risk Assessment, Journal of the American College of Cardiology Vol. 49, No. 3, 2007

(10) http://archinte.ama-assn.org/cgi/content/full/164/12/1285
Using the Coronary Artery Calcium Score to Predict Coronary Heart Disease Events. A Systematic Review and Meta-analysis Mark J. Pletcher, MD et al. Arch Intern Med. 2004;164:1285-1292. Vol. 164 No. 12, June 28, 2004

(11) http://www.heartscan.com/
Dr. John Rumberger. Heart Scan 2161 Ygnacio Valley Road Suite #100 Walnut Creek, CA 94598

(12) http://www.heartscan.com/Budoff_EBCT.pdf
Why EBCT? by Matthew Budoff, MD, FACC, FAHA Assoc. Professor of Medicine, Director, Cardiac CT Harbor-UCLA Medical Center, Torrance, CA

(13) http://www.heartscan.com/Clinton_heart_disease.pdf
Clinton Heart Disease Reveals Misconceptions about Testing Colorado Heart & Body Imaging says "Clinton Syndrome" reveals limitations of stress tests and promise of EBT heart scans

(14) http://www.ajronline.org/cgi/content/abstract/95/3/667
THE SIGNIFICANCE OF CORONARY CALCIFICATION. Joseph Jorgens et al. A J R, Vol 95, 667-672, 1965 by American Roentgen Ray Society

(15) http://www.ajronline.org/cgi/content/full/187/1/73
How Predictive Is Breast Arterial Calcification of Cardiovascular Disease and Risk Factors When Found at Screening Mammography? AJR 2006; 187:73-80

(16) http://circ.ahajournals.org/cgi/content/full/94/5/1175.
Coronary Artery Calcification: Pathophysiology, Epidemiology, Imaging Methods, and Clinical Implications. Circulation. 1996;94:1175-1192.

(17) http://www.sciencedirect.com/science?_ob=ArticleURL&_udi=B6T18-3RTYDN3
Clinical Studies Arterial Calcification and Not Lumen Stenosis Is Highly Correlated with Atherosclerotic Plaque Burden in Humans: A Histologic Study of 723 Coronary Artery Segments Using Nondecalcifying Methodology. Journal of the American College of Cardiology Volume 31, Issue 1, January 1998, Pages 126-133

(18) http://content.onlinejacc.org/cgi/content/abstract/27/2/285
Prognostic value of coronary calcification and angiographic stenoses in patients undergoing coronary angiography R Detrano et al. J Am Coll Cardiol, 1996; 27:285-290.

(19) http://aje.oxfordjournals.org/cgi/content/full/162/5/421
Coronary Artery Calcium Score and Coronary Heart Disease Events in a Large Cohort of Asymptomatic Men and Women. Michael J. LaMonte et al. American Journal of Epidemiology 2005 162*(5)*:421-429

(20) http://content.onlinejacc.org/cgi/content/abstract/49/18/1860
Long-Term Prognosis Associated With Coronary Calcification Observations From a Registry of 25,253 Patients. Matthew J. Budoff, MD et al. J Am Coll Cardiol, 2007; 49:1860-1870,

(21) http://content.onlinejacc.org/cgi/content/full/49/3/378
ACCF/AHA 2007 Clinical Expert Consensus Document on Coronary Artery Calcium Scoring By Computed Tomography in Global Cardiovascular Risk Assessment and in Evaluation of Patients With Chest Pain. J Am Coll Cardiol, 2007; 49:378-402.Philip Greenland, MD, et al.

(22) http://circ.ahajournals.org/cgi/content/full/114/5/e83
Circulation. 2006;114:e83.*)* Correspondence Response to Letter Regarding Article, "Coronary Artery Calcium: Should We Rely on This Surrogate Marker?" Rita F. Redberg, MD, MSc

(23) http://www.pubmedcentral.nih.gov/pagerender.fcgi?artid=458849&pageindex=1
Incidence and significance of coronary artery calcification. J H McCarthy and F J Palmer. Br Heart J. 1974 May; 36*(5)*: 499–506.

(24) http://circ.ahajournals.org/cgi/content/abstract/104/4/412
Long-Term Prognostic Value of Coronary Calcification Detected by Electron-Beam Computed Tomography in Patients Undergoing Coronary Angiography. Paul C. Keelan, MB. Circulation. 2001;104:412.

(25) *http://tech.snmjournals.org/cgi/content/full/36/1/18*
Cardiac CT: Indications and Limitations. Susanna Prat-Gonzalez et al. Journal of Nuclear Medicine Technology Volume 36, Number 1, 2008 18-24

(26) *http://circ.ahajournals.org/cgi/content/abstract/96/6/1755*
Active Serum Vitamin D Levels Are Inversely Correlated With Coronary Calcification. Karol E. Watson, MD et al. Circulation. 1997;96:1755-1760.

(26A) *http://circ.ahajournals.org/cgi/content/short/117/4/503*
Vitamin D Deficiency and Risk of Cardiovascular Disease. Thomas J. Wang MD et al. Circulation. 2008;117:503-511.

(27) *http://content.onlinejacc.org/cgi/content/abstract/19/6/1167*
Fluoroscopic coronary artery calcification and associated coronary disease in asymptomatic young men. TH Loecker et al. J Am Coll Cardiol, 1992; 19:1167-1172

(28) *http://diabetes.diabetesjournals.org/cgi/content/abstract/51/6/1949*
Lipoprotein Subclasses and Particle Sizes and Their Relationship With Coronary Artery Calcification in Men and Women With and Without Type 1 Diabetes. Helen M. Colhoun et al. Diabetes 51:1949-1956, 2002

(29) *http://jcem.endojournals.org/cgi/content/full/88/10/4525*
Low-Density Lipoprotein Size and Cardiovascular Disease: A Reappraisal, CLINICAL REVIEW 163: CARDIOVASCULAR ENDOCRINOLOGY Frank M. Sacks and Hannia Campos

(30) *http://www.masson.fr/masson/portal/bookmark?Global=1&Page=18&MenuIdSelected=106&MenuItemSelected=0&MenuSupportSelected=0&CodeProduct4=535&CodeRevue4= DM&Path=REVUE/DM/1999/25/3/ARTICLE11106159681.xml&Locations=* The small, dense LDL phenotype and the risk of coronary heart disease: epidemiology, patho-physiology and therapeutic aspects. Lamarche B, Lemieux I, Després JP. Diabetes & Metabolism Vol 25, NO 3,1999, p. 199.

(31) *http://content.nejm.org/cgi/content/short/358/13/1336*
Coronary Calcium as a Predictor of Coronary Events in Four Racial or Ethnic Groups. Robert Detrano ET AL. NEJM Volume 358:1336-1345 March 27, 2008 Number 13

(32) *http://www.nytimes.com/2008/03/12/business/12cnd-scan.html*
Medicare to Keep Paying for Heart Scans By REED ABELSON Published: March 12, 2008. New York Times.

(33) *http://jeffreydach.com/2008/01/27/cholesterol-lowering-statin-drugs-for-women-just-say-no-by-jeffrey-dach-md.aspx* Cholesterol Lowering Statin Drugs for Women Just Say No to Statin Drugs

(34) *http://jeffreydach.com/2007/05/14/lipitor-and-the-dracula-of-modern-technology-by-jeffrey-dach-md.aspx*
Lipitor and The Dracula of Modern Technology by Jeffrey Dach MD

(35) *http://nobelprize.org/nobel_prizes/medicine/laureates/1998/press.html*
Nobel Prize in Physiology or Medicine for 1998 jointly to Robert F. Furchgott, Louis J. Ignarro and Ferid Murad for their discoveries concerning "nitric oxide as a signalling molecule in the cardiovascular system". L-Arginine is converted to Nitric Oxide.

Fish Oil

(36) *http://www.purecaps.com/itemdy00.asp?T1=ED11*
Pure Encapsulations information on EPA/DHA.

Linus Pauling Protocol Vitamin C

(37) *http://www.internetwks.com/pauling/short.html*
Linus Pauling Protocol SHort Version for prevention, reversal of heart disease

Essential Phospholipid

(38) *http://www.phoschol.com/about_phoschol/*
Essential Phospholipid, PhosChol is 100 percent pure polyenylphosphatidylcholine (PPC), with up to 52% DLPC. In fact, PhosChol delivers the highest available concentrated source of dilinoleoylphosphatidylcholine (DLPC).

(39) *http://nutrasalpharmaceuticals.stores.yahoo.net/phoschol9001.html*
ource for PPC, 3 PhosChol capsules delivers 2700mgs of purified PPC.

(40) *http://www.jbc.org/cgi/content/full/270/10/5151*
Effect of the Cholesterol Content of Reconstituted LpA-I on Lecithin:Cholesterol Acyltransferase Activity. Daniel L. Sparks et al. J. Biol. Chem. Sparks et al. 270 (10): 5151.

(40b) Dobasiova M, Stribrna J, Matousovic K. Effect of polyenoic phospholipid therapy on lecithin cholesterol acyltransferase activity in the human serum. Physiol-Bohemoslov. 1988;37(2):165–172.

Magnesium

(41) *http://www.pubmedcentral.nih.gov/pagerender.fcgi?artid=1345822&pageindex=1#page*
A clinical approach to common electrolyte problems: Hypomagnesemia.

C Berkelhammer and R A Bear. Can Med Assoc J. 1985 February 15; 132(4): 360–368.

(42) http://www.pubmedcentral.nih.gov/articlerender.fcgi?tool=pmcentrez&artid=2146789

Muscle cramps and magnesium deficiency: case reports. D. L. Bilbey and V. M. Prabhakaran Can Fam Physician. 1996 July; 42: 1348–1351.

(43) http://www.ncbi.nlm.nih.gov/pubmed/3282851

Magnesium metabolism in health and disease. Elin RJ. Dis Mon. 1988 Apr;34*(4)*:161-218.

Slo Niacin

(44) http://www.cvs.com/CVSApp/cvs/gateway/detail?prodid=846063

Slo-Niacin at CVS drugs costs $14.99 for 100 tablets of 500 mg

DHEA

(45) http://jama.ama-assn.org/cgi/content/full/292/18/2243

Effect of DHEA on Abdominal Fat and Insulin Action in Elderly Women and Men A Randomized Controlled Trial Dennis T. Villareal, MD; John O. Holloszy, MD JAMA. 2004;292:2243-2248.

ESTROGEN

(46) http://content.nejm.org/cgi/content/short/356/25/2591

Estrogen Therapy and Coronary-Artery Calcification JoAnn E. Manson, M.D., Volume 356:2591-2602 June 21, 2007 Number 25. Results: The mean coronary-artery calcium score was lower among women receiving estrogen *(***83.1***)* than among those receiving placebo *(***123.1***)*.

Testosterone

(47) http://care.diabetesjournals.org/cgi/content/full/26/6/1929

Testosterone and Atherosclerosis Progression in Men. Shalender Bhasin, MD and Karen Herbst, MD, PHD, Diabetes Care 26:1929-1931, 2003

(48) http://www.hormoneandlongevitycenter.com/nss-folder/pictures/TestosteroneDecreasesHeartDisease.pdf

Low Levels of Endogenous Androgens Increase the Risk of Atherosclerosis in Elderly Men: The Rotterdam Study A. Elisabeth Hak et al. The Journal of Clinical Endocrinology & Metabolism. Aug 2002. Vol. 87, No. 8 3632-3639. Optimal testosterone levels in men have been shown to decrease the risk of coronary artery disease by 60%

Tom Levy MD and Vitamin C

(49) *http://www.livonlabs.com/cgi-bin/htmlos.cgi/LV/apps/stop-americas-killer.html*
STOP AMERICA'S #1 KILLER! Reversible Vitamin C deficiency found to be cause of heart disease. by Thomas E. Levy, MD JD

(50) *http://www.tomlevymd.com/*
Tom Levy MD Web site

(51) *http://www.livonbooks.com/*
Tom Levy MD author of two books on Vitamin C

Linus Pauling and Vitamin C

(52) *http://www.paulingtherapy.com/*
Linus Pauling Protocol for prevention and reversal of heart disease

(53) *http://www.newmediaexplorer.org/chris/5278189.pdf*
Patent: PREVENTION AND TREATMENT OF OCCLUSIVE CARDIOVASCULAR DISEASE WITH ASCORBATE AND SUBSTANCES THAT INHIBIT THE BINDING OF LIPOPROTEIN *(A)*
Inventors: Matthias W. Rath, 7141 Kirchberg/Murr Linus C. Pauling, Big Sur, CA 93920
Patent Application Number: 557,516

(54) *http://www.nutrienthealth.net/library/jom/1992/pdf/1992-v07n01-p005.pdf*
Linus Pauling Unified Theory of Heart Disease

(55) *http://www.pubmedcentral.nih.gov/articlerender.fcgi?artid=54501.*
Hypothesis: lipoprotein*(a)* is a surrogate for ascorbate. M Rath and L Pauling. Proc Natl Acad Sci U S A. 1990 August; 87*(16)*: 6204–6207.

(56) *http://www.pubmedcentral.nih.gov/articlerender.fcgi?artid=55170.*
Immunological evidence for the accumulation of lipoprotein*(a)* in the atherosclerotic lesion of the hypoascorbemic guinea pig. M Rath and L Pauling. Proc Natl Acad Sci U S A. 1990 December; 87*(23)*: 9388–9390.

(57) Solution to the puzzle of human cardiovascular disease: its primary cause is ascorbate deficiency leading to the deposition of lipoprotein(a) and fibrinogen/fibrin in the vascular wall. Pauling L, Rath M. J Orthomol Med. 1992;6:125-133.

(58) *http://jeffreydach.com/2007/05/05/jeffreydachdrdachvitaminc.aspx*
Vitamin C and Stroke Prevention by Jeffrey DACH MD

(59) *http://www.amazon.com/review/RVRC3UKH8XQ22/ref=cm_cr_rdp_perm*
Hypothyroidism the Unsuspected Illness, by Broda Barnes MD, book review by Jeffrey Dach MD on Amazon.

(60) *http://jeffreydach.com/2007/06/10/vitamin-d-deficiency--by-jeffrey-dach-md.aspx*
Vitamin D Deficiency by Jeffrey Dach MD

(61) *http://www.heartfixer.com/CHC - Treatments - PC.htm*
James Roberts MD FACC 3110 W. Central Ave.Toledo, Ohio 43606 Phone (419) 531-6254

Chapter 26

Heart Disease Part Two - Atherosclerosis: How Does it Happen?

A Brief Review of Part I

The previous chapter discussed the Coronary Calcium Score, which is useful because it provides an estimate of total plaque burden. The previous chapter also contains the shocking statement that the conventional lipid panel is now obsolete. It has been replaced by the more sophisticated lipoprotein panel called the NMR or the VAP, which gives truly useful information of risk markers such as the LDL particle size and Lipoprotein *(a)*. Also discussed were treatment strategies with dietary modification and various nutritional supplements such as niacin, fish oil, and L-arginine which can slow or reverse plaque formation. Two previous chapters have discussed the role of statin drugs and their adverse side effects.*(7)(8)* Previously, it was explained how plaque formation is the cause of heart disease, and how enlarging plaques eventually cause heart attack by either occlusion, or plaque rupture with thrombosis. Although there is usually some warning such as chest pain or shortness of breath, sudden plaque rupture with thrombosis may cause a heart attack without warning.

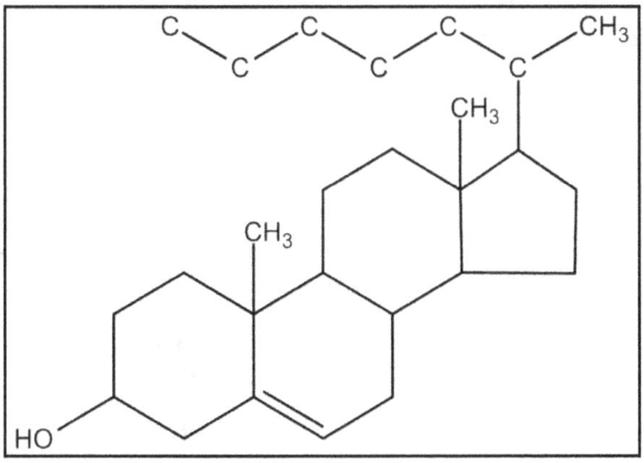

Image: cholesterol molecule chemical structure

Part Two - A Closer Look at Plaque Formation

In Part II we take a closer look at the individual steps leading to plaque formation in the artery wall. Based on this knowledge, we will then suggest additional strategies for preventing and reversing plaque formation in the arteries. There is an excellent review article on the detailed mechanism of atherosclerotic plaque formation by Navab from UCLA.*(2)*

Understanding the Events Leading to Atherosclerosis - The Fatty Streak

Atherosclerotic plaque formation is a series events. The very first event is the deposition of lipoproteins in called the Fatty Streak which eventually becomes the lipid core of the plaque. We know the fatty streak is the first step because it has been observed in the human fetus.*(18)* That is really early. The fatty streak is composed of LDL cholesterol, short for low density lipoprotein. Formation of the Fatty Streak precedes the next step in plaque formation which is infiltration with cells called Monocytes.

The Linus Pauling Theory - Vitamin C Deficiency -Cholesterol Patches

Linus Pauling and others, suspected that the LDL deposition in the wall serves as patching material to repair small cracks in the arterial wall at sites of mechanical stress from pulsations and flow turbulence. Pauling theorized that, because of a subclinical vitamin C deficiency, the normal repair mechanisms are ineffective, so that an alternate repair mechanism with LDL cholesterol evolved. The LDL cholesterol serves as a sort of rubber cement to patch up the cracks in arteries, just like patching the inner tube of our tires.

Since the appearance of the fatty streak appears so early in the fetus, it is highly likely that there is a constant ebb and flow of lipoprotein material in and out of the arterial wall. We now know there is a transport mechanism for cholesterol to travel in the blood stream to the arterial wall in the form of LDL particles. And, there is a reverse cholesterol transport mechanism which transports cholesterol back from the artery wall to the liver in the form of HDL particles using the LCAT enzyme *(*Lecithin-Cholesterol Acetyl Transferase*)*.

Cholesterol Transport – the Good *(*HDL*)* and Bad *(*LDL*)* and the Ugly Cholesterol

The LDL particles are transported from the liver out to the body tissues in the blood stream and delivers cholesterol to the Fatty Streak in the artery wall. The HDL particles carry cholesterol from the Fatty Streak in the artery wall back to the liver where it is metabolized and excreted as bile.

Calling LDL "bad", and HDL "good" is like calling the ambulance that comes from the hospital to your home the "bad" one, and the ambulance that takes you back to the hospital , the "good" one. Perhaps this is a useful analogy for children, but is overly simplistic for adults.*(4)*

Oxidized Cholesterol – the Ugly

The reality is that LDL cholesterol itself is not the culprit, rather it is oxidized LDL that is the "bad" guy. Lowering plain LDL cholesterol will also lower the oxidized fraction of LDL cholesterol, but this is a rather crude way to do it. Cholesterol is a building block for membranes and sex steroids, is important for over-all health, and lower cholesterol is associated with increased mortality from cancer, liver disease and mental disease.(5)(6) Perhaps this is the reason why lowering cholesterol with statin drugs can reduce "cardiac events", but sadly, statin drugs have little or no benefit in terms of all-cause mortality. (7)(8) It would be much more beneficial to selectively reduce only the Oxidized LDL cholesterol. Researchers have tests to measure oxidized LDL cholesterol, but this is not yet available to clinicians, and should be.

The Role of Anti-Oxidants

Selectively reducing Oxidized LDL is exactly what is done with anti-oxidants like vitamin C, E, Carotenoids, and Red wine polyphenols. These dietary supplements as well as a healthy diet and lifestyle are clearly beneficial.*(9)* However, many people are confused by the opposing views in the medical literature and the media. These views oppose the use of dietary supplements to prevent heart disease. Some have even proposed the bizarre notion that vitamins increase mortality. Of course, these anti-vitamin views represent the interests of the pharmaceutical industry which could lose billions from reduction in heart disease and reduced demand for drugs.*(10)(11)(12)(13)(14)* It is clear that dietary antioxidants like carotinoids in fresh vegetables as well as red wine polyphenols inhibit LDL oxidation and reduce heart disease.*(15)* We will later look at novel anti-oxidants such as liposomal glutathione *(16)* and Boswellia.

Infiltration by Monocytes- Macrophages and Inflammation

The next step in plaque formation is the infiltration of cells into the wall of the artery. Current thinking is that oxidized LDL attracts the influx of monocytes. These are cells in the blood stream which have the ability to transform themselves into large scavenger cells called macrophages which serve as the garbage trucks for pick up and disposal. They engulf, digest and dispose of the old toxic stuff the body needs to get rid of. These macrophages engulf the LDL cholesterol, and try to dispose of it. During the disposal process more of the LDL is oxidized. Something goes wrong at this step, and the macrophages continue to accumulate more and more oxidized LDL until the poor cell looks like an over inflated balloon ready to burst. This becomes the Foam Cell.

The Foam Cell- The Culprit is Oxidized LDL

This new over-stuffed macrophage is now called a "Foam Cell" because it looks foamy under the microscope. It is clear that the culprit is the oxidized or rancid form of LDL cholesterol. If the LDL is not oxidized, there seems to be no problem and the LDL can be transported out of the artery back to the liver in the form of HDL using the LCAT enzyme for reverse cholesterol transport. The Foam Cells accumulate, and send out more chemical messages which invoke an inflammatory cascade that attracts more macrophages and other cells in an inflammatory reaction. This inflammation in the wall of the artery causes the thickening in the wall called plaque formation.

The Fibrous Cap

The last step in plaque formation is the fibrous cap which creates a seal between the puddle of oxidized LDL and its inflammatory cells and the flowing blood at the interior of the artery. Rupture of the fibrous cap is the final event which exposes the thrombogenic material in the plaque to the blood stream causing clot formation and a heart attack.

How to Prevent Oxidation of LDL cholesterol

Now that we know the events leading to plaque formation and rupture, we can create a logical plan to prevent and reverse this process. Even after LDL becomes oxidized, it can be converted back to its original form with the use of anti-oxidants in a process called reduction. There are a number of anti-oxidants which have been shown effective. The most important and most powerful intracellular antioxidant is glutathione, a simple chemical structure composed of three amino acids, and sulfur.

What is Glutathione?

Glutathione is the most powerful naturally occurring antioxidant in all human cells. It is a small simple compound composed of three amino acids, glutamic acid, cysteine and glycine. Cysteine contains sulfur accounting for its sulfur taste and smell. Glutathione is found in all cells in the body, and the highest concentration in the liver, important for detoxification and elimination of toxins and products of oxidation called free radicals. For the past 10 years, Glutathione has been available only as an intravenous agent. David Perlmutter MD in Naples, Florida has been pioneering the use of IV glutathione in Parkinson's Disease patients for the past 10 years with dramatic results. These Parkinson's patients have immediate improvement in their symptoms after Glutathione IV infusion. In addition, inhaled glutathione in the form of a nebulizer has been beneficial for chronic obstructive lung disease patients.

Liposomal Glutathione Reduces Plaque by 30%

A recent 2007 publication from the Technion in Haifa showed that Liposomal Glutathione reduced plaque formation by 30% in genetically modified Apo-E mice. *(16)* These are mice that have accelerated atherosclerosis, the mouse equivalent of familial hypercholesterolemia in humans. They also found the enzyme, glutathione peroxidase in the LDL particle itself. This enzyme converts the oxidized LDL back to its original reduced form. How convenient this enzyme is already in place on the LDL particle. This was an important discovery. At the recent ACAM meeting in Orlando (April 2008), Tim Guilford MD presented the data on Liposomal Glutathione reversing plaque in Apo-E mice. The studies were done by Technion researchers using Dr. Guilford's liposomal glutathione product called *Readisorb*.

What is Boswellia ?

Oxidation of the LDL cholesterol involves the Lipoxygenase pathway which can be inhibited by Boswellia. Boswellia works by suppressing inflammation by inhibiting an enzyme called 5-lipoxygenase (5 L-OX) and its by products called leukotrienes. This pathway is important in chronic inflammatory diseases such as arthritis, colitis, asthma, allergies, osteoporosis, eczema and psoriasis. Boswellia is also useful in preventing the inflammation inside the arterial tree associated with atherosclerotic plaque formation. In mice where the 5-lipoxygenase is absent there is a 26 fold reduction in atherosclerotic plaque compared to controls.*(17)*

Currently mainstream medicine has no drug to control the 5-L-OX enzyme, because up to now the pharmaceutical industry has not been able to make such a drug without major adverse side effects. However, Boswellia is a safe, natural gum resin of the frankincense tree, which powerfully suppresses the 5-lipoxygenase enzyme like no other substance known. Ancient traditional uses and more recent studies have shown significant improvements in asthma, arthritis, colitis, allergies, and heart disease.

The most active of Frankincense component is called AKBA (acetyl-11-keto-beta-boswellic acid). Unfortunately, currently available Boswellia extracts contain only a small amount of AKBA in the range of 1-3%. This small amount makes it virtually impossible to attain plasma levels needed for any real clinical benefit. Fortunately, a new Boswellia extract contains the more active 90% AKBA and is available from *True Botanica* and Ross Rentea MD.

References

(1) http://www.lipid.org/clinical/patients/1000005.php

ATHEROSCLEROSIS - A STORY OF CELLS, CHOLESTEROL, AND CLOTS John R. Guyton, M.D. Excellent Review Article

(2) http://www.jlr.org/cgi/content/full/45/6/993

Thematic review series: The Pathogenesis of Atherosclerosis The oxidation hypothesis of atherogenesis: the role of oxidized phospholipids and HDL. Mohamad Navab et al. Journal of Lipid Research, Vol. 45, 993-1007, June 2004

(3) *http://physrev.physiology.org/cgi/content/full/84/4/1381*
Role of Oxidative Modifications in Atherosclerosis. Roland Stocker and John F. Keaney, Jr. Physiol. Rev. 84: 1381-1478, 2004;.

(4) *http://www.jpands.org/vol10no3/colpo.pdf*
LDL Cholesterol:Bad Cholesterol, or Bad Science? Anthony Colpo, Journal of American Physicians and Surgeons Volume 10 Number 3 Fall 2005. p 83.

Low Serum LDL is not Healthy

(5) *http://www.annclinlabsci.org/cgi/content/abstract/37/4/343 Low Serum LDL Cholesterol Levels and the Risk of Fever, Sepsis, and Malignancy. Renana Shor et al. Annals of Clinical & Laboratory Science 37:343-348 (2007). In summary, low serum LDL cholesterol level was associated with increased risks of hematological cancer, fever, and sepsis.*

(6) *http://www.ncbi.nlm.nih.gov/pubmed/15006277*
Why Eve Is Not Adam: Prospective Follow-Up in 149,650 Women and Men of Cholesterol and Other Risk Factors Related to Cardiovascular and All-Cause Mortality. Hanno Ulmer et al. Journal of Women's Health. January 1, 2004, 13*(1)*: 41-53.

Jeffrey Dach MD Previous Statin Drug Articles

(7) *http://jeffreydach.com/2008/01/27/cholesterol-lowering-statin-drugs-for-women-just-say-no-by-jeffrey-dach-md.aspx*
Cholesterol Lowering Drugs for Women, Just say No, by Jeffrey Dach MD

(8) *http://jeffreydach.com/2007/05/14/lipitor-and-the-dracula-of-modern-technology-by-jeffrey-dach-md.aspx*
Lipitor and the Dracula of Medical Technology by Jeffrey Dach MD

Dietary Anti-Oxidants- Pro

(9) *http://circ.ahajournals.org/cgi/content/abstract/107/7/947*
Six-Year Effect of Combined Vitamin C and E Supplementation on Atherosclerotic Progression - The Antioxidant Supplementation in Atherosclerosis Prevention *(*ASAP*)* Study. Riitta M. Salonen, MD et al., PhD. Circulation. 2003;107:947.

Opposition to Anti-Oxidants in Heart Disease Prevention

(10) *http://www.ajcn.org/cgi/content/full/84/4/680*
American Journal of Clinical Nutrition, Vol. 84, No. 4, 680-681, October 2006 EDITORIAL The dubious use of vitamin-mineral supplements in relation to cardiovascular disease Donald B McCormick

Slamming Vitamins with Bad Science

(11) http://www.healthfreedom.net/index.php?option=com_content&task=view&id=425
The Truth Behind the Cochrane Slam on Dietary Supplements. HealthFreedom.Net

(12) http://www.alliance-natural-health.org/_docs/ANHwebsiteDoc_270.pdf
Poor methodology in meta-analysis of vitamins. Dr Steve Hickey, Dr Len Noriegai and Dr Hilary Roberts

(13) http://www.ajcn.org/cgi/content/full/85/1/293S
What is the Efficacy of Single Vitamin and Mineral Supplement Use in Chronic Disease Prevention? Heart disease and single-vitamin supplementation1,2,3,4 Maret G Traber. American Journal of Clinical Nutrition, Vol. 85, No. 1, 293S-299S, January 2007

(14) http://www.ajcn.org/cgi/content/full/81/4/736
Vitamins E and C are safe across a broad range of intakes. American Journal of Clinical Nutrition, Vol. 81, No. 4, 736-745, April 2005 John N Hathcock et al.

(15) http://www.ncbi.nlm.nih.gov/pubmed/16596803
Dietary antioxidants and paraoxonases against LDL oxidation and atherosclerosis development. Aviram M et al. Handb Exp Pharmacol. 2005;*(170)*:263-300.

Liposomal Glutathione

(16) http://www.ncbi.nlm.nih.gov/pubmed/17588583
Anti-oxidant and anti-atherogenic properties of liposomal glutathione: studies in vitro, and in the atherosclerotic apolipoprotein E-deficient mice. Rosenblat M et al. Atherosclerosis. 2007 Dec;195*(2)*:e61-8.

Inhibition of 5-LOX Reduces Aorta Plaque 26 fold

(17) http://circres.ahajournals.org/cgi/content/full/91/2/120
Molecular Medicine Identification of 5-Lipoxygenase as a Major Gene Contributing to Atherosclerosis Susceptibility in Mice. Margarete Mehrabian et al. Circulation Research. 2002;91:120.

Fatty Streak in Fetal Aortas

(18) http://www.pubmedcentral.nih.gov/articlerender.fcgi?tool=pubmed&pubmedid=9389731
Fatty streak formation occurs in human fetal aortas. C Napoli et al. J Clin Invest. 1997 December 1; 100*(11)*: 2680–2690.

Oxidized LDL Cholesterol, Not LDL Cholesterol

http://atvb.ahajournals.org/cgi/content/abstract/20/3/708
Oxidized Cholesterol in the Diet Accelerates the Development of Atherosclerosis in LDL Receptor– and Apolipoprotein E–Deficient Mice, Ilona Staprans et al. Arteriosclerosis, Thrombosis, and Vascular Biology. 2000;20:708.

http://atvb.ahajournals.org/cgi/content/abstract/18/6/977
Oxidized Cholesterol in the Diet Accelerates the Development of Aortic Atherosclerosis in Cholesterol-Fed Rabbits Ilona Staprans; Xian-Mang Pan et al. Arteriosclerosis, Thrombosis, and Vascular Biology. 1998;18:977-983.

http://www.specialtylabs.com/books/display.asp?id=1095
Oxidized Low Density Lipoproteins and their Autoantibodies. James B. Peter et al.

http://www.fasebj.org/cgi/content/full/15/12/2073
Oxidized LDL and HDL: antagonists in atherothrombosis, ANN MERTENS et al. FASEB Journal. 2001;15:2073-2084.

Foam Cells and Oxidized LDL

http://bme.virginia.edu/ley/lab/publications/Shashkin.pdf
Macrophage Differentiation to Foam Cells Pavel Shashkin et al. Current Pharmaceutical Design, 2005, 11, 3061-3072 3061

5-Lipoxygenase implicated in Heart Disease

http://circres.ahajournals.org/cgi/content/full/91/2/120?ijkey=1a2f5d238a615afeac88628298ba9514369f40c9 Identification of 5-Lipoxygenase as a Major Gene Contributing to Atherosclerosis Susceptibility in Mice. Margarete Mehrabian et al. Circulation Research. 2002;91:120

http://www.jlr.org/cgi/content/full/43/1/26
Induction of monocyte differentiation and foam cell formation in vitro by 7-ketocholesterol. John M. Hayden et al. Journal of Lipid Research, Vol. 43, 26-35, January 2002

Oxidized Cholesterol in Plasma Strong Predictor of Heart Attack

http://circ.ahajournals.org/cgi/content/full/112/5/651
Plasma Oxidized Low-Density Lipoprotein, a Strong Predictor for Acute Coronary Heart Disease Events in Apparently Healthy, Middle-Aged Men From the General Population. Christa Meisinger et al. Circulation. 2005;112:651-657.

http://www.blackwell-synergy.com/doi/full/10.1111/j.1365-2796.2004.01402.x
Oxidized low-density lipoprotein in plasma is a prognostic marker of subclinical atherosclerosis development in clinically healthy men. K. Wallenfeldt et al. Journal of Internal Medicine 256 *(5)*, 413–420, 2004

Measuring Oxidized LDL in Blood

http://diabetes.diabetesjournals.org/cgi/content/full/53/4/1068
The Metabolic Syndrome, Circulating Oxidized LDL, and Risk of Myocardial Infarction in Well-Functioning Elderly People in the Health, Aging, and Body Composition Cohort. Paul Holvoet et al. Diabetes 53:1068-1073, 2004

APO A1 and APO B Proteins

http://en.wikipedia.org/wiki/Apolipoprotein_A1
Apolipoprotein A1

http://en.wikipedia.org/wiki/Apolipoprotein_B
Apolipoprotein B *(*APO-B is the primary apolipoprotein of low density lipoproteins *(*LDL or "bad cholesterol"*)*, which is responsible for carrying cholesterol to tissues.

APO -E

http://en.wikipedia.org/wiki/Apolipoprotein_E
Defects in apolipoprotein E result in familial dysbetalipoproteinemia, or type III hyperlipoproteinemia *(*HLP III*)*, in which increased plasma cholesterol and triglycerides are the consequence of impaired clearance of chylomicron and VLDL remnants.[1]

More on Glutathione

http://www.ebmonline.org/cgi/content/full/230/1/40
Glutathione Preconditioning Attenuates Ac-LDL–Induced Macrophage Apoptosis via Protein Kinase C–Dependent Ac-LDL Trafficking. Rene S. Rosenson-Schloss et al. Experimental Biology and Medicine 230:40-48 *(*2005*)*

http://content.onlinejacc.org/cgi/content/full/47/5/1005
The Relationship Between Plasma Levels of Oxidized and Reduced Thiols and Early Atherosclerosis in Healthy Adults, Salman Ashfaq et al. J Am Coll Cardiol, 2006; 47:1005-1011

http://circ.ahajournals.org/cgi/content/full/100/22/2244
Serum Glutathione in Adolescent Males Predicts Parental Coronary Heart Disease. John A. Morrison et al. Circulation. 1999;100:2244.

Tim Guilford MD

http://www.cancercontrolsociety.com/bio2005/guilford.html

TIM GUILFORD, M.D.,

http://www.readisorb.com Readisorb Liposomal Glutathione Web Site

Boswellia

http://www.truebotanica.com/boswellia_science.html

Cardio-vascular Diseases: The role of the 5-Lipoxygenase in atherosclerosis is particularly interesting.

Articles by Ross Rentea MD on Boswelia etc.

http://www.satyacenter.com/health-plant_medicine-gold-frankincense-myrrh

Gold, Frankincense and Myrrh - Companions for overcoming work-related stress? by Ross Rentea, M.D.

http://www.lilipoh.com/articles/2005/summer/sensory_overload.aspx

Sensory Overload Author: An Interview with Ross Rentea, M.D. Issue: LILIPOH #40 - Summer 2005: HEALTH & THE SENSES

*http://www.lilipoh.com/articles/2006/winter/anthroposophical_aspects_of_diabetes_treatment.aspxAnthroposophical Aspects of Diabetes Treatment Author: Ross Rentea, M.D..Issue:LILIPOH#46-Issue 11 Winter2006http://www.truebotanica.com/*TrueBotanica Web Site

Boswellia References

http://ajrccm.atsjournals.org/cgi/content/full/161/2/S1/S120

5-Lipoxygenase and Leukotrienes, Transgenic Mouse and Nuclear Targeting Studies. COLIN D. FUNK and XIN-SHENG CHEN, Am. J. Respir. Crit. Care Med., Volume 161, Number 2, February 2000, S120-S124

C-Reactive Protein *(***CRP***)*

http://health.ucsd.edu/news/2002/09_09_Chang.html

UCSD Team Identifies Potential Role of CRP In Development of Atherosclerosis, Sept. 9, 2002 by Proceedings of the National Academy of Sciences. Mi-Kyung Chang, M.D.,

http://www.emedicine.com/med/TOPIC446.HTM

Coronary Artery Atherosclerosis Vibhuti N Singh, MD

http://www.thirdage.com/ebsco/files/21509.html#ref40

L- Arginine

IV Glutathione in Parkinson's Video

http://www.glutathioneexperts.com/benefits-glutathione.html

Benefits of Glutathione, The information in the following video describes the use of intravenous glutathione in Parkinson's disease at the Perlmutter Health Center, Naples, Florida with Dr. David Perlmutter. We see videos of Parkinson's patients before and after glutathione is administered. You can noticeably see the improvement in each patient after IV glutathione. The video should not be used in and of itself to diagnose or treat any specific medical condition.

http://www.glutathioneexperts.com/parkinsons.html

IV Glutathione Articles - Parkinson's Disease

http://www.glutathioneexperts.com/index.html

Reduced L-glutathione, most commonly called glutathione or GSH, is the most powerful naturally occurring antioxidant in all human cells.

http://www.drperlmutter.com/

Pioneered use of IV Glutathione for Parkinson's. David Perlmutter, MD, FACN is a Board-Certified Neuroland Fellow of the American College of Nutrition who received his M.D. degree from the University of Miami School, and he serves as Medical Director of the Perlmutter Health in Naples Florida

Chapter 27

Reversing Heart Disease without Drugs

Heart Disease, also called clogged arteries, is today's number one killer in America, and is the reason why 16 million Americans are taking a statin anti-cholesterol drugs. In this chapter, we will examine the current knowledge about what causes heart disease and how to prevent and reverse heart disease without drugs or surgery.

Most everyone will tell you that high cholesterol and fat in the diet causes heart disease, and you will see this type of information prominently mentioned on television and in newspapers. However, if you actually look at the data, you will find a number of disturbing facts. Most heart attack victims admitted to the hospital have normal cholesterol blood levels. People who consume mostly animal fat such as the Greenland Eskimos show virtually no heart disease. In America before the 1920's, we consumed plentiful amounts of eggs, butter and lard, yet heart disease was relatively rare at that time. Only after the 1920's did heart disease became an epidemic in the US, about the same time as the introduction of processed vegetable oils *(*also called Trans Fats*)* and refined sugar products.

How can something as American as refined sugar which has nothing to do with fat or cholesterol cause our current epidemic of heart disease? The answer is that it is not the sugar that is the culprit because sugar is the brain's primary fuel. It is the resulting high Insulin level provoked by the blood sugar that is the bad guy. The high Insulin leads to Insulin resistance, Obesity and Diabetes, and it activates an important enzyme in the body which turns on a little switch causing chronic inflammation. If the chronic inflammation attacks the lining of the arteries, you get heart disease. If it attacks your joints, you get arthritis.

Yes, cholesterol is a major part of the atherosclerotic plaque that clogs the artery along with calcium. However, cholesterol is not the cause. It is deposited in the artery wall to repair damage from the inflammation which is the real cause. Cholesterol is essential for life. It is an important substance used by the body to make hormones such as estrogen, and testosterone and it accounts for one half the dry weight of the brain. Cholesterol is present in all the cell membranes. What happens when your cholesterol is reduced too low? You get blood sugar problems, edema, mineral deficiencies, chronic inflammation, and difficulty in healing, allergies, asthma, reduced libido, infertility and various reproductive problems.

Statin drugs work very well at reducing cholesterol measurements in the blood. They also are successful at reducing cardiac events such as heart attacks. However a critical examination of the data on the numerous medical studies again raises some disturbing questions. Firstly, none of the Statin Drug studies has ever shown a mortality benefit for women. Secondly, in the elderly over age 65, lowering the cholesterol is associated with a higher mortality.

In middle aged men who have known heart disease, the benefits of a Statin anti-cholesterol drug are not related to the degree in which they lower the blood cholesterol level. Instead, the Statin Drug seems to work as a crude anti-inflammatory drug.

Adverse side effects of the Statin Drugs include muscle damage, nerve damage, and transient global amnesia. These are all related to depletion of an essential vitamin called Coenzyme Q-10 manufactured by the same liver enzyme that also makes cholesterol. So if you are taking a Statin drug and your doctor hasn't recommended that you also supplement with Coenzyme Q-10, please give this article to him or her, as well as an invitation to call me for the references on this subject.

If you would like to avoid the adverse side effects of drug treatment listed above, then what can you do to prevent or even reverse heart disease? I have revealed some of the secrets revealed below:

1. Low Glycemic Diet. This is a diet which does not raise your blood sugar and insulin levels. Consult a Glycemic Index chart and you will be surprised to discover that certain foods such as bread, potatoes and pasta which contain dense carbohydrates will raise your blood sugar level the same at eating pure refined sugar. This is the main cause of our current epidemic of Obesity and Type Two Diabetes. The Lyon Diet Heart Study which followed heart attack survivors who ate a low glycemic diet, found a 70% reduction in fatal heart attacks compared to the high glycemic group.

2. Omega -3 Fatty Acids in the form of Fish Oil. The Italian GISSI study showed a 45% reduction in sudden death from heart attack and 20% reduction in mortality in the group taking fish oil supplements. This benefit is better than any Statin Drug study. Fish oils are anti-inflammatory and work better than NSAIDs, which are over-the-counter non-steroidal anti-inflammatory drugs like Aleve or Motrin, without their side effects. One problem, though, is that most fish are contaminated with Mercury and PCBs, so make sure you use a purified pharmaceutical grade fish oil with all contaminants removed. Molecular distilled fish oil is a good choice.

3. Exercise program. The New USDA Food Guidelines now include exercise steps along side the food pyramid diagram. Exercise reduces chronic inflammation and makes you feel good. See your doctor for a treadmill EKG test before you start your exercise program to see if you can tolerate it.

4. Fiber products: Profibe, a grapefruit fiber product developed by Dr. James Cerda at the University of Florida was found to reverse atherosclerosis in an animal model

and is available on the internet at www.profibe.com. Anther fiber product is ground flax seeds which is very popular and I personally take every day.

5. Essential Phospholipids was a patented drug in Europe for many years and many research studies were completed showing it works very well at reversing heart disease. This is a nutritional supplement available without a prescription from Nutrasal called phosphatidyl-choline.

6. Niacin, also called Nicotinic Acid is one of the B vitamins and the subject of the Coronary Drug Project (CDP) which was published in the Journal of the American College of Cardiology in 1986. In the group taking Niacin, they found a 27% decrease in heart attacks and a 10% reduction in total deaths, results better than any statin drug study.

7. Avoid Trans-Fats found in processed vegetable oils and margarine as recommended by the new USDA Food Guidelines. These are toxic to the heart.

8. Have your blood homocysteine level checked. This is a marker for inflammation in the arteries of the heart. If elevated, this can be simply remedied with B vitamins. Everyone over 50 should be taking vitamin-B12 supplements as recommended by your government, USDA Food Guidelines.

9. Lastly, this may be the most important piece of information on the page: The Unified Theory of Heart Disease, proposed by Linus Pauling and Mathias Rath suggests that subclinical vitamin C deficiency (scurvy), Lipoprotein small (a) and mechanical stress at key arterial sites (such as bifurcations) are the major players in causation of heart disease. The mechanical damage to the endothelium causes lysine and proline in collagen to be exposed. Lp(a) has lysine and proline receptors which allow attachment to the exposed collagen forming a "patch" over the exposed area.

Drs. Pauling and Rath obtained a U.S. patent on the use of Vitamin C (6-18 grams/day) and Lysine (6 grams/day) for the prevention and reversal of heart disease. Dr. Rath has added Proline and Coenzyme Q-10 to this formula. In 1992, before his death, Linus Pauling made a video describing this discovery. The real culprit is not cholesterol or the LDL fraction, the real culprit is a "sticky" relative of LDL called *lipoprotein(a)* or Lp(a). The VAP lipid panel can show your Lp(a) level. Note: **LDL combined with apoprotein(a) makes Lp(a).**

The VAP Test by Atherotec goes beyond the routine cholesterol panel (HDL, calculated LDL, triglycerides, and total cholesterol), by providing measurements of HDL, LDL, and VLDL (very low-density lipoprotein), and also measuring other important lipoprotein subclasses, including Lp(a), HDL subtypes, and IDL (intermediate-density lipoprotein). The test also measures LDL pattern density – important because patients with small, dense LDL *(*Pattern B*)* have a four-fold increased risk of developing heart disease.

References

Recommended Reading for Statin Drugs, Cholesterol, and Heart Disease:

Lipitor: Thief of Memory, Statin Drugs and the Misguided War on Cholesterol, by Duane Graveline, M.D.(c) 2004

The Cholesterol Myths : Exposing the Fallacy that Saturated Fat and Cholesterol Cause Heart Disease, by *Uffe Ravnskov,MD, PhD,*

The Heart Revolution : The Extraordinary Discovery That Finally Laid the Cholesterol Myth to Rest by Kilmer McCully, M.D. *(c)* 2000

Heart Frauds: Uncovering the Biggest Health Scam in History by Charles T. McGee, M.D.

The Myth of Cholesterol: Dispelling the Fear and Creating Real Heart Health - Dugliss Paul, M.D. *(c)* 2005

The Truth About the Drug Companies: How They Deceive Us and What to Do About It - Marcia Angell, M.D. *(c)* 2004 Random House

Overdosed America: The Broken Promise Of American Medicine - John Abramson, M.D.*(c)* 2004 HarperCollins

Track Your Plack by William Davis MD

Chapter 28

Remembering Interventional Radiology Days

Back in 2002, saving a life was just part of my routine work day. As the Interventional Radiologist, one of my jobs in the hospital was to fish out the lost catheters and IV lines inside the patient that float back to the heart and get lodged in the pulmonary artery.

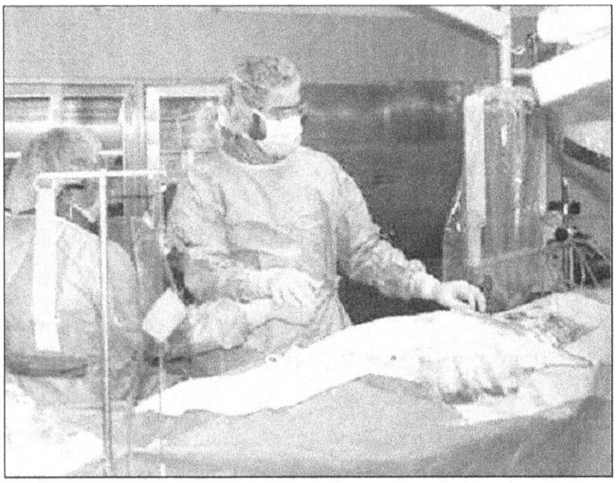

Jeffrey Dach MD Performing a Percutaneous Nephrostomy Procedure in Radiology

The photo at left shows me in 2001, wearing a sterile surgical gown performing a percutaneous nephrostomy in the Interventional Radiology Suite. Note the plexiglass radiation shield suspended above the patient on the right, and the x-ray fluoroscope machine is at the upper right corner. The plastic bag at the lower right collects the urine from the nephrostomy tube in place in the kidney. Note that the urine in the bag is dark indicating blood in the urine which is quite common immediately after puncturing the kidney. The urine clears to a more suitable amber color after a few hours of drainage. My assistant at the left was later promoted to administrative head of the radiology department.

A Fragment Lost in the Pulmonary Artery

One day I while reading films, I noticed an unusual finding in a chest x-ray which showed a swan ganz catheter fragment. This had broken loose and ended up in the right pulmonary artery, representing a foreign body, and if allowed to remain in place, causes infection, sepsis and ultimately death. Such a catheter fragment must be removed or the patient will eventually die of infection.

How to Remove the Foreign Body

There are two methods used for removal. The first rather extreme method is open heart surgery performed under general anesthesia in the operating room. The chest is opened, pulmonary artery clamped, an incision made into the artery, and the catheter fragment retrieved. Alternatively, they call the Interventional

Radiologist to remove the lost catheter fragment in a much simpler procedure. This is done percutaneously, through a skin incision in the groin under local anesthesia in the X-Ray Department using the Snare Technique while the patient is awake and talking.*(1)*

The Snare Technique for Intravascular Foreign Body Removal

The Wire-Snare Technique for intravascular foreign body removal was well known. It involves a percutaneous approach by puncturing the large vein at the right groin (the femoral vein), advancing a long angiographic catheter from there to the heart, through the heart and into the right pulmonary artery. Going through the heart was the tricky part because of all the pulsations and cardiac movement.*(1)*

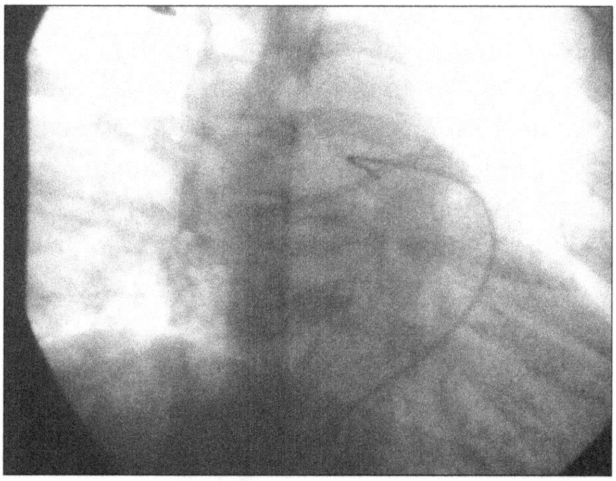

Swan Ganz catheter with snare attached

Once the catheter tip is in the pulmonary artery in the vicinity of the foreign body, a wire snare can be advanced through the angiographic catheter. This wire snare forms a loop as it protrudes from the end of the angiographic catheter, and this loop can be manipulated around the foreign body. Once in position around the foreign body, the wire snare can then be pulled back which then closes the loop tightly upon the foreign body, and the whole thing can be pulled out safely.*(4)*

Removing a Wire Lost inside the Patient

I remember another patient who came from another hospital with a diagnosis of infection in the blood with positive blood cultures. The chest x-ray had been repeatedly read as "normal" by many other doctors. However, when I looked at the chest x-ray, I saw a small white line over the right pulmonary artery that looked like a scratch on the x-ray film. This wasn't a scratch, it was a thin metal wire lodged in the artery which had been cut off and lost in the patient after a removing a central line at the previous hospital. This foreign body was causing the sepsis and positive blood cultures. We brought the patient down to the x-ray department into the Interventional Angiographic Suite and did a percutaneous removal with the snare technique. This was successful, and the patient had an uneventful recovery and shortly went home.*(2)*

Removing The Knotted Swan Ganz Catheter - Inventing a New Technique

Another problem I encountered while doing my fellowship in angiography at Jackson Memorial hospital in 1980-1981 involved a patient who had a "knotted" swan ganz catheter. Occasionally in the ICU, the CVP catheters become so coiled up while in the pulmonary circulation, they loop and form a knot which prevents the ICU doctor from removing the catheter. This is a special problem called the "knotted swan ganz catheter", and after trying a few ideas, the knotted catheter was removed using a large polyethylene sheath which protected the soft tissues as the catheter knot was pulled out. I later published an article describing the invented technique which allowed removal of knotted catheters without major surgery.*(7)*

Gallbladder Drainage in the ICU

I recall a totally different case involving an old man who was septic in the ICU from a severely infected gallbladder. This was usually treated with a surgical operation which removes the gallbladder. However, in this case, the surgeon was unwilling to operate because of the patient's poor clinical condition made it unlikely the patient would survive surgery. As the interventional radiologist on call, it was my task to place a drainage tube into the gallbladder which could drain off the infected material and save the patient's life. Normally this procedure is done with combined ultrasound and fluoroscopic guidance in the X-ray department, in the interventional suite with benefit of all the imaging equipment. However, the patient was much too sick to leave the intensive care unit, so we had to get by with limited imaging at the bedside.

The gall bladder drainage procedure had to be done in the ICU, and the only available imaging equipment was a bedside portable ultrasound machine. I had been doing gallbladder ultrasound studies for 20 years, using ultrasound hands-on for many interventional procedures to guide needle placement for biopsies and drainage procedures. This past experience made me more comfortable doing the procedure in the ICU with limited imaging.

The ultrasound machine allowed visualization of the gallbladder fairly easily and it was not difficult advancing the needle into the gallbladder. Correct needle placement was confirmed by returning green/black bile from the needle hub. Once bile was obtained from the needle, it was fairly straight forward to advance a guidewire through the needle into the gallbladder. The only problem was making sure the wire would stay inside the gallbladder while the larger drainage catheter was advanced over it. There was a risk that the guidewire would become dislodged and the drainage catheter slide out of the gallbladder into the subhepatic space. This, of course, would mean disaster because the leaking bile would cause bile peritonitis, and the patient's demise.

This disastrous bile leakage was avoided by advancing enough wire so that it coiled nicely into the gallbladder. Normally this was done under fluoroscopic guidance, but in the ICU, there was no fluoroscope, so this had to be done "blind" without imaging going by the "feel" of the guidewire. I had enough experience over the years, so I knew the distinctive feel for each step. Luckily everything went well, and when the guidewire was removed from the drainage catheter, green bile was aspirated from the catheter indicating correct placement, later confirmed with a portable radiograph. The surgeon congratulated me for a procedure well done which saved the patient's life. For me, it was all in a day's work.

My Second Medical Career in Natural Medicine

Do I miss the excitement and challenge of the Interventional Radiology days? Of course I do. However, because of my detached retina and multiple eye surgeries to correct the detachment, I no longer have the eagle eye required for my old job in radiology. I took this "time out" opportunity to attend meetings and retrain in a second medical career, which is natural medicine and bio-identical hormone therapy. I then founded the TrueMedMD Clinic in Hollywood, Florida, devoted to the practice of natural medicine. Gratefully, the response of the community has been overwhelming with a schedule now booked well in advance. Our product is simple, we deliver a level of health care surpassing conventional mainstream medicine. Our medical practice is indeed, "The Revolution in Modern Medicine", which would make an excellent title for a new book. The success of this new medical practice is due in large part to the efforts of my wife, Judith Fine, who has a PhD degree in anthropology and serves as the patient advocate. Judith guides the patient through the office process from the first telephone inquiry to the later follow-up telephone call.

References

(1) http://www.ajronline.org/cgi/content/full/176/6/1509
percutaneous Retrieval of Lost or Misplaced Intravascular Objects
Andreas Gabelmann1, Stefan Kramer and Johannes Gorich University Clinics of Ulm Germany. AJR 2001; 176:1509-1513

(2) http://bja.oxfordjournals.org/cgi/content/full/88/1/144
British Journal of Anaesthesia, 2002, Vol. 88, No. 1 144-146
Loss of the guide wire: mishap or blunder? W. Schummer1, C. Schummer2, E. Gaser2 and R. Bartunek3

(3) http://www.cookmedical.com/di/dataSheet.do?id=391
Needle's Eye Snare For use in the percutaneous retrieval of indwelling catheters, cardiac leads, fragments of catheter tubing or wire guides, and other foreign objects.

A transfemoral grasping tool that forms a basket snare around the lead body. It is delivered to the vicinity of the lead through a long, flexible 12 Fr cannula that is placed coaxially within a larger outer cannula which has a hemostasis valve at its proximal end. *(*Two sizes of grasping tip. Requires no extra handle. 16 French Straight Femoral Introducing Equipment included.*)*

(4) http://www.hemodinamiadelsur.com.ar/journals/journal_124.asp
Transfemoral Snaring of Broken Catheters From the Right Heart in Small Infants
Kyung J. Chung, MD, Harvey L. Chernoff, MD, Lucian L. Leape, MD, and Marshall B. Kreidberg, MD

(5) http://content.nejm.org/cgi/content/full/352/4/e3/DC1#a2
Video Clip of Intravascular Foreign Body Removal with snare technique
Supplement to: Morguet AJ and Schultheiss H-P. Embolization of the Tip of a Central Venous Catheter into the Pulmonary Artery. N Engl J Med 2005;352*(4)*:e3.

(6) http://content.nejm.org/cgi/content/full/352/4/e3
Embolization of the Tip of a Central Venous Catheter into the Pulmonary Artery
NEJM Volume 352:e3 January 27, 2005 Number 4 Andreas J. Morguet, M.D. Heinz-Peter Schultheiss, M.D. Charité–Campus Benjamin Franklin
12200 Berlin, Germany

(7) http://www.ajronline.org/cgi/reprint/137/6/1274
AJR Am J Roentgenol. 1981 Dec;137*(6)*:1274-5. The knotted Swan-Ganz catheter: new solution to a vexing problem.Dach JL, Galbut DL, LePage JR.

(8) http://www.mirs.org/rounds/ir_retrievefrm.htm
Endovascular Retrieval of a Central Venous Catheter Fragment Todd Bostwick, MD

(9) http://journals.tubitak.gov.tr/medical/issues/sag-99-29-1/sag-29-1-17-97171.pdf
Percutaneous Retrieval of Broken Port Catheter Entrapped in the Right Atrium

(10) http://www.cookmedical.com/di/dataSheet.do?id=60
Curry Intravascular Retriever Sets Used to snare a foreign body and withdraw it to a peripheral vascular location. The special wire guide snare "folds" at midpoint and forms a loop when passed through the catheter.

Chapter 29

The Untold Message of Breast Cancer Awareness Month

Breast Cancer Awareness Month Fails to Disclose Limitations of Mammography

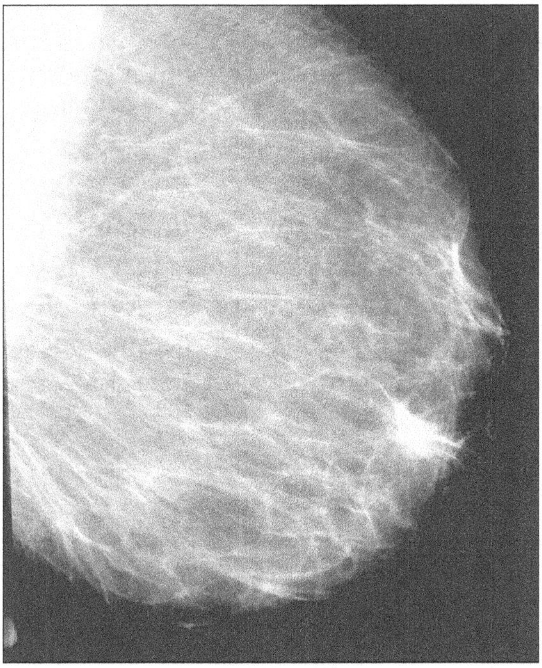

Screening Mammogram

October Breast Cancer Awareness Month is actually an advertising campaign for national mammography screening.*(1)* An eminent radiologist, Leonard Berlin MD says this advertising campaign fails to disclose that screening mammography has limitations. Mammography misses 30-70% of breast cancers, and leads to over diagnosis and over treatment. Dr. Berlin also says mammography warnings and disclosures should be mandated, just like the warnings on cigarette and drug ads.*(2)* Otherwise, we create unrealistic expectations for mammography which cannot be met. The public expects every breast cancer to be detected. They are not. This translates into increased medical malpractice payouts for the missed cancer, which is now the most prevalent medical malpractice case against all physicians.*(3)(4)(5)(6)*

The fact is that mammograms are difficult to interpret, cancers can be hidden, and many are missed. This cancer miss is not from lack of training or competency on the part of the radiologist. It is inherent in the mammogram technique itself. The American College of Radiology says that 30-70% of breast cancers are missed on the initial mammogram, and are seen in retrospect a year later by going back to the previous mammogram interpreted as normal. Considering this kind of legal environment, it is a miracle that mammography has survived at all.*(7)(8)*

Screening Mammography is Not Prevention.

Leonard Berlin points out that 57% of the American women believe that mammograms prevent breast cancer, a misleading message from Breast Awareness Month.*(3)* Mammograms are designed to detect cancer, not prevent it. Thinking that a mammogram can prevent breast cancer is like thinking that checking your house annually for broken windows, prevents robberies.

Secondly. the most likely outcome of a positive mammogram is an unnecessary biopsy, causing emotional distress, breast deformity and scarring. 80% of all breast biopsies done for a positive finding on a mammogram are negative for cancer.*(7)*

My Own Experience with Mammography

When I began residency training in radiology at Rush Presbyterian Hospital in Chicago in 1971, the state of the art was Xeromammography. This was a machine made by the Xerox Company which was prone to mechanical failure, and always breaking down. It produced a blue photo on paper with blue toner powder.*(9)*

In those days, *Franklin S Alcorn MD,(10)* was the only brave soul willing to read the Xerox images, and the book was Xeroradiography by John N. Wolfe. In 1972, the consensus in the department was that mammography was an orphan procedure and might never become acceptable. Some docs thought xeromammography was bordering on quackery, and screening mammogram had not been invented yet.*(11)*

Useful to the Surgeon

In those early days, the surgeon's criteria for doing a breast biopsy was a palpable mass. Many women have palpable lumps and bumps called fibrocystic breast disease which is quite common, and now known to be caused by iodine deficiency.*(12)*

Cyst or Solid Breast Mass?

In those days, the surgeon approached a breast mass with needle aspiration to differentiate between a fluid containing cyst or a solid mass. Nowadays, ultrasound determines this easily.

Back to the surgeon and his needle aspiration procedure; if the lesion is a cyst, the fluid is removed and the mass disappears. If no fluid can be obtained, then the mass is solid, and surgical removal is the next step. This is where the surgeons found the xeromammogram useful, occasionally showing a second occult mass or calcification which alerts the surgeon to remove additional tissue.

Invention of Needle Localization

Sometimes the surgeon had trouble actually finding the tiny calcifications at surgery since they could not feel them, so needle localization was invented. The radiologist placed a needle in the breast tissue near the calcifications which guided the surgeon to the spot to be removed. The surgically excised breast tissue was returned to the X-ray department for another mammogram of the specimen to determine if the lesion had been removed.

The Switch from Blue Paper to Gray X-ray Film

Grey X-Ray film mammograms replaced the blue Xerox paper images around 1982. By that time, I had joined a radiology group in Hollywood, Florida, but they were still using the Xerox machine even though the whole country had already made the switch to regular x-ray film. This inevitable switch-over to X-ray film made possible the large scale national breast screening programs, since the mammogram could be done at any hospital x-ray department.*(9)*

Finally, We All Learn Mammography

My radiology group made the plunge into film mammography. None of us had prior training or experience reading mammograms, so we traveled to expensive meetings and teaching courses on mammography from leaders in the field, such as Marc Homer MD and Laszlo Tabar MD *(*Sweden*)*, and then we started reading on our own.*(57)(13)*

From Breast Needle Biopsy to the Creation of a New Department

Soon we were doing the needle localizations using the Marc Homer needle, and needle biopsies in the radiology department. Initially, biopsies were done simply with a standard 20 gauge needle and 10 cc disposable syringe. A few years later, the radiology industry came out with spring loaded and vacuum assisted biopsy guns, and later invented dedicated biopsy tables using stereo-tactic guidance. This stereo guided machine allows the operator to take two x-rays at different angles, and uses a computer to calculate the exact depth and angle to advance the biopsy needle into the breast lesion.

By 2005, the cranky unreliable blue toner xeromammogram had been replaced with a shiny new department on the third floor with all the new modalities of hi-resolution digital mammography, stereotactic biopsy, breast ultrasound, and breast MRI. There is no question that the combination of these modalities makes a powerful and useful tool for diagnosis, treatment and follow up of breast cancer cases.

Screening is Quite Different from the Diagnostic Mammogram

However, screening mammography is quite different from diagnostic mammography as discussed below. Diagnostic mammography deals with a known abnormality in the breast, a mass or a palpable lump or even an abnormality on a breast thermogram or any suspicious area. In this case, the mammogram is quite useful in evaluating the abnormality to determine if it represents cancer. Screening mammography, on the other hand, takes a population of the worried well, and submits them to a mammogram to screen for any abnormality which might turn out to be cancer.

Victimization of Women?, No, Merely Good Medical Care.

When the screening mammogram program started years ago, many of the suspicious findings were false positive meaning they looked like something, but were in fact nothing. The radiologist would send a report of "suspicious requires biopsy" to the doctor who would tell the patient it might be cancer, and the terrorized woman would then not only submit to surgical biopsy under anesthesia, she would become hysterical and insist on the biopsy immediately. A negative biopsy would be then be a relief to the patient, also turning the surgeon into a hero. Feminists call this victimization of women, and healthcare professionals would call this good medical care.

Occasionally, about 10-20% of the time, a real cancer would be found at surgery. These were typically spiculated masses or fine branching calcifications. In the early days, the punctate calcifications and the milk-of calcium *(*teacup calcium*)* were called benign and did not require biopsy, and the branching calcifications indicated malignancy requiring biopsy and further treatment. However, nowadays, even the benign calcifications are routinely sent for biopsy, sometimes showing a controversial non-aggressive cancer called DCIS. *(14)(15)*

What's Your Track Record ?

At first, we had no idea how many of our mammogram readings of suspicious for cancer were actually found to be cancer by surgical biopsy and pathology evaluation. So to answer this question, we started compiling the pathology data and attended monthly conferences to review the data and our track record. We found that on average, one cancer for every 5 biopsies, but each radiologist and hospital may have more or less. Optimally, this information should be posted on the wall of the waiting room. Unfortunately, this type of data is rarely available to the patient.

Questioning Screening Mammography

In the 1980s everyone in health care believed that mammography was capable of early detection of breast cancer, and that mass screening programs were capable of reducing breast cancer mortality. I also believed in this, and to show my loyalty, I wrote an editorial in the Miami Herald praising the merits of screening mammography, which won the admiration of my colleagues in the radiology department.

However, beginning in 1995, I began to have doubts and misgivings and began to question the value of screening mammography. Right from beginning days, a debate raged between the advocates and the critics of screening mammography, arguing that medical studies of the technique either did, or did not show reduction in breast cancer mortality. Some critics of mammography screening such as Samuel Epstein MD say that mammograms cause harm from overtreatment with unnecessary breast biopsies, and the radiation exposure increases breast cancer risk.*(24)(25)(26)(27)(28)* Other outspoken critics such as Nortin Hadler*(37)* , Michael Baum *(46)(47)(48)(49(50))* and David Plotkin *(39)* have said screening mammography is so blunt that it approaches being useless, finding very few cancers that are truly treatable, and missing many of these, and it produces too many false positives. They seriously doubt that screening mammography has any impact on breast cancer mortality.

Luck of the Draw - Mammography Malpractice

One of radiologists in my group had the misfortune of being sued for malpractice. He missed a cancer on a mammogram that was visible in retrospect a year later. Remember, this routinely happens 30-70% of the time. This event happened early in his career, just out of his training period, before I met him. The story I heard was that the insurance company quickly settled the case by paying the woman a settlement of a million dollars, with no attempt at defending the case. As you can imagine, this was a major event which changed how my partner interpreted mammograms. After that event, it was understandable that he was gun shy, and almost always called the patient back for additional mammograms, and always recommended biopsy for any vague density. The problem is that almost every mammogram has vague densities, and almost all of the biopsies recommended under such circumstances are unnecessary for the patient, but are quite necessary for the radiologist, considering the medico-legal climate aptly described by Dr. Leonard Berlin.*(3)*

It quickly evolved into a game in which the x-ray technologists learned to bring the mammograms over to my side of the room to my reading area for a quick negative report, rather than to the other side of the reading room, where they can bet on doing additional mammogram views, and then have the patient sent for a biopsy of a questionable area. We played this game many years, and even with all these negative reports, I was never sued for malpractice for a mammogram reading during my entire career. I consider this "the luck of the draw".

Realizing the high rate of false positive biopsies and the emotional impact on women, I did my best to call the negative mammograms negative, all the while acknowledging there could be a cancer hiding on the mammogram somewhere, perhaps underneath an area of vague density. That was just one of the limitations of mammography. At the same time, when I did see abnormalities that had a high probability of cancer, these bonafide cases were sent for breast biopsy for good reason.

Biopsy Everything and Anything

The reality of a hostile medico-legal malpractice climate and the financial pressures dictates the practice of mammography in most community hospitals. This basically means that the usual practice is to biopsy anything and everything that shows up on the mammogram, as long as the patient is compliant. It is not difficult getting compliance by telling patient that it might be cancer, we just can't be sure. That usually is enough to make the woman hysterical and submit to biopsy. The radiologist is happy because he thinks he is reducing his chances of being sued for malpractice. His partners and the hospital administrators are happy because the procedures bring in more income. If cancer is found, the surgeons are happy because they have more lumpectomies and cancer operations to keep them busy.

DCIS, the Controversial Non-Aggressive Cancer

Over half of the cancers detected with mammography are DCIS *(*ductal carcinoma in situ*)*. This is a non-aggressive form of cancer which has a 98% survival after 5 years even with no treatment, although when found, the DCIS cases are treated with surgery just like any other cancer.*(31)* Some consider this detection and treatment of DCIS a form of overtreatment, others consider it good medical care.

Some critics have said that increased mammographic detection of DCIS has skewed the statistics, falsely reducing breast cancer mortality. This makes it **look like** we are reducing breast cancer mortality, while in reality there is no reduction in mortality from the real breast cancers.*(33)*

Without mammography, most of these DCIS cases would go undetected, and probably never cause a problem. Autopsy studies of women dying from car accidents have shown occult DCIS in up to 15% of the population.*(16)(17)* The actual incidence of cancer mortality is 0.4 per cent, not 15 per cent, suggesting that 96% of DCIS cases never go on to clinical disease. Yet, when DCIS is detected on the mammogram, these cases are treated with the same mastectomy or lumpectomy. A third of the time, pathologists will disagree on the diagnosis of DCIS while looking at the same case.*(16)(17)*

Lung Cancer Screening

Screening tests in radiology have been tried before. For example chest x-ray screening for lung cancer was tried, studied and abandoned. It was found that when you do a chest X-ray on smokers every 6 months, find the cancers and send the patient to surgery for treatment, there is no change in mortality figures. No lives are saved. In addition to make matters worse, when you go back to the earlier films 6 months before, on the film that was read as negative or normal in retrospect the lesion is visible 90% of the time.*(18)*

We thought these problems would be solved by moving up to CAT scans, a more advanced imaging technique. However, now we have a problem with seeing too many "suspicious" lesions and the false positive diagnosis. The net result is that lung cancer screening even with CAT scanning has not caught on.*(19)*

Mammogram screening in the under 50 age group NOT recommended by all other countries.

Current guidelines recommend a screening mammogram every 2 years for the 40-50 year age group. No other western country does this, as these women have dense breast tissue difficult to image and are most prone to a false positive reading, or a diagnosis of DCIS, the controversial less aggressive form of cancer. Most European countries restrict screening to post-menopausal women, after 50, when breast tissue involutes to fat and the cancers become more conspicuous.

Efficacy of Breast Cancer Screening - Does It Reduce Mortality?

The public perception is that breast cancer screening reduces breast cancer mortality. The reality is that this is a fiercely debated question in the medical literature with no clear winner. Leonard Berlin's articles summarize this debate in the medical literature.*(5)*

The debate is best shown by one example mentioned Dr. Berlin in the Sept 2002 issue of the Annals of Internal Medicine in which two conflicting articles appeared in the same issue, one stating that mammography has no mortality benefit, and the other saying it does.

Here are the Two Opposing Views on Mortality Benefit:

(1) Canadian researchers concluded that mammography screening did not reduce breast cancer mortality.*(20)(21)*

(2) United States Preventive Services Task Force concluded mammography reduces breast cancer mortality among women 40-74 years old.*(22)(23)*

Another excellent *review* of major Mammography Screening Studies can be found at the National Breast Cancer Coalition.*(59)(24)*

Bottom line, the debate rages on with no clear winner.

One observation which might clarify the debate is this: in two countries with socialized medicine, Canada and Sweden, careful studies of mammography screening were found to have **NO Mortality Benefit** compared to breast clinical exam.

Here in the US, however, with a 4 billion dollar fee-for-service screening mammogram industry, the mammography studies are interpreted to show that **Yes, there is a Mortality Benefit of about 15-20%**.

The influence of money and politics over medical science is pervasive, and mammography is certainly not immune. A few MD PhD's from Canada or Sweden are **not** about to derail a 4 billion dollar industry in the US.

Conflict of Interest in Sponsoring Breast Cancer Awareness Month?

Screening mammography critic, Samuel Epstein MD, irritates the establishment every time he points out that in 1984, the American Cancer Society created the October National Breast Cancer Awareness Month sponsored by money from the Astra-Zeneca Company, the maker of Tamoxiphen, the best selling breast cancer drug. In addition, Astra-Zeneca also manufactures industrial chemicals that cause breast cancer. Some consider this a conflict of interest.

Epstein also points out that past ACS advertisement promised early detection results in a cure nearly 100% of the time. Even more seriously, the Awareness Month advertisements avoid any reference to information on avoidable causes and prevention of breast cancer.*(24)(25)*

What is breast cancer prevention?

A previous chapter discusses *Iodine* supplementation as the most effective way to prevent breast cancer. Iodine tablets are safe, inexpensive and readily available. This is true prevention.*(12)*

Samuel Epstein's landmark book, "The Politics of Cancer" discusses carcinogenic chemicals in our food supply, home and workplace. Removing them can reduce breast cancer. This is true prevention.*(26)(27)*

The Untold Message of Breast Cancer Awareness Month:

To summarize, here is the untold message of Breast Cancer Awareness Month:

1) mammography screening is detection, not prevention and has several limitations, namely 30-70% missed cancers, and a tendency towards over diagnosis and over treatment.*(7)*

2) Many different carcinogenic chemicals cause breast cancer, and removing these chemicals from the workplace or home can reduce breast cancer rates. *(26)(27)*

3*)* Iodine deficiency causes fibrocystic disease, and Iodine supplementation prevents breast cancer.*(12)*

4*)* Synthetic hormones like Provera increase breast cancer risk. *(*WHI Study*)(29)*

5*)* Bio-Identical Hormone programs are safe, and do not increase risk of breast cancer. *(*French Cohort Study*)(30)*

Will mainstream medicine ever endorse Dr. Leonard Berlin's Truth-in-Mammography disclaimers? I predict this will never happen. Instead, the public's unrealistic expectation that a breast cancer nodule will be detected 100% of the time will continue, and the high cost of medical malpractice will simply be absorbed into "the cost of doing business". The screening mammogram is here to stay. As for my opinion, I am not opposed to the status quo of mammogram screening in the over 50 age group. However, we should educate the public to be realistic in their expectations of mammography. Unfortunately this task of educating the public is thwarted by the unrealistic expectations created by false and deceptive advertising about screening mammography. Perhaps that is the real untold message of October Breast Cancer Awareness Month.

References

(1) http://www.cancer.org/docroot/PED/content/PED_2_3X_ACS_Cancer_Detection_Guidelines_36.asp?sitearea=PED
American Cancer Society Breast Cancer Prevention Page: Yearly mammograms are recommended starting at age 40 and continuing for as long as a woman is in good health.

(2) http://www.rnsmc.org/news_article.asp?ID=41
Leonard Berlin, M.D, FACR, Chairman of Radiology at Rush North Shore Medical Center, Skokie, was awarded the Distinguished Service Gold Medal Award of the Chicago Radiological Society, its highest honor on April 21, 2005 in Chicago, IL. The Gold Medal is awarded annually to an individual who has rendered unusual service to the science of radiology and will be presented to Dr. Berlin by his son, radiologist Jonathan W. Berlin, M.D. Berlin is Chairman of Skokie Valley Hospital Department of Radiology.

(3) http://radiology.rsnajnls.org/cgi/reprint/233/3/641
Mammography Screening Can Survive Malpractice . . . If Radiologists Take Center Stage and Assume the Role of Educator by Leonard Berlin, MD. Radiology December 2004.

(4) http://www.ajronline.org/cgi/content/full/176/5/1131
The missed breast cancer redux: time for educating the public about the limitations of mammography? Berlin L. AJR 2001; 176:1131-1134

(5) *http://www.ajronline.org/cgi/content/full/180/5/1229*
Malpractice Issues in Radiology, Breast Cancer, Mammography, and Malpractice Litigation: The Controversies Continue Leonard Berlin, *AJR* 2003; 180:1229-1237, Excellent discussion of controversy of screening mammography and impact on mortality figures.

(6) *http://www.ajronline.org/cgi/content/full/176/5/1123*
Perspective on Dot Size, Lead Time, Fallibility, and Impact on Survival Continuing Controversies in Mammography Leonard Berlin MD. AJR 2001; 176:1123-1130

(7) *http://www.fda.gov/ohrms/dockets/ac/03/briefing/3945b1_05_Berlin%20testimony.pdf*
STATEMENT of Leonard Berlin, M.D. To the U.S. Senate Committee on Health, Education Labor and Pensions Re: Mammography Quality Standards Act Reauthorization April 8, 2003. Leonard Berlin: "Suffice it to say that research studies performed at some of the most prestigious medical institutions in the United States reveal that as many as 90% of lung cancers, and 70% of breast cancers, can at least partially be observed on previous studies read as normal."

(8) *http://www.imagingeconomics.com/issues/articles/2004-11_02.asp*
A Manifesto for Truth-in-Mammography Advertising by Leonard Berlin MD Imaging Economics, November 2004. "From cigarettes to pharmaceuticals to financial services, all advertisements feature a disclaimer: Why not those for mammography? Of all medical malpractice lawsuits filed in the United States that allege a delay in the diagnosis of breast cancer, radiologists are the most frequently sued specialists. Of all medical malpractice lawsuits lodged against radiologists, the most frequent cause is the allegation of a missed breast cancer on mammography. Why has "missed breast cancer" risen to first place in the medical malpractice standings? I suggest that it is because we have oversold mammography. We have marketed mammography without informing the American public all that we know about not only the benefits, but more important the limitations and potential harms of mammography." Endquote Dr. Berlin.

(9) *http://radiology.rsnajnls.org/cgi/content/full/215/1/1*
Breast Imaging: From 1965 to the Present Edward A. Sickles, MD, Radiology. 2000;215:1-16.*)* Examples of xeromammograms and film mammograms, speculated lesion, needle localization.

(10) *http://www.chi-rad-soc.org/illinois.html*
History: Narratives Radiology in Illinois By Franklin Alcorn, M.D. Dr. Alcorn's history appearedintheprogramoftheChicagoRadiologicalSocietyattheCentennialofRadiology in 1995.

(11) *http://www.chi-rad-soc.org/illinois.html*
History: Narratives Radiology in Illinois By Franklin Alcorn, M.D. Dr. Alcorn's history appeared in the program of the Chicago Radiological Society at the Centennial of Radiology in 1995.

(12) *http://jeffreydach.com/2007/05/05/jeffreydachdrdachiodine.aspx*
Breast Cancer Prevention and Iodine Supplementation by Jeffrey Dach MD, Iodine Supplementation Prevents Breast Cancer by Jeffrey Dach MD

(13) *http://www.sma.org/AM2005/ANM2004pdfs/Saturday/S21_Otto_P.pdf*
Screening mammogram Swedish Study by Dr. Laszlo Tabar (1977- 1984) Population-based randomized controlled study showed 31% reduction in breast cancer mortality in women 50 plus. Breast Cancer Screening Southern Medical Association's 98th Annual Scientific Assembly November 13, 2004 Pamela M. Otto, MD Associate Professor UTHSCSA, Dept of Radiology

(14) *http://sprojects.mmi.mcgill.ca/mammography/calcifications1.htm*
INTERACTIVE MAMMOGRAPHY ANALYSIS WEB TUTORIAL. Images of benign calcifications, secretory disease, milk of calcium, etc. Molson Medical Informatics Project 1999. McGill University.

(15) *http://sprojects.mmi.mcgill.ca/mammography/calcifications3.htm*
Tutorial 2 : CALCIFICATIONS ASSOCIATED WITH A HIGH PROBABILITY OF MALIGNANCY. Molson Medical Informatics Project 1999. McGill University. Fine linear branching calcifications are high probability for malignancy.

(16) *http://www.moffitt.org/moffittapps/ccj/v6n3/article5.htm*
Ductal Carcinoma In Situ of the Breast by Elisabeth L. Dupont, MD; Ni Ni K. Ku, MD; Christa McCann, BA; and Charles E. Cox, MD, FACS. Moffitt Cancer Center. DCIS, 60% of DCIS cases are discovered solely by mammography. Seven major autopsy studies of women not known to have had breast cancer have provided insight. Six studies found an incidence of 4% to 18%. DCIS now accounts for nearly half of mammographically detected cases of cancer.

(17) *http://www.annals.org/cgi/content/full/127/11/1023*
Using Autopsy Series To Estimate the Disease "Reservoir" for Ductal Carcinoma in Situ of the Breast: How Much More Breast Cancer Can We Find? H. Gilbert Welch, MD, MPH, and William C. Black, MD Annals of Internal Medicine December 1997 Volume 127 Issue 11 Pages 1023." **Conclusions:** A substantial reservoir of DCIS is undetected during life. How hard pathologists look for the disease and, perhaps, their threshold for making the diagnosis are potentially important factors in determining how many cases of DCIS are diagnosed. The latter has important implications for what it means to have the disease."

(18) *http://www.respiratoryreviews.com/apr00/rr_apr00_lungcancer.html*
DOES LUNG CANCER SCREENING SAVE LIVES? by Janis Kelly, Respiratory Reviews April 2000.

(19) *http://www.bcbsnc.com/services/medical-policy/pdf/lung_cancer_screening_ct_scanning_or_chest_radiographs.pdf*
Corporate Medical Policy Lung Cancer Screening, CT Scanning or Chest Radiographs, Blue Cross Blue Shield of N Carolina. No Policy coverage for Lung cancer screening with chest CAT or Xrays.

(20) *http://www.annals.org/cgi/content/full/137/5_Part_1/305*
The Canadian national breast screening study. 1. Breast cancer mortality after 11 to 16 years of follow-up. Miller AB, To T, Baines CJ, Wall C. Ann Intern Med 2002;137:305 312. "After 11 to 16 years of follow-up, four or five annual screenings with mammography, breast physical examination, and breast self-examination **had not** reduced breast cancer mortality compared with usual community care after a single breast physical examination and instruction on breast self-examination. The study data show that true effects of 20% or greater are unlikely. Controversy will persist because other studies suggest that screening causes small reductions in breast cancer mortality."

(21) *http://jnci.oxfordjournals.org/cgi/content/abstract/92/18/1490*
Canadian National Breast Screening Study-2: 13-Year Results of a Randomized Trial in Women Aged 50-59 Years. Anthony B. Miller, Teresa To, Cornelia J. Baines, Claus Wall, Journal of the National Cancer Institute, Vol. 92, No. 18, 1490-1499, September 20, 2000. "**Conclusion: In women aged 50 - 59 years, the addition of annual mammography screening to physical examination has no impact on breast cancer mortality."**

(22) *http://www.annals.org/cgi/content/full/137/5_Part_1/344*
Screening for Breast Cancer: Recommendations and Rationale, U.S. Preventive Services Task Force. Humphrey LL, Helfand M, Chan BKS, Woolf SH. Ann Intern Med 2002;137:347 -360 The U.S. Preventive Services Task Force recommends screening mammography, with or without clinical breast examination, every 1 to 2 years for women aged 40 and older.

(23) *http://www.ahrq.gov/clinic/3rduspstf/breastcancer/brcanrr.pdf*
United States Preventive Services Task Force concluded mammography reduces breast cancer mortality among women 40-74 years old.

Samuel Epstein MD

(24)(25)(26)(27)(28)

http://www.preventcancer.com/patients/mammography/ijhs_mammography.htm
Dangers and Unreliability of Mammography: Breast Examination is a Safe, Effective, and Practical Alternative by Samuel S. Epstein, Rosalie Bertell, and Barbara Seaman. International Journal of Health Services, 31*(3)*:605-615, 2001. Breast Cancer Coalition.

(25) http://findarticles.com/p/articles/mi_m1525/is_5_84/ai_62896172
Cancer, Inc and National Breast Cancer Awareness Month. by Sharon Batt, Liza Gross. Sierra, Sept, 1999" THEY MAKE THE CHEMICALS, THEY RUN THE TREATMENT CENTERS, AND THEY'RE STILL LOOKING FOR "THE CURE"--NO WONDER THEY WON'T TELL YOU ABOUT BREAST CANCER PREVENTION". Blistering Criticism.

(26) http://www.preventcancer.com/work/
Cancer Prevention Coalition. Samuel S. Epstein, MD founder and Chairman of the Cancer Prevention Coalition, and is professor emeritus of Environmental and Occupational Medicine at the University of Illinois School of Public Health. He has published some 260 peer reviewed articles, and authored or co-authored 11 books including: the prize-winning 1978 The Politics of Cancer; the 1995 Safe Shopper's Bible; the 1998 Breast Cancer Prevention Program; the 1998 The Politics of Cancer, Revisited.

(27) http://www.preventcancer.com/press/books/poc.htm
The Politics of Cancer, Revisited 1998 By Samuel S. Epstein, M.D. Foreword by Congressman David Obey, Introduction by Congressman John Conyers In this book, world-cancer expert Dr. Samuel Epstein indicts the National Cancer Institute and the American Cancer Society for responsibility in losing the cancer war.

http://www.stopbreastcancer.org/
Stop Breast Cancer Dot Org

(29) http://jama.ama-assn.org/cgi/content/abstract/288/7/872
Postmenopausal Hormone Replacement Therapy Scientific Review Heidi D. Nelson, MD, MPH; Linda L. Humphrey, MD, MPH; Peggy Nygren, MA; Steven M. Teutsch, MD, MPH; Janet D. Allan, PhD, RN JAMA. 2002;288:872-881.

French Cohort Study

(30) http://www.ncbi.nlm.nih.gov/pubmed/12626212
Combined hormone replacement therapy and risk of breast cancer in a French cohort study of 3175 women. de Lignières B et al., Climacteric. 2002 Dec;5(4):332-40. French Cohort Study shows no increased risk of breast cancer from bio-identical human hormones.

DCIS

(31) http://radiology.rsnajnls.org/cgi/content/full/221/3/770
Case 41: Ductal Carcinoma in Situ, by Alanna T. Harris, MD. "The detection of ductal carcinoma in situ has increased markedly in recent years secondary to the widespread use of screening mammography, and it now accounts for 25 to 40% of mammographically detected breast cancers."

(33) *http://jnci.oxfordjournals.org/cgi/content/abstract/94/20/1546*
Detection of Ductal Carcinoma In Situ in Women Undergoing Screening Mammography by Virginia L. Ernster, Journal of the National Cancer Institute, Vol. 94, No. 20, 1546-1554, October 16, 2002. "Conclusions: Overall, approximately 1 in every 1300 screening mammography examinations leads to a diagnosis of DCIS. Given uncertainty about the natural history of DCIS, the clinical significance of screen-detected DCIS needs further investigation."

(34) *http://www.allbookstores.com/Mammography_p4sd.html*
Mammography Books available.

(35) *http://www.blogher.com/pink-ribbon-madness-say-no-breast-cancer-exploitation-corporate-profit*
Pink Ribbon Madness: Say No to Breast Cancer Exploitation for Corporate Profit by Suzanne Reisman 10/06/2007

(36) *http://www.naturalnews.com/022115.html*
October is Breast Cancer Propaganda Month: Pinkwashing, Breast Cancer Action and Vitamin D. Thursday, October 11, 2007 by: Mike Adams. Critical of mammography.

NORTIN HADLER. M.D.

(37) *http://abcnews.go.com/Health/OnCallPlus/story?id=3196417&page=1*
Does Screening Mammography Save Lives? Numbers May Not Justify Practice for Routine Mammograms, OPINION By **NORTIN HADLER. M.D.** May 21, 2007, ABC News. Dr. Nortin Hadler is professor of medicine and microbiology/immunology at the University of North Carolina at Chapel Hill, and an attending rheumatologist at University of North Carolina Hospitals.

"In the United States, radiologists are so hesitant to read a mammogram as "normal" that false positive rates can reach 80 percent. This hedging on the readings is driven by the fact that "missing a breast cancer" on mammography is the most frequent reason for malpractice litigation in the United States.

But screening mammography is so terribly blunt that it approaches useless: It finds very few cancers that are truly treatable, it misses many of these and it is awash in false positives. Norway, Sweden, Australia and the United Kingdom are re-examining their national experience with screening mammography because of appraisals similar to mine.

If a woman's life was saved because of early detection of an evil breast cancer, she should thank her lucky stars rather than her mammographer. I would relegate mammograms to the archives of false starts, next to radical mastectomy" Endquote.

(38) *http://jnci.oxfordjournals.org/cgi/content/full/92/20/1630*

After 40 Years, Mammography Remains as Much Emotion as Science by Judith Randal, Journal of the National Cancer Institute, Vol. 92, No. 20, 1630-1632, October 18, 2000 "For the better part of a century, it would have been unthinkable to treat primary breast cancer with anything but the operation pioneered in the 1890s by William Halsted, M.D., one of the most prominent surgeons of his day. Beginning in the 1970s, the Halsted era drew gradually to a close when randomized controlled trials found that the operation generally known as radical mastectomy was no more effective than less drastic surgery *(*sometimes in combination with radiation*)*. Could a similar fate await the current gold-standard status of screening mammography? Will a time come when its popularity dwindles, too?...Mammography now a $4 billion a year industry in the United States alone...Absent unforeseen developments, it is probably safe to predict that mammography for screening will continue to be as much about strongly held opinions and political pressures as about science."endquote Judith Randall.

David Plotkin MD

(39) *http://www.theatlantic.com/doc/199806/breast-cancer*

Good News and Bad News About Breast Cancer by **David Plotkin M.D.** The Atlantic Monthly, June 1998,"Breast cancer is a major public-health concern; it kills 0.04 percent of all American women yearly...Most of the time the news is reassuring; two thirds to four fifths of all biopsies reveal that the abnormality is not malignant. *(*Women in their forties are more likely than older women to have negative biopsies, because mammograms of their naturally lumpier breasts are harder to interpret.*)*...An official nationwide mammography program would be a huge commitment: 51.5 million American women are aged forty or above. And one must bear in mind the cost of needless medical procedures generated by the huge number of false-positive mammograms...two to four false positives for every true positive, according to some measures.

On balance, then, I reluctantly support the status quo. When my patients come in for their mammograms, I do not try to dissuade them. But I tell them that the most optimistic interpretation of the available evidence suggests that **routine mammography has only a marginal effect on a woman's chances of surviving breast cancer, and that it may have no effect at all."** endquote

(40) *http://jco.ascopubs.org/cgi/content/full/21/1/41*

High Prevalence of Premalignant Lesions in Prophylactically Removed Breasts From Women at Hereditary Risk for Breast Cancer by N. Hoogerbrugge et al.J ournal of Clinical Oncology, Vol 21, Issue 1 *(*January*)*, 2003: 41-45. Full text.

"Conclusion: Many women at high risk of hereditary breast cancer develop high-risk histopathologic lesions, especially after the age of 40 years. Surveillance does not detect such high-risk histopathologic lesions."

(41) *http://content.nejm.org/cgi/content/full/348/17/1672*

Mammographic Screening for Breast Cancer Suzanne W. Fletcher, M.D., and Joann G. Elmore, M.D., M.P.H. NEJM Volume 348:1672-1680 April 24, 2003 Number 17

(42) *http://www.hsph.harvard.edu/causal/publications/mammography.pdf*
POINT COUNTERPOINT On the efficacy of screening for breast cancer by David A Freedman, Diana B Petitti, and James M Robins, International Journal of Epidemiology 2004;33:4355. Review of studies concludes mammography screening is effective.

(43) *http://www.hsph.harvard.edu/causal/publications/rejoinder.pdf*
Rejoinder,by David A Freedman, Diana B Petitti and James M Robins. International Journal of Epidemiology 2004;33:6973. More on effciacy of screening mammography.

(44) *http://jama.ama-assn.org/cgi/content/full/293/10/1245*
Screening for Breast Cancer. Joann G. Elmore, MD, MPH; Katrina Armstrong, MD; Constance D. Lehman, MD, PhD; Suzanne W. Fletcher, MD, MSc JAMA. 2005;293:1245-1256. "All major US medical organizations recommend screening mammography for women aged 40 years and older. Screening mammography reduces breast cancer mortality by about 20% to 35% in women aged 50 to 69 years and slightly less in women aged 40 to 49 years at 14 years of follow-up.

Approximately 95% of women with abnormalities on screening mammograms do not have breast cancer with variability based on such factors as age of the woman and assessment category assigned by the radiologist. Studies comparing full-field digital mammography to screen film have not shown statistically significant differences in cancer detection while the impact on recall rates *(*percentage of screening mammograms considered to have positive results*)* was unclear."endquote

(45) *http://cebp.aacrjournals.org/cgi/content/full/13/4/501*
Fear, Anxiety, Worry, and Breast Cancer Screening Behavior: A Critical Review Nathan S. Consedine, Carol Magai, Yulia S. Krivoshekova, Lynn Ryzewicz and Alfred . Neugut. Cancer Epidemiology Biomarkers & Prevention Vol. 13, 501-510, April 2004.

Michael Baum

(46) *http://www.healthy.net/scr/article.asp?Id=2717*
Cancer: When it isn't a killer DCIS: Precancer, benign cancer or what? What Doctors Don't Tell You *(*Volume 13, Issue 10*)*. "The cancer establishment was recently rocked to its core when Professor Michael Baum, an eminent and well-respected breast surgeon and researcher, claimed that screening for breast cancer should be scrapped because it caused hundreds of healthy women to undergo risky, mutilating and unnecessary treatments even when they may never develop the disease. His comments, made at a meeting of the Royal Society of Medicine, cut even more deeply because Baum was one of the physicians who helped set up the 50-million-a-year breast-screening service *(*Frith M, Scrap Breast Cancer Screening, Evening Standard, 10 December 2002, p 1*)*. **Baum** has stated publicly that the most dramatic consequence of the rise in the numbers of routine mammographies has been a huge increase in the incidence of small, well-contained, relatively benign breast cancers known as ductal carcinoma in situ *(*DCIS*)* *(*BMJ Rapid Responses at bmj.com/cgi/eletters/325/ 7361/418#24945, 24 August 2002*)*." endquote

(47) *http://www.bmj.com/cgi/eletters/325/7361/418#24945*
Re: Screening and Mastectomy rates, Letter to the editor of BMJ by **Michael Baum**, Emeritus Prof. of Surgery University College London The Portland Hospital, 212-214 Great Portland Street, London W1W 5QN.

(48) *http://www.thisislondon.co.uk/news/article-2407684-details/'Scrap+breast+cancer+screening'/article.do*
'Scrap breast cancer screening' By Maxine Frith, Health Correspondent, Evening Standard 10.12.02

The man who helped to set up the NHS breast screening programme claims today that it does more harm than good.

Professor Michael Baum, a leading expert in the field, said that screening for the disease causes hundreds of healthy women to have risky, mutilating and unnecessary treatments even when they may never develop the disease.

Fifteen years after he established one of the first screening centres in the UK, Professor Baum has now called for the Â£50million a year service to be shut. He believes the techniques used for screening are not accurate enough and lead to too many false alarms.

Professor Baum, who is to address the Royal Society of Medicine in London today, has been a long-standing critic of screening but has never before gone so far as to say it should be scrapped entirely,

He is one of the most eminent breast surgeons in the country and a respected researcher into the disease. His comments have sparked a furious row among experts over the benefits of the NHS breast screening programme

(49) *http://news.bbc.co.uk/2/hi/health/6061652.stm*
Breast screen 'wrong care' fears, BBC News, 18 October 2006. "Breast screening may produce false positives. Concerns have been raised that breast cancer screening might lead to some women undergoing unnecessary treatment. Researchers looked at international studies on half a million women. They found that for every 2,000 women screened over a decade, one will have her life prolonged, but 10 will have to undergo unnecessary treatment. UK experts said women over 50 should go for their breast checks, but a screening pioneer raised doubts about the NHS programme's future. The report, published in the Cochrane Library, involved a review of breast cancer research papers from around the world."endquote.

(50) *http://www.telegraph.co.uk/news/uknews/1531694/Doubts-raised-by-the-pioneer-of-screening.html*
Doubts raised by the pioneer of screening By Nic Fleming, Medical Correspondent 18/10/2006 .Prof Michael Baum set up one of the first breast cancer screening programmes in England in 1987.

Cochrane Report

cochrane.org/reviews/en/ab001877.html
Screening for breast cancer with mammography. Gotzsche PC, Nielsen M Cochrane Reviews

(52) http://www.cochrane.dk/research/Screening for breast cancer with mammography (Cochrane review).pdf
Screening for breast cancer with mammography Gotzsche PC, Nielsen M cochrane collaboration 2006 full text pdf

(53) http://findarticles.com/p/articles/mi_m3225/is_2_68/ai_105645316
Should we offer routine breast cancer screening with mammography? - Cochrane For Clinicians: Putting Evidence Into Practice. by Sean P. David. American Family Physician, July 15, 2003

(54) http://www.bmj.com/cgi/content/full/323/7319/956
Row over breast cancer screening shows that scientists bring "some subjectivity into their work Susan Mayor, London, BMJ 2001;323:956 *(*27 October*)*.

"The review claimed that there was no reliable evidence to support the value of mammography screening in reducing deaths from breast cancer and alleged an association with increased rates of breast surgery.

Ole Olson and Peter Gotsche from the Nordic Cochrane Centre, Righospitalet, Copenhagen, Denmark, reassessed as part of a Cochrane review a meta-analysis of seven randomised trials of screening mammography which they had previously carried out. This confirmed their original conclusion, that there was no evidence of a reduction in either total or breast cancer mortality in two of the trials that they considered to be of sufficient quality to analyse.

They added:"We have also confirmed that screening leads to more aggressive treatment, increasing the number of mastectomies by about 20% and the number of mastectomies and tumourectomies by about 30%" *(*Lancet 2001;358:1340-2 *)*."endquote.

(55) http://www.bmj.com/cgi/content/full/324/7338/677/b
Letters Breast screening seems driven by belief rather than evidence. Hazel Thornton, independent advocate for quality in research and healthcare. BMJ 2002;324:677.16 March

(56) http://www.bmj.com/cgi/content/full/323/7321/1131/a
Letters. Office of NHS cancer screening programme misrepresents Nordic work in breast screening row by Peter C Gotzsche, director. Nordic Cochrane Centre, Rigshospitalet, DK-2100 Copenhagen Ã¸, BMJ 2001;323:1131 *(*10 November 2001*)*

(57) *http://www.mammographyed.com/docs/2007/Melbourne-schedule2.pdf*
LÃzlo Tabar, M.D. Professor of Radiology Course Director 2007 BREAST SEMINAR SERIES Covering the world of breast diagnosis.

Opposed to Screening

(58) *http://www.annieappleseedproject.org/natbreascanc3.html*
National Breast Cancer Coalition (NBCC) The Mammography Screening Controversy: Questions and Answers February 8, 2002

(59) *http://www.stopbreastcancer.org//index2.php?option=com_content&do_pdf=1&id=133*
Position Statement on Screening Mammography Updated May 2007. National Breast Cancer Coalition 1707 L Street, NW, Suite 1060 Washington, D.C. 20036 (202) 296-7477 voice (202) 265-6854 fax

(60) *http://www.breastcancerchoices.org/iodineindex.html*
BreastCancerChoices.org cancer advocacy Iodine Supplement Information
contact lynne. Breast Cancer Choices, Inc., a nonprofit organization helping patients make informed choices about breast screening, diagnostic procedures and treatment.

(61) *http://www.newamerica.net/publications/articles/2002/search_and_destroy*
Search and Destroy, Why Mammograms Are Not the Answer, By Shannon Brownlee, New America Foundation, The New Republic April 22, 2002

Section Ten

Medical Meetings Reports

Chapter 30

Pulsed Electromagnetic Devices for Healing Sports Injuries

Roger Federer, Member of the Swiss Tennis Team

The number one ranked tennis player, Roger Federer, swept the Australian Open, Wimbledon and the U.S. Open in all three years, 2004, 2006 and 2007. Federer is also a member of the Swiss Tennis Team.*(1)(2)* Of course, top tennis players are gifted athletes, but could some of them have a secret weapon that gives an edge on the tennis court? You might be surprised to know that the Swiss Tennis Team uses of gadget called a BEMER. This is a portable pulsed magnetic field device which speeds healing of muscle and tendons after tough tennis matches. According to the BEMER web site, the Swiss Tennis Team and many other athletes have been using a portable pulsed magnetic therapy unit regularly.*(3)*

Horse Racing and Pulsed Magnetic Wave Devices

Pulsed magnetic therapy for sports injuries is nothing new, and has been used in horse racing for many years. There is big money in Horse Racing, and trainers give their horses pulsed magnetic therapy to gain an edge on the track. Benefits include faster recovery time from sports injuries, improved blood flow, improved nerve regeneration, and faster wound and fracture healing.*(4)(5)(6)(7)(9)(10)*

Dan Clark MD and the BioEnergetic Medicine Conference

I learned about Pulsed Electromagnetic Fields *(*pulsed EMF*)* for healing of sports injuries at Dan Clark's BioEnergetic Medicine Conference in Orlando, September 2007.*(15)* Electromagnetic radiation as a therapeutic device wasn't accepted by mainstream medicine until 1985 when Robert O Becker, M.D. discovered that non-united bone fractures heal with pulsed EMF electrical stimulation. This is now standard practice in all hospitals. Becker's books, The Body Electric in 1985, and Cross Currents in 1990, broke new ground, and the 3 decades of research since then have shown pulsed EMF to be effective for non-united bone fractures, relief of musculo-skeletal pain, migraine headaches, low back pain, depression, wound healing, improvement in blood flow and nerve regeneration, to mention a few. Robert Becker discovered that weak electric currents recruit stem cells which differentiate into the body part requiring healing. Becker also discovered a second nervous system in the body which corresponds to the Chinese acupuncture meridians. *(11)(12)(13)(14)* There are numerous therapeutic uses of pulsed EMF published in the medical literature. *(69)(70)(71)(72)(73)(74)(75)*

Electromagnetic Waves are the Basis of the Chemical Bond

Although modern science began with Isaac Newton's laws of mechanics in 1687, Michael Faraday's principles of electromagnetic induction were discovered only recently in 1831.*(16)(17)(18)* Since then, Albert Einstein and quantum mechanics further changed our understanding of matter, energy, and the universe. *(19)(20)(21)(22)* Paradoxically, the electron and all electromagnetic energy are both particle and wave, and the electron's wave function derived from quantum mechanics is the basis of the chemical bond, first described by Linus Pauling.*(23)* The chemical bond is now understood as sharing electrons (electromagnetic energy wave forms) between two atoms or molecules.

Electro-Magnetic Energy Use in Diagnosis

We have been using electromagnetic energy for medical diagnosis since the beginning of modern medicine. For example, the Electrocardiogram (EKG) and Electroencephalogram (EEG) record electrical activity from body parts. The CAT scan image is created by passing electromagnetic radiation through a body part and recording the transmitted radiation. The MRI scanner makes an image by pulsing electromagnetic energy through the body and then "listening" for the emitted energy signal. The mass spectrograph, a primitive form of MRI machine is used daily in the hospital lab for routine blood testing.

Electromagnetic Energy is Essential for Life

When we bask in the sun, and our skin makes vitamin D from sun light, this is electromagnetic radiation driving a bio-chemical reaction in our body. Photosynthesis is another example of absorption of electromagnetic radiation to form carbon bonds in plants. As a matter of fact, all biochemistry can be explained as electrical interactions between outer shell electrons. Electromagnetic energy is a basic part of the biochemistry of life.

BEMER and ONDAMED Devices

One elementary problem with pulsed electro magnetic therapy as a treatment is: how do we determine the exact pulse frequency to be used? The BEMER device steps through a series of pre-set frequencies. Another device called the Ondamed uses a more sophisticated method of diagnosis before applying the treatment.*(24)* With the Ondamed device, the operator scans though a frequency range while palpating the radial pulse. When the pulse becomes palpably stronger, this indicates a vascular autonomic response (VAS), and that frequency is selected as the treatment frequency

(25) Our understanding of pulsed magnetic field treatment is still in its infancy, and the next few decades will see more research and refinement of technique, and greater acceptance into mainstream medicine.

Shari Lieberman

Dr. Shari Lieberman presented three cases of plantar fasciitis treated with the Ondamed device, all with prompt recovery. Dr. Lieberman is currently compiling additional Ondamed cases of trigeminal neuralgia, reflex sympathetic dystrophy, bell's palsy, and others.*(26)(27)*

Poly-MVA

Dr. Shari Lieberman also presented Poly-MVA case studies. Poly MVA, available since 1995, is a non-toxic nutritional supplement containing palladium, which has been used for nutritional support for cancer patients. Dr. Lieberman presented cases of clinical improvement with Poly MVA. These cases included multiple myeloma, lung cancer, and prostate cancer. *(28)(29)(30)(31)(32)(33)(34)*

Merrill Garnett

Merrill Garnett, the inventor of Poly MVA, is a brilliant researcher and author of the book, First Pulse, which describes the electrical pulsations inside every cell, and how Poly MVA manipulates these electrical pulsations to cause the death of cancer cells without injuring normal cells. Garnett's life-long search for an anti-cancer agent culminated in his discovery of Poly MVA. One hundred years from now, I predict that the history of science will place Merrill Garnett in the same company with Faraday, Einstein, and Becker.*(35)(36)(37)(38)*

Patricia Kane PhD

Patricia and Ed Kane of the Haverford Wellness Center, Havertown, PA presented their treatment protocol and case studies. They use IV phospholipid therapy for ALS, Stroke, Environmental illness, Hypercoagulation, Parkinson's, Cardiovascular Disease, Hepatitis C and Autism. This is the original IV phospholipid formulation from Natterman in Germany, and they showed case photos before and after treatment which were simply amazing, and by far the most impressive at the meeting.*(39)(40)(41)(42)(43)*

Ed Kane, cell membrane phospholipid bilayers, the key to health.

Phospholipids are long chain carbon molecules which form microscopic tuning forks that oscillate and resonate at set electromagnetic frequencies. The phospholipid unit which forms the membrane bilayer has two long chain fatty acids joined at the "head" by phosphate group which resembles a tuning fork. The CIS double bond is the "kink" in one of the long chains. This "kinked"chain is not stationary, as the molecular structure wobbles back and forth allowing it to absorb energy and synchronize its vibrations with other "tuning forks" in the membrane.

These phospholipid bilayers are not only located at the outer cell membrane, they are also present as folded layers throughout the cell cytoplasm providing surfaces for all biochemical reactions to take place. Energy absorption by these bilayers speeds up biochemical reactions at the membrane surfaces. Mitochondria inside the cells have membrane bilayers where energy production takes place. The membrane bilayers are made of tuning fork phospholipids which absorb and emit electromagnetic energy.

Sangeeta Pati, M.D.

Sangeeta Pati, M.D. discussed bio-identical hormones, reviewing the medical literature which demonstrates that bio-identical hormones are safe and do not increase risk of breast cancer as shown in the French Cohort study.*(47)* In addition, bio-identical hormones are protective and reduce risk of heart disease as shown in a recent NEJM coronary calcium score study.*(48)* On the other hand, the synthetic progestins are the bad guys which should be avoided. Don't miss Dr. Sangeeta Pati explaining bio-identical hormone therapy in a *video interview* on the Wellness Hour viewable on the internet.*(44)(45)(46)*

Adrenal Fatigue

A diagnosis of adrenal fatigue can be made with salivary cortisol testing, and treatment with cortisol or phosphatidyl serine. Chronic daily stress eventually causes exhaustion, and this means reduced adrenal production of cortisol, which is the definition of adrenal fatigue. I had a recent phone conversation with an old time friend who is also an endocrinologist. She informed me that adrenal fatigue simply doesn't exist as a real medical diagnosis. Mainstream medicine doesn't believe in it. The adrenal gland is normal, functioning at 100%, or nonfunctional *(*Addison's' Disease*)*, with nothing in between. For these doubting mainstream docs, the medical literature shows that adrenal fatigue is indeed caused by cortisol deficiency which can be measured with salivary testing, and the condition can be cured with bio-identical natural cortisol. *(49)(50)(51)(52)(53)(54)(55)(56)(57)(58)(59)(60)*

A more complete treatment involving lifestyle modification and nutritional supplements to relieve adrenal fatigue is described in the book, Adrenal Fatigue by James C. Wilson.*(61)* The book, The Safe Use of Cortisol by McJefferies is also a useful reference on low dose cortisol treatment for adrenal fatigue.*(62)*

Russell Jaffe MD

Russell Jaffe MD discussed how vitamin and nutritional deficiencies are prevalent and cause chronic diseases such as cardiovascular disease, cancer, and osteoporosis.*(62)(63)* Russell Jaffe is the founder of the Perque Company, a unique vitamin and nutritional supplement company which is miles ahead of the competition. At our office, we use exclusively the Perque Vitamin C because it is 100% L-ascorbate, fully buffered with no fillers, and is the superior product. Dr. Jaffe *(*Russ*)* has solved a number of nutritional supplement problems. His choline citrate solves the magnesium uptake block issue. His glucosamine joint product provides more rapid pain relief, his bioflavonoids provide more pain relief, and a new fiber which is better tolerated. Russ also has a new adrenal stress product containing Relora which was unveiled at the meeting, and the samples I tried were incredible. Russ has continued to improve the Perque line. For example, Strontium is now included in the Bone Guard supplement for osteoporosis prevention. Always the showman, Dr. Jaffe made the closing comments at the meeting describing how Louis Pasteur triumphed over his rival Bechamp with superior marketing, rather than with superior technology.*(64)(65)*

References

(1) http://www.rogerfederer.com/en/index.cfm
Roger Federer Official Web Site.

(2) http://en.wikipedia.org/wiki/Roger_Federer
Roger Federer Wikipedia listing

(3) http://www.bemerclinics.com.au/public/html/sports.html
Listing of athletes using the BEMER pulsed magnetic device at the BEMER web site.

Race Horses

(4) http://www.horsemagneticpulser.com/HMPstory.pdf
History of Pulsed Magnetic Fields for Treatment of Horses *(*PDF / Adobe Acrobat*)*. horsemagneticpulser.com. By Gary Wade, Physicist 6/03/2007

(5) http://www.tgselectronics.com.au/vetpmft.html
Veterinary Application of Pulsed Magnetic Field Therapy. by Dr. D. C. Laycock Ph.D. Australian Pulsed Magnetic Fields for Treatment of Horses. TSG Electronics Australia.

(6) http://www.equi-stimlegsaver.com/history.htm
Horses and pulsed magnetic fields, EQUI-STIM LEG SAVER Web Site.

(7) http://en.wikipedia.org/wiki/List_of_historical_horses
List of historial and famous race horses on Wikipedia

(8) *http://commons.wikimedia.org/wiki/Image:Muybridge_race_horse_animated.gif*
Animated sequence of a race horse galloping. Photos taken by Eadweard Muybridge (died 1904), first published in 1887 at Philadelphia. Animation by Waugsberg, 2006-9-24. Courtesy of Wikimedia Commons.

Therapeutic Uses of Pulsed EMF Review Article

(9) *http://www.ursi.org/RSBissues/RSBdecember2003.pdf*
Therapeutic Uses of Pulsed EMF, Review Article. Naomi M. Shupak, Radio Science Bulletin No 307 Dec 2003.

(10) *http://www.curatronic.com/pdf/PEMF therapeutic uses.pdf*
Therapeutic Uses of Pulsed EMF, Review Article. Naomi M. Shupak, Radio Science Bulletin No 307 Dec 2003. Same article as *(9)* but different url source.

Robert Becker MD

(11) *http://www.earthpulse.net/Becker.htm*
Robert O. Becker, MD; a research bibliography. A lifetime of brilliant medical research by a man that was far ahead of his time. The father of electromedicine and electrochemically induced cellular regeneration.

(12) *http://en.wikipedia.org/wiki/The_Body_Electric*
The Body Electric: Electromagnetism and the Foundation of Life is a book by Robert O. Becker and Gary Selden in which Dr. Becker, an orthopedic surgeon.

(13) *http://www.harpercollins.com/books/9780688069711/The_Body_Electric/excerpt.aspx*
Exerpt from the Body Electric The Body Electric Electromagnetism And The Foundation Of Life Copyright 1985 By Robert Becker, Gary Selden Described as "the greatest scientific work of the 20th century, with the POSSIBLE exception of Einstein's "Collected Works on Relativity". Yes, Becker is that good."

(14) *http://www.amazon.com/gp/reader/0874776090/ref=sib_dp_pt/104-6967425-7603934#reader-link*
Amazon Online Reader for portions of book CrossCurrents by Robert O Becker Copyright 1990.

(15) *http://www.bioenergeticseminars.com/*
Daniel Clark, MD, The 11th Annual International Congress Of BioEnergetic Medicine September 6-9th 2007

(16) *http://en.wikipedia.org/wiki/Isaac_Newton*
Sir Isaac Newton, 1643 – 1727, was an English physicist, mathematician, astronomer, natural philosopher, alchemist and theologian. His Philosophiæ Naturalis Principia

Mathematica, published in 1687, is said to be the greatest single work in the history of science.

(17) *http://en.wikipedia.org/wiki/Image:GodfreyKneller-IsaacNewton-1689.jpg*
The portrait of Newton is a copy of one printed in 1689 by Sir Godfrey Kneller

(18) *http://en.wikipedia.org/wiki/Michael_Faraday*
Michael Faraday on Wikipedia. Faraday discovered the relationship between magnetism and electricity, and he initiated the widespread use of electricial and magnetic devices.

(19) *http://hyperphysics.phy-astr.gsu.edu/hbase/mod1.html*
Light-Particle/Wave duality

(20) *http://web.jjay.cuny.edu/~acarpi/NSC/index.htm*
Matter and Energy

(21) *http://en.wikipedia.org/wiki/Matter*
Definition of matter on Wikipedia

(22) *http://en.wikipedia.org/wiki/Energy*
Definition of energy on Wikipedia

(23) *http://osulibrary.oregonstate.edu/specialcollections/coll/pauling/bond/narrative/page46.html*
Linus Pauling, 1939, The Nature of the Chemical Bond and the Structure of Molecules and Crystals: An Introduction to Modern Structural Chemistry became an instant classic.

OndaMed

(24) *http://www.ondamed.net/*
Ondamed Web Site. 'ONDAMED is a battery-powered biofeedback device that a medical practitioner uses to determine which frequencies of sound, as well as the accompanying weak pulsed electromagnetic fields, cause a response in a patient's autonomic nervous system

(25) *http://www.iaam.nl/_fundamental/00080000.htm*
The Biophysics of the Vascular Autonomic Signal and Healing, John M. Ackerman, M.D., Reprinted from: Frontier Perspectives, Center for Frontier Sciences at Temple University, Vo. X, No. 2, Fall, 2001. Research of orthopedic surgeon, Joseph H. Navach, M.D.

Shari Lieberman

(26) *http://www.drshari.net/*
Shari Lieberman Official Web Site.

(27) *http://www.ondamed.net/shari_lieberman.php*
Shari Lieberman joins as head of Ondamed research team.

Poly MVA

(28) *http://www.polymva.com/*
PolyMVA

(29) *http://www.facr.org/pdf/Case-studies-for-prostate-8-05.pdf*
Poly MVA for treating Prostate Cancer, a report of three cases by Shari Lieberman PhD and James Forsyth M.D.

(30) *http://www.polymva.com/pdf/MultipleMyeloma-final-revision.pdf*
Poly-MVA in an Integrative Approach to the Treatment of Multiple Myeloma: A Case Report, Shari Lieberman, PhD, CNS, FACN and Frank Antonowich, PhD, Townsend Letter; Aug/Sept 2007 issue.

(31) *http://www.liebertonline.com/doi/abs/10.1089/act.2006.12.77*
Poly-MVA for Treating Non–Small-Cell Lung Cancer: A Case Study of an Integrative Approach by Shari Lieberman, James W. Forsythe. Alternative & Complementary Therapies. April 1, 2006, 12*(2)*: 77-80.

(32) *http://www.townsendletter.com/FebMar_2003/polymva0203.htm*
The Medical Journalist Report of Innovative Biologics: Cancer Remission Rates Increase from Use of the Safe and Effective Lipoic Acid Palladium Complex Poly-MVA by Morton Walker, DPM From the Townsend Letter for Doctors & Patients February/March 2003

(33) *http://www.facr.org/*
Foundation for the Advancement of Cancer Research . 2514 Jamacha Road #502-196 El Cajon, CA 92019. Dr. Albert Sanchez, 1320 Seacoast Drive Suite A, Imperial Beach, CA 91932 Phone: *(619)* 575-9474. Poly MVA information.

(34) *http://www.polymvasurvivors.com/index.html*
Cancer Survivors, Poly MVA information web site." Our purpose is to alert everyone about the positive results our members & others are receiving. Many of our members are now in remission and many others are experiencing a greatly improved quality and extension of life."

Merrill Garnett

(35) *http://www.electrogenetics.net/*
Merrill Garnett, SELECTED ABSTRACTS + TECHNICAL WRITINGS. Electrogenetics is the basis for designing medicines that can short circuit the electrical charges in cancer cells and produce their selective electrocution.

(36) *www.firstpulseprojects.com/Publications.html*

First Pulse Book by Merrill Garnett, describes how Garnet discovered PolyMVA and how Poly MVA Works.

(37) *http://www.firstpulseprojects.com/firstpulsereview.html*
Book Review of First Pulse by Brian Thomas Carroll.

(38) *http://www.explorepub.com/articles/summaries/13_1_garnett.html*
TheFireintheGenes, Copyright2004byMerrillGarnett,ExploreIssue:Volume13,Number1 "The palladium-lipoic acid polymer known as palladium DNA reductase (Poly-MVA) carries current from membrane fatty acids to DNA at the resonant frequencies of DNA. This current is disruptive to anaerobic cell systems including certain tumors. In the absence of oxygen, the strong polarization force of the current dissociates membrane proteins."

Ed and Patricia Kane

(39) *http://www.bodybio.com/index.htm*
Body Bio, Ed and Patricia Kane web site.

(40) *http://www.bodybio.com/main/products/detoxxbook.htm*
Detoxx Book, Patricia Kane

(41) *http://www.haverfordwellness.com/*
LIPID EXCHANGE UTILIZING PHOSPHATIDYLCHOLINE. Phosphatidylcholine (PC) is one of the most groundbreaking therapies now available which was originated by Patricia Kane, Ph.D. PC supports positive outcomes of patients with states of toxicity and neurological disorders. Patricia Kane. Haverford Wellness Center 2010 West Chester Pike, Suite 310 Havertown, PA 19083

(42) *http://explorepub.com/articles/nutrition1.html*
Essential Fatty Acids, Lorenzo's Oil and Beyond. Copyright 1997 by Patricia Kane, Ph.D., Millville, New Jersey, U.S.A. Explore Issue: Volume 7, Number 6

PhosChol

(43) *http://www.phoschol.com/physicians/*
PhosChol. PhosChol contains: Highly purified Essential Phospholipids (EPL) or Polyunsaturated Phosphatidylcholine / Polyenylphosphatidylcholine (PPC) (active principle: diglyceride esters of cholinephosphoric acid of natural origin, with excess of unsaturated fatty acids, predominantly linoleic acid [approximately 70%] with 1,2- dilinoleoylphosphatidylcholine [(DLPC) up to 52%], linolenic acid and oleic acid).

Sangeeta Pati, M.D

(44) *http://www.sajune.com/*
Sangeeta Pati, M.D. SaJune Spa and Medical Center Orlando

(45) *http://www.wellnesshour.com/features/hormone_replacement/pati_sangeeta.html*
Sangeeta Pati MD Video Interview on the Wellness Hour with Randy Alvarez

(46) *http://www.youtube.com/watch?v=hxOvbBI-FRQ*
Sangeeta Pati, MD Video Interview on the Wellness Hour with Randy Alvarez on U-Tube

(47) *http://www.ncbi.nlm.nih.gov/pubmed/12626212*
Combined hormone replacement therapy and risk of breast cancer in a French cohort study of 3175 Women. De Lignières B. et al. Climacteric. 2002 Dec;5*(4)*:332-40. Paris, France. French Cohort Study showing no increased risk of breast cancer from bio-identical hormones.

(48) *http://content.nejm.org/cgi/content/short/356/25/2591*
Estrogen Therapy and Coronary-Artery Calcification. JoAnn E. Manson, M.D. et al. NEJM Volume 356:2591-2602 June 21, 2007 Number 25 NEJM study which shows that estrogen therapy prevents heart disease.

Adrenal Fatigue

(49) *http://www.ncbi.nlm.nih.gov/pubmed/6316831*
Salivary cortisol: a better measure of adrenal cortical function than serum cortisol. Vining RF, McGinley RA, Maksvytis JJ, Ho KY. Ann Clin Biochem. 1983 Nov;20 *(*Pt 6*)*:329-35."Salivary cortisol is a more appropriate measure for the clinical assessment of adrenocortical function than is serum cortisol."

(50) *http://www.ncbi.nlm.nih.gov/pubmed/2828410*
Salivary cortisol measurement: a practical approach to assess pituitary-adrenal function. J Clin Endocrinol Metab. 1988 Feb;66*(2)*:343-8. Laudat MH, Cerdas S, Fournier C, Guiban D, Guilhaume B, Luton JP.

(51) *http://www.ncbi.nlm.nih.gov/pubmed/11164057*
Salivary cortisol patterns in vital exhaustion. Nicolson NA, van Diest R. J Psychosom Res. 2000 Nov;49*(5)*:335-42.

(52) *http://bjp.rcpsych.org/cgi/content/full/184/2/136*
Salivary cortisol response to awakening in chronic fatigue syndrome.Roberts AD, Wessely S, Chalder T, Papadopoulos A, Cleare AJ. Br J Psychiatry. 2004 Feb;184:136-41. *(*FULL TEXT*)*

(53) *http://jcem.endojournals.org/cgi/content/full/86/8/3545*
Hypothalamo-Pituitary-Adrenal Axis Dysfunction in Chronic Fatigue Syndrome, and the Effects of Low-Dose Hydrocortisone Therapy. The Journal of Clinical Endocrinology & Metabolism Vol. 86, No. 8 3545-3554 A. J. Cleare, J. Miell, E. Heap, S. Sookdeo, L. Young, G. S. Malhi and V. O'Keane *(*FULL TEXT*)* "In conclusion, this study provides evidence that

there may be impaired adrenal cortical function in CFS on some measures and that low-dose hydrocortisone therapy is associated with a reversal of this HPA axis dysfunction."

(54) *http://www.annalsnyas.org/cgi/content/abstract/1057/1/466*
Stress-Induced Hypocortisolemia Diagnosed as Psychiatric Disorders Responsive to Hydrocortisone Replacement, SUZIE E. SCHUDER Ann. N.Y. Acad. Sci. 1057: 466–478 (2005). "By correcting underlying hormonal insufficiencies, many patients improved, with some patients having a total reversal of psychiatric symptoms."

(55) *http://edrv.endojournals.org/cgi/content/full/24/2/236*
The Neuroendocrinology of Chronic Fatigue Syndrome. Anthony J. Cleare. Endocrine Reviews 24 (2): 236-252, 2003, Full Text.

(56) *http://www.adrenalfatigue.org/*
The official web site for the book, Adrenal Fatigue by James L Wilson D.C., N.D., Ph.D. The 21st Century Syndrome.

(57) *http://www.cocoonnutrition.org/catalog/page_adrenal_cortical.php*
The Use Of Adrenal Cortical Extracts In Adrenal Fatigue By James L. Wilson DC, ND, PhD

(58) *http://crobm.iadrjournals.org/cgi/content/full/13/2/197*
THE DIAGNOSTIC APPLICATIONS OF SALIVA— A REVIEW, The Monitoring of Hormone Levels, Eliaz Kaufman,Ira B. Lamster. Crit Rev Oral Biol Med 13(2):197-212 (2002)

(59) *http://www.biodia.com/TechnicalCharts/SALIVARY_REFERENCES.pdf*
Listing of about one hundred medical references on salivary hormone testing with hyperlinks.

(60) *http://coastherbal.com/web_standard/adrenal_stress.html*
Adrenal Stress: Measuring and Treating, by Thomas G. Guilliams Ph.D. The Standard, Volume 3, No. 1. Excellent review article on diagnosis, treatment of adrenal fatigue with salivary cortisol testing.

(61) *http://www.amazon.com/review/R1QNDLO1R9EX3U/ref=cm_cr_rdp_perm*
Adrenal Fatigue by James L Wilson D.C., N.D., Ph.D. The 21st Century Syndrome reviewed by Jeffrey Dach MD.

(62) *http://www.amazon.com/review/R2IPB7XGMO20NE/ref=cm_cr_rdp_perm*
Safe Uses of Cortisol (Cortisone, Hydrocortisone) by William McK., M.D. Jefferies (Author) reviewed by Jeffrey Dach MD.

Russell Jaffe MD PhD

(62) *http://jama.ama-assn.org/cgi/content/full/287/23/3116*
Vitamins for Chronic Disease Prevention in Adults, Scientific Review , Kathleen M. Fairfield, MD,DrPH; Robert H. Fletcher, MD,MSc, JAMA. 2002;287:3116-3126.

(63) *http://jeffreydach.com/2007/07/08/americas-healthcare-system-found-critically-ill-by-russell-jaffe-md.aspx*
SICKO, America's healthcare system found 'critically ill' by Russell Jaffe MD PhD, July 4, 2007

(64) *http://www.perque.com/*
Perque, Russell Jaffe MD PhD, Two of the Perque LifeGuard Multivitamins have more nutritional value than 100 Centrum Silver, or 100 Theragram vitamins.

(65) *http://www.perque.com/pdfs/DrGuyersOctNewsletter.pdf*
One on One Interview with Russell Jaffe MD October 2005 by Dale Guyer MD

Robert Becker -Silver

(66) *http://www.rexresearch.com/becker/becker1.htm*
Dr. Robert O. Becker, Silver Ionotophoresis, Healing & Regeneration, US Patent # 5,814,094 Iontopheretic System for Stimulation of Tissue Healing and Regeneration *(*9-29-1998*)* Becker, Robert O., et al.

BOOKS on BioElectric Medicine

(67) *http://www.amazon.com/Bioelectromagnetic-Healing-Rationale-its-Use/dp/0964107058*
Bioelectromagnetic Healing: A Rationale for its Use by Thomas Valone 2003

(68) *http://www.amazon.com/Energy-Medicine-Scientific-James-Oschman/dp/0443062617*
Energy Medicine: The Scientific Basis by James L. Oschman 2000

Therapeutic Uses of Pulsed EMF

(69)(70)(71)(72)(73)(74)(75) *http://ajp.psychiatryonline.org/cgi/content/full/163/1/88*
A Randomized, Controlled Trial of Sequential Bilateral Repetitive Transcranial Magnetic Stimulation for Treatment-Resistant Depression, Am J Psychiatry 163:88-94, January 2006

(70) *http://www.ondamed.net/publication/html/en/article15.html*
Impulse magnetic-field therapy for migraine and other headaches: a double-blind, placebo-controlled study. Adv Ther. 2001 May-Jun;18*(*3*)*:101-9 Pelka RB, Jaenicke C, Gruenwald J. Seventy-six percent of active-treatment patients experienced clear or very clear relief of their complaints.

(71) *http://www.thefreelibrary.com/Pulsed+microamperage+stimulation:+a+controll ed+*
study+of+healing+of+...-a014944034
Pulsed microamperage stimulation: a controlled study of healing of surgically induced wounds in Yucatan pigs. Byl NN, McKenzie AL, West JM, et al. Phys Ther. 1994,74:201-219.]

(72) *http://www.biomedcentral.com/1471-2121/7/37*
Nanoelectropulse-driven membrane perturbation and small molecule permeabilization Gundersen BMC, Cell Biology 2006. Electric pulses produce membrane disturbances that are associated with phospholipid rearrangements and the influx of small molecules from the medium into the cytoplasm.

(73) *http://www.pubmedcentral.nih.gov/articlerender.fcgi?tool=pubmed&pubmedid= 16545779*
Nanosecond pulsed electric fields cause melanomas to self-destruct. Richard Nuccitelli et al. Biochem Biophys Res Commun. 2006 May 5; 343*(2)*: 351–360.

(74) *http://www.ncbi.nlm.nih.gov/pubmed/17714104*
Prospective, randomized, single-blind, sham treatment-controlled study of the safety and efficacy of an electromagnetic field device for the treatment of chronic low back pain: a pilot study. Harden RN et al. Pain Pract. 2007 Sep;7*(3)*:248-55. TEMF may be effective and safe for the treatment of chronic low back pain disorders.

(75) Pulsed magnetic fields accelerate cutaneous wound healing in rats. Strauch B, Patel MK, Navarro JA, Berdichevsky M, Yu HL, Pilla AA. Plast Reconstr Surg. 2007 Aug;120*(2)*:425-30.The authors successfully demonstrated that exposing wounds to pulsed magnetic fields of very specific configurations accelerated early wound healing in this animal model, as evidenced by significantly increased wound tensile strength at 21 days after wounding.

Chapter 31

Orthomolecular Medicine Meeting in Toronto Honoring Abram Hoffer, MD

Highlights of the Orthomolecular Medicine Meeting

After returning from the Orthomolecular Medicine Meeting in Toronto April 2007, I immediately felt the need to write a summary report on this historic meeting.*(1)* The evening before the scientific sessions, we attended the black-tie tribute dinner honoring the 90 year old Abram Hoffer, MD, the original founder of the orthomolecular medical society, and a prolific writer and researcher.*(2)(3)* My wife and I were lucky to be seated at a family table with Garry Vickar, M.D. Hoffer's nephew. Garry Vickar is an orthomolecular psychiatrist from St. Louis, and proudly reported that the Hoffer family had endowed the Hoffer-Vickar chair of orthomolecular psychiatry at Ben Gurion University.*(4)*

What is Orthomolecular Medicine? *(5)*

You probably never heard of this word, "orthomolecular". It was coined by Linus Pauling 50 years ago and means substances in the human body like vitamins, minerals, and hormones used to treat disease.*(5)(5A)* It sounds a lot like natural medicine, holistic medicine, and integrative, complementary medicine, doesn't it? In actuality, all of these definitions are blurred together, and we are really talking about the use of non-toxic natural substances, instead of patented drugs which can be toxic and produce adverse side effects. Abram Hoffer, Linus Pauling and Humphrey Osmond founded the orthomolecular medical society in the 1950's, and Hoffer is still active as editor-in-chief of its journal.*(6)*

Gala Dinner Honoring Abram Hoffer MD

The April 2007 award dinner in Toronto was a touching and moving tribute to a great pioneer and scientist. Dr. Hoffer graciously allowed us to introduce ourselves and speak with him briefly, and I can report to you that he is charming, pleasant, and has the intellect of much younger person. He was the final speaker at the podium, and spoke for about 10 minutes recapping the highlights of his career and thanking everyone involved in the dinner.

The actress Margot Kidder was the master of ceremonies at the dinner. Remember, she played Lois Lane in the superman movies. Kidder was successfully treated by Hoffer after having her own personal problems in 1996. She is now a grateful recovered Abram Hoffer patient, and also a political activist for orthomolecular medicine as the first line of treatment of mental illness. *(7)*

Abram Hoffer is well known for his research investigating the use of high dose niacin, vitamin B3, as a treatment for schizophrenia. Hoffer noticed the association of pellagra *(*niacin deficiency*)* and dementia, and speculated some people needed higher niacin *(*B3*)* intakes to avoid mental illness. Hoffer found niacin *(*B3*)* to be quite effective and treated 4,000 schizophrenics with three grams of B3 per day with a 90% success rate. His original paper was published in Lancet in 1962, Massive Niacin Treatment in Schizophrenia. Review of a nine-year study.*(8)*

A new study of niacin *(*B3*)* for schizophrenia is underway at Ben Gurion University, entitled, Treatment of Acute Schizophrenia With Niacin Vitamin Therapy. This study is currently recruiting patients at Beersheva Mental Health Center. The director is RH Belmaker, MD, who is also the Hoffer-Vickar chair in orthomolecular psychiatry.*(9)*

Over his long career, Abram Hoffer has touched the lives of many Canadians, and many of the people at the meeting were there because Hoffer had treated family members with dramatic improvements. Dr. Hoffer's autobiography, "Adventures in Psychiatry: The Scientific Memoirs of Dr. Abram Hoffer", is a must read. We were all given gift copies of the book, personally autographed by Dr. Hoffer.*(10)(11)(12)(12A)(13)*

First Day of Meeting, I.V. Vitamin C Treatment for Cancer

The scientific meeting started the next day bright and early. And the first day was devoted to Vitamin C as a treatment for cancer, and all the big names were there. *Steve Lawson* from the *Linus Pauling Institute* appeared first.*(14)* He gave a short history of the original Cameron-Pauling Clinical Trials of Vitamin C treatment for cancer, which showed that cancer patients who received vitamin C lived 4 times longer than those who didn't. One hundred terminal cancer patients were given 10 grams of vitamin C daily *(*2.5 grams four times per day*)* and followed clinically until they succumbed to their underlying cancer. The Vitamin C group lived 4.2 times longer *(*210 days*)*, compared to 1,000 "matched controls" who averaged only 50 days till death from cancer. *(15)(16)(17)*

In spite of these encouraging results by Linus Pauling, Vitamin C research was halted early on because of subsequent negative studies at the Mayo Clinic. Some say the Mayo Clinic studies were intentionally designed to fail and discredit vitamin C. The Mayo Clinic docs changed the Pauling protocol and failed to demonstrate the beneficial findings. *(18)*

Jeanne Drisko MD

However, after all these years, interest in vitamin C as an adjunctive cancer treatment appears to be reviving. One of those responsible for this renewed interest in Vitamin C as a treatment for cancer is *Jeanne Drisko, MD*, Professor of Orthomolecular Medicine at University of Kansas who discussed her ongoing clinical trial investigating intravenous vitamin C as a treatment for ovarian, uterine and cervical cancer at the University of Kansas.*(19)(20)*

John Hoffer, MD *(*Abram Hoffer's son*)* from the Jewish General Hospital of Montreal reported three well-documented cases of advanced cancers, confirmed by pathology biopsy. All three patients had unexpectedly long survival times after treatment with intravenous vitamin C.*(21)*

Mark Levine MD

Mark Levine, MD, (22) Section Chief for Vitamin C Research at the NIH, presented his work showing intravenous Vitamin C kills cancer cells and infectious agents by producing Hydrogen Peroxide in the extracellular space. *(23)(24)(25)(26)(27)* Dr Levine also studied vitamin C in volunteers and then recommended increasing the current RDA of 60 mg daily to 200 mg daily*(27)*. Steve Hickey, PhD. author of Ascorbate, the Science of Vitamin C also spoke at the meeting.*(28)*.

Second Day of Meeting, Bio-Identical Hormones for Women

Phyllis Bronson PhD

The second day of the meeting was devoted to Women's Bio-Identical Hormone Replacement, *Phyllis Bronson, PhD (29)* discussed the biochemistry of estradiol and progesterone and their effects on mood, depression and brain function. She explained how hormonal imbalance causes PMS which can be treated with supplemental progesterone rather than SSRI anti-depressants.

Dr. Bronson discussed I3C and DIM for the beneficial effect on estrogen metabolism, and as nutritional supplements for breast cancer prevention. *Indole 3 Carbinol (I-3-C)* and *Di-Indole Methane (DIM)* and Iodine are the basic breast cancer prevention program that we use in our office.*(30)* We have discussed the role of Iodine as a cancer preventive agent in a previous chapter on Breast Cancer Prevention and Iodine Supplementation.*(31)*

Kenton Bruice MD

Dr. Bronson was followed by *Kenton Bruice MD,(32)* a practicing OB/Gyne doc who routinely prescribes bio-identical hormones. He summarized the medical literature showing safety of bio-identical hormone replacement. Dr. Kenton Bruice cited the French Cohort study which showed no increased risk of breast cancer from bio-identical hormones. *(*The RR = 1.005, which is identical to the control group.*) (33)* He also discussed the medical literature on heart disease risk, and showed that women using bio-identical hormones *(*estradiol and progesterone*)* have actually less heart disease risk.*(34)*

Mark Starr MD

Mark Starr, M.D. presented his talk on Type Two Hypothyroidism, and announced the new edition of his book.*(35)* His information on hypothyroidism was covered in my previous article, Hypothyroidism Type Two and Thyroflex.*(36)* I had previously heard his talk and met him at an ICIM *(*Integrative Medicine*)* meeting in Grand Rapids, MI, so it was a pleasure meeting him again, and I was glad he remembered me from the last meeting. One change he mentioned in his office protocol: He is now giving iodine supplementation along with natural thyroid and having better results.

Third Day of Meeting Orthomolecular Treatment for

Obsessive-Compulsive Disorder *(*OCD*)*

James Greenblatt MD

James Greenblatt MD (37) from *Waldon Behavioral Care (38)* gave a very good talk discussing orthomolecular treatment of Obsessive Compulsive Disorder *(*OCD*)*. What is OCD? This is a fairly common mental disorder which affects kids and adults who have obsessive thoughts such as phobias, or fears *(*such as fear of contamination*)*, and in order to deal with these thoughts they have repeating behaviors called compulsions such as handwashing, counting, hoarding, etc.

Kids who are interrupted from their compulsive activities can become violent. The standard treatment is SSRI antidepressants, which may work initially, however, they come with a price of well known side effects. Dr. Greenblatt has had dramatic success in OCD patients using non-toxic supplements such as 5-HTP, and Inositol *(*18 grams per day*)*. *(39)(40)*. 5-HTP is an amino acid precursor to serotonin, and Inositol is a non-toxic sugar like molecule.

William Shaw Great Plains Lab

Dr. Greenblatt discussed the use of lab testing for the opiate peptides, Gliadorphin and Casomorphin, which can be done on urine samples sent to the *Great Plains Laboratory (41)* run by *William Shaw.(42)(43)* Apparently the cause for OCD, depression, bulimia, panic disorders etc. has been found to be these Gliadorphin and Casomorphin peptides which mimic neurotransmitters in the brain. Fortunately, these unwanted peptides can be degraded by digestive enzymes, and Greenblatt uses a digestive enzyme product called Serenaid with much success.

Dr. Greenblatt presented cases showing dramatic clinical improvement in kids with OCD with the use of orthomolecular medicine, 5HTP, Inositol, digestive enzymes and probiotics. These children recovered dramatically from their OCD symptoms of hoarding, repeating activities, handwashing, phobias and social withdrawal etc. This is orthomolecular medicine at its best.

References

(1) *http://www.orthomed.org/NMT/nmt.html*
Orthomolecular Medicine Society Presents 36th Annual Meeting Nutritional Medicine Today May 11, 2007 Toronto Canada and gala dinner Honoring Abram Hoffer MD/

(2) *http://en.wikipedia.org/wiki/Abram_Hoffer*
Abram Hoffer MD Wikipedia Entry Biography. Abram Hoffer (born 1917) is a Canadian psychiatrist known for the use of nutrition and vitamins in the treatment of schizophrenia, orthomolecular psychiatry.

(3) *http://www.orthomed.org/tribute.pdf*
The International Schizophrenia Foundation Lifetime Achievement Gala Dinner honoring Abram Hoffer, MD, PhD with Margot Kidder as Master of Ceremonies, Thursday, April 19, 2007, The Fairmont Royal York Hotel Toronto, Canada

(4) *http://iffohs.med.ad.bgu.ac.il/people/PDetails.asp?StaffID=11129*
R.H. Belmaker, M.D., Hoffer-Vickar Professor of Psychiatry, Ben-Gurion University. Beer-Sheva.

(5) *http://lpi.oregonstate.edu/f-w99/orthomolecular.html*
What is Orthomolecular Medicine? Stephen Lawson, Administrative Officer Linus Pauling Institute The word "orthomolecular" was introduced by Linus Pauling in "Orthomolecular Psychiatry", his seminal 1968 article published in the journal Science.

(5A) *http://orthomolecular.org/library/articles/orthotheory.shtml*
On the Orthomolecular Environment of the Mind: Orthomolecular Theory by Linus Pauling, Ph.D. Journal Of Orthomolecular Medicine Vol. 7, No. 1, 1995 "Varying the concentrations of substances normally present in the human body may control mental disease." - Linus Pauling

(6) *http://www.orthomed.org/*
Orthomolecular Medicine is the practice of preventing and treating disease by providing the body with optimal amounts of substances which are natural to the body. The key idea in orthomolecular medicine is that genetic factors affect not only the physical characteristics of individuals, but also to their biochemical milieu. Biochemical pathways of the body have significant genetic variability and diseases such as atherosclerosis, cancer, schizophrenia or depression are associated with specific biochemical abnormalities which are causal or contributing factors of the illness.

(7) *http://en.wikipedia.org/wiki/Margot_Kidder*
Margot Kidder born October 17, 1948 is a Canadian-American film and television actress best known for playing Lois Lane in the Superman movies of the 1970s and 1980s.

(8) *http://www.ncbi.nlm.nih.gov/pubmed/14482545*
Massive niacin treatment in schizophrenia. Review of a nine-year study. OSMOND H, HOFFER A. Lancet. 1962 Feb 10;1(7224):316-9.

(9) *http://clinicaltrials.gov/ct/show/NCT00140166;jsessionid=CC8103A221364A096728C7BE7C6788FD?order=46*
Treatment of Acute Schizophrenia With Vitamin Therapy, This study has been completed.

Sponsors and Collaborators: Beersheva Mental Health Center. Supported by a Hilton Family Foundation grant to International Schizophrenia Foundation. Therefore, this proposal is to study in a controlled manner carefully defined first onset schizophrenic patients using the protocol advocated by Osmond and Hoffer (1962) (high dose niacin).

(10) *http://findarticles.com/p/articles/mi_m0ISW/is_275/ai_n16675820*
Adventures in Psychiatry: The Scientific Memoirs of Dr. Abram Hoffer by Dr. Abram Hoffer, Kos Publishing Inc

(11) *http://www.doctoryourself.com/review_hoffer_B3.html*
Vitamin B-3 and Schizophrenia: Discovery, Recovery, Controversy by Abram Hoffer, MD Quarry Press, Kingston, Ontario Canada (1998) Review by Andrew W. Saul

(12) *http://www.islandnet.com/~hoffer/*
Hoffer's Home Page -Orthomolecular Treatment of Cancer.

(12A) *http://www.islandnet.com/~hoffer/hofferhp.htm*
Hoffer's Home Page -The Schizophrenias

(13) *http://members.aol.com/pbchowka/hoffer.html*
Abram Hoffer MD, PhD Interviewed by Peter Barry Chowka On Orthomolecular Medicine.

(14) *http://lpi.oregonstate.edu/*
Linus Pauling Institute

(15) *http://www.pnas.org/cgi/content/abstract/73/10/3685*
Supplemental Ascorbate in the Supportive Treatment of Cancer: Prolongation of Survival Times in Terminal Human Cancer. Ewan Cameron and Linus Pauling. PNAS, October 1, 1976, vol. 73, no. 10, p3685-3689.

(16) *http://www.pnas.org/cgi/content/abstract/75/9/4538*
Supplemental Ascorbate in the Supportive Treatment of Cancer: Reevaluation of Prolongation of Survival Times in Terminal Human Cancer. Ewan Cameron and Linus Pauling. PNAS, September 1, 1978, vol. 75, no. 9, 4538-4542.

(17) *http://www.sciencedirect.com/science?_ob=ArticleURL&_udi=B6T56-479DHBR-3H&_user=4420034*
The orthomolecular treatment of cancer II. Clinical trial of high-dose ascorbic acid supplements in advanced human cancer, Ewan Cameron and Allan Campbell, Chemico-Biological Interactions Volume 9, Issue 4, October 1974, Pages 285-315.

(18) *http://www.ncbi.nlm.nih.gov/pubmed/384241*
Failure of high-dose vitamin C (ascorbic acid) therapy to benefit patients with advanced cancer. A controlled trial. Creagan ET, Moertel CG, O'Fallon JR, Schutt AJ, O'Connell MJ, Rubin J, Frytak S.N Engl J Med. 1979 Sep 27;301(13):687-90.

(19) *http://integrativemed.kumc.edu/bio-drisko.htm*
Jeanne A. Drisko, MD Riordan Endowed Professor of Orthomolecular Medicine, Director, Program in Integrative Medicine

(20) *http://clinicaltrials.gov/ct/show/NCT00284427?order=10*
Safety of Antioxidants During GYN Cancer Care. University of Kansas, June 2008

Principal Investigator:Jeanne Drisko, MD University of Kansas

(21) *http://www.pubmedcentral.nih.gov/articlerender.fcgi?artid=1405876*
Intravenously administered vitamin C as cancer therapy: three cases
Sebastian J. Padayatty, Hugh D. Riordan, Stephen M. Hewitt, Arie Katz, L. John Hoffer, and Mark Levine.CMAJ. 2006 March 28; 174(7): 937–942.

(22) *http://intramural.niddk.nih.gov/research/faculty.asp?People_ID=1492*
Mark A. Levine, M.D.Molecular and Clinical Nutrition Section, Chief Digestive Diseases Branch. NIDDK, National Institutes of Health Building 10, Room 4D52 Bethesda, MD 20892-1372

(23) *http://www.medscape.com/viewarticle/512724*
Study: Vitamin C May Fight Cancer Sept. 12, 2005 -- Vitamin C may have some cancer-fighting potential, new research shows.

(24) *http://www.annals.org/cgi/content/abstract/140/7/533*
Vitamin C Pharmacokinetics: Implications for Oral and Intravenous Use. Sebastian J. Padayatty and Mark Levine, MD. Ann Intern Med. 2004 Volume 140 Issue 7, Pages 533-537.

(25) *http://www.annals.org/cgi/reprint/140/7/533.pdf*
Vitamin C Pharmacokinetics: Implications for Oral and Intravenous Use Sebastian J. Padayatty, MRCP, PhD; He Sun, PhD, CBS; Yaohui Wang, MD; Hugh D. Riordan, MD; Stephen M. Hewitt, MD, PhD; Arie Katz, MD; Robert A. Wesley, PhD; and Mark Levine, MD Ann Intern Med. 2004;140:533-537.

(26) *http://www.jacn.org/cgi/content/full/19/4/423*
Reevaluation of Ascorbate in Cancer Treatment: Emerging Evidence, Open Minds and Serendipity . Sebastian J Padayatty, MRCP, PhD and Mark Levine, MD, FACN
Journal of the American College of Nutrition, Vol. 19, No. 4, 423-425 (2000)

(27) *http://www.pnas.org/cgi/content/abstract/93/8/3704*
Vitamin C pharmacokinetics in healthy volunteers: Evidence for a recommended dietary allowance (ascorbic acid / bioavailability) Mark Levine et al. Vol. 93, Issue 8, 3704-3709,

April 16, 1996, "the current RDA of 60 mg daily should be increased to 200 mg daily, which can be obtained from fruits and vegetables. Safe doses of vitamin C are less than 1000 mg daily, and vitamin C daily doses above 400 mg have no evident value."

(28) http://www.amazon.com/Ascorbate-Science-Vitamin-Steve-Hickey/dp/1411607244
The Science of Vitamin C by Steve Hickey

(29) http://aspenphilanthropist.com/directory_detail.php?oid=34
Phyllis Bronson, Ph.D., the primary researcher Aspen Philanthropist.

(30) http://findarticles.com/p/articles/mi_m0ISW/is_2001_August/ai_78177206
The Cruciferous Choice: DIM or 13C? Phytonutrient Supplements for Cancer Prevention and Health Promotion - diindolyl-methane, indole-3-carbinol. Townsend Letter for Doctors and Patients, August, 2001 by Michael A. Zeligs

(31) http://jeffreydach.com/2007/05/05/jeffreydachdrdachiodine.aspx
Breast Cancer Prevention and Iodine Supplementation by Jeffrey Dach MD

(32) http://www.kentonbruicemd.com/index.php
Bruice Kenton MD Board Certified Gynecologist. Natural Hormone Replacement Therapy with Bio-Identical Hormones

(33) http://www.ncbi.nlm.nih.gov/pubmed/12626212
Combined hormone replacement therapy and risk of breast cancer in a French cohort study of 3175 Women. De Lignières B. et al. Climacteric. 2002 Dec;5(4):332-40. Paris, France. French Cohort Study showing no increased risk of breast cancer from bio-identical hormones.

(34) http://content.nejm.org/cgi/content/short/356/25/2591
Estrogen Therapy and Coronary-Artery Calcification. JoAnn E. Manson, M.D. et al. NEJM Volume 356:2591-2602 June 21, 2007 Number 25 NEJM study which shows that estrogen therapy prevents heart disease.

(35) http://www.type2hypothyroidism.com/
Mark Starr MD Type Two Hypothyroidism

(36) http://jeffreydach.com/2007/05/05/jeffreydachdrdachthyroid.aspx
Hypothyroidism Type Two and Thyroflex by Jeffrey Dach MD

(37) http://www.naturaladd.com/about/index.htm
Dr. Greenblatt is a dually board certified in child and adult psychiatry.

(38) http://www.waldenbehavioralcare.com/about_walden_leadership.asp
About Walden Since its founding in 2003, Walden Behavioral Care has become a national leader in the treatment of eating disorders and psychiatric disorders.

(39) *http://ajp.psychiatryonline.org/cgi/content/abstract/153/9/1219*
Inositol treatment of obsessive-compulsive disorder. M Fux, J Levine, A Aviv and RH Belmaker . Ministry of Health Mental Health Center, Faculty of Health Sciences, Ben Gurion University of the Negev, Beersheva, Israel. Am J Psychiatry 1996; 153:1219-1221

(40) *http://westsuffolkpsych.homestead.com/inositol_and_ocd.html*
Inositol and OCD By Frederick Penzel, Ph.D.

(41) *http://www.greatplainslaboratory.com/home/eng/home.asp*
The Great Plains Laboratory helps children and adults with conditions such as autism & PDD, ADD/ADHD, Down's Syndrome with autistic-like symptoms, Fibromyalgia, Chronic Fatigue, MS or MS-like symptoms, Irritable Bowel Syndrome, Brain Fog, Depression, Psychosis, GI disorders, and many other diseases and conditions.

(42) *http://www.greatplainslaboratory.com/aboutus.html*
Dr. William Shaw received a Ph.D. Great Plains Lab.

(43) *http://www.greatplainslaboratory.com/autismbook.html*
Biological Treatments for Autism and PDD, by William Shaw, Ph.D.

Abram Hoffer B3 Niacin for Schizophrenia

(44) *http://www.doctoryourself.com/hoffer_krypto.html*
The Discovery of Kryptopyrrole and its Importance in Diagnosis of Biochemical Imbalances in Schizophrenia and in Criminal Behavior by Abram Hoffer, M.D., Ph.D. Journal of Orthomolecular Medicine: The Discovery of Kryptopyrrole and its Importance. Vol. 10, No. 1, 1995

(45) *http://www.hdfoster.com/Foster_Schizophrenia.pdf*
What really Causes Schizophrenia? by Harold Foster

(46) *http://books.google.com/books?id=wT4HUH3Vgg8C*
Orthomolecular Treatment for Schizophrenia By Abram Hoffer Published 1999 McGraw-Hill Professional Schizophrenia

(47) *http://findarticles.com/p/articles/mi_m0ISW/is_2001_April/ai_72297151/pg_1*
Schizophrenia & Orthomolecular Treatment Townsend Letter for Doctors and Patients, April, 2001 by Jule Klotter

Section Eleven Case Reports and LDN

Chapter 32

Low Dose Naltrexone *(*LDN*)*

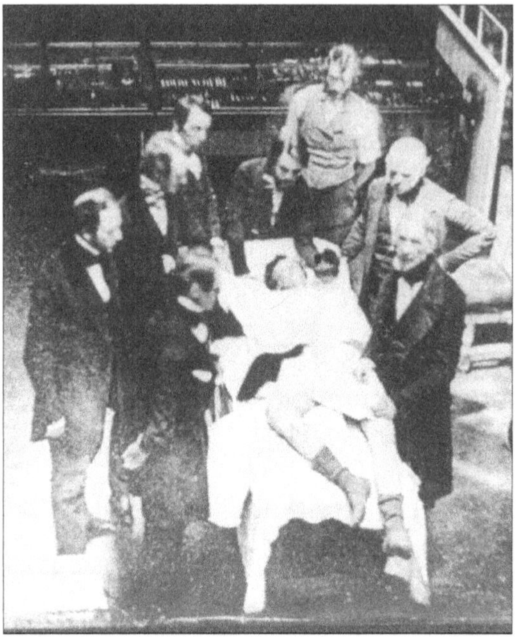

Image: First demonstration of anesthesia 1846. Courtesy Library of Congress.

Imagine a drug addict slumped over from a lethal heroin overdose. He has shallow breathing and will die unless he receives prompt medical care in the emergency room. If he is lucky enough to make the trip to the ER, the doctors will give him an IV injection of Narcan *(*Naloxone*)*, the drug of choice to reverse narcotics overdose, waking the victim and snatching him from the jaws of death. Narcan is available in the hospital operating room where anesthesiologists use it to wake up the patient after the operation. It reverses the sedating effect of opiates by binding to the opioid receptors in the brain. A close cousin of Naloxone is Naltrexone, another opioid antagonist used as treatment for narcotics and alcohol addiction.

FDA approved since 1984

Naltrexone has been FDA approved since 1984 for treatment of narcotics and alcohol addiction. Naltrexone is another opioid antagonist and has a similar chemical structure to Narcan and Morphine. It was a surprise for me to find out that Naltrexone has other important uses at a much lower dosage as an oral capsule. Medical scientists have been carefully studying its effect of Naltrexone on the immune system, and its clinical benefits for a host of disease states for the past 20 years.

Low Dose Naltrexone, *(*LDN*)*, How Does it Work?

The beneficial effect of low dose naltrexone, LDN, was discovered by Bernard Bihari, MD *(1)(1A)*, a physician in New York City who found that a small dose *(*3 mg*)* of naltrexone taken as a capsule at bedtime blocks the opiate receptors in the brain for a few hours during sleep, which then stimulates the brain to increase production of endorphins over the next 24 hours. These endorphins then stimulate the immune system. Although Bihari did much of the early clinical work, Zagon did much of the groundwork with animal research studies at Pennsylvania State University.*(*3-17*)*

LDN Cures Crohn's Disease

A recent publication in the Jan 2007 Journal of Gastroenterology on the use of LDN in Crohn's Disease, was the first breakthrough publication to appear entitled, Low-Dose Naltrexone Therapy Improves Active Crohn's Disease by Jill Smith MD.*(2)*

Crohn's disease is a severe inflammatory condition of the small bowel which can be difficult to treat. Not difficult for LDN however. Jill Smith, M.D. reported that two-thirds of her 17 Crohn's patients went into remission, and 90% of the group had some benefit. Her article showed impressive colonoscopy photos before and after LDN treatment with complete clearing of the inflammatory changes in the bowel mucosa. Dr. Smith concluded that "LDN therapy appears effective and safe in subjects with active Crohn's disease."*(2)*

Other Conditions Which Benefit from LDN

The major therapeutic action of LDN is the restoration of normal endorphin production by the brain. This is beneficial for any condition in which there is a deficiency in endorphin production, such as autoimmune disease, cancer and HIV/AIDS. Bernard Bihari, MD, who discovered the LDN protocol has used it in hundred of patients in the following categories:

LDN for Cancer

LDN is useful for cancers of the Bladder, Breast, Colon & Rectal Cancer , Glioblastoma, Lung Cancer *(*Non-Small Cell*)*, Lymphocytic Leukemia *(*chronic*)*, Lymphoma Hodgkin's and Non-Hodgkin's*)* Malignant Melanoma, Multiple Myeloma , Ovarian Cancer, Pancreatic Cancer, Prostate Cancer *(*untreated*)*, Renal Cell Carcinoma, Uterine Cancer.

LDN is useful for Autoimmune and other Diseases:

LDN treatment has benefited these diseases: ALS *(*Lou Gehrig's Disease*)*, Autism Spectrum Disorders, Chronic Fatigue Syndrome, Crohn's Disease, Fibromyalgia, HIV/AIDS, Multiple Sclerosis *(*MS*)*, Parkinson's Disease, Psoriasis, Rheumatoid Arthritis, Scleroderma, Systemic Lupus *(*SLE*)*, Ulcerative Colitis, Wegener's Granulomatosis.

LDN Has Virtually No Side Effects:

Occasionally, during the first week's use of LDN, patients may complain of some difficulty sleeping. This rarely persists after the first week. Should it do so, dosage can be reduced from 4.5mg to 3mg nightly.

Caution About Narcotics Withdrawal

Because LDN blocks opioid receptors throughout the body for three or four hours, people using narcotics pain pills such as Ultram *(tramadol)*, morphine, Percocet, Duragesic, Oxycontin or codeine, should not take LDN until after complete withdrawal from their narcotic drugs. The use of LDN may induce narcotics withdrawal.

Although naltrexone is FDA approved, the LDN protocol is what is called "off-label use", and it is unlikely that any company will spend the millions needed to fund studies for FDA approval of the LDN protocol. However, off-label use of an FDA approved drug such as naltrexone is commonplace and widely accepted. The naltrexone capsules are inexpensive, about 20 dollars a month. The treatment is safe, with no adverse side effects.

Pharmacies that offer compounded LDN capsules:

The Compounder Pharmacy 340 Marshall Ave Unit 100, Aurora, IL 60506-2956 Phone: 630-859-0333 Fax: 630-859-0114. *(22)*

Skip's Pharmacy 21000 Boca Rio Rd Suite A-29 Boca Raton, Florida 33433, telephone 561-218-0111 800-553-7429 Fax: 561-218-8873 *(24)*

Thanks to *Larry Frieders, the Compounder* for bringing LDN to my attention, and for making low cost LDN capsules available to the public. *(22)*

References:

(1) http://www.ldninfo.org/index.htm
Web site for low dose naltrexone information.

(1A) http://www.ldninfo.org/bbihari_cv.htm
Curriculum Vitae, BERNARD BIHARI, M.D. 29 West 15th Street New York, N.Y. 10011, *(212)* 929-4196 **retired as of March 2007.**

(2) http://www.ncbi.nlm.nih.gov/pubmed/17222320
Low-dose naltrexone therapy improves active Crohn's disease. Smith JP, Stock H, Bingaman S, Mauger D, Rogosnitzky M, Zagon IS. Am J Gastroenterol. 2007 Apr;102*(4)*:820-8. Department of Medicine, Pennsylvania State University College of Medicine, Hershey, Pennsylvania 17033, USA.

(3) http://www.ncbi.nlm.nih.gov/pubmed/6640516
Cancer Lett. 1983 Nov;21*(1)*:89-94. Opioid antagonists inhibit the growth of metastatic murine neuroblastoma.Zagon IS, McLaughlin PJ.

(4) http://www.ncbi.nlm.nih.gov/pubmed/6316064
Life Sci. 1983 Dec 12;33*(24)*:2449-54.
Naltrexone modulates growth in infant rats.Zagon IS, McLaughlin PJ.

(5) http://www.ncbi.nlm.nih.gov/pubmed/10592296
Brain Res. 1999 Dec 4;849*(1-2)*:147-54. Cloning, sequencing, expression and function of a cDNA encoding a receptor for the opioid growth factor, [Met*(5)*]enkephalin. Zagon IS, Verderame MF, Allen SS, McLaughlin PJ.

(6) http://www.ncbi.nlm.nih.gov/pubmed/11029512
Opioid growth factor regulates the cell cycle of human neoplasias.Zagon IS, Roesener CD, Verderame MF, Ohlsson-Wilhelm BM, Levin RJ, McLaughlin PJ.

(7) http://www.ncbi.nlm.nih.gov/pubmed/8620464
Cancer Lett. 1996 Mar 29;101*(2)*:159-64. Inhibition of human colon cancer by intermittent opioid receptor blockade with naltrexone.Hytrek SD, McLaughlin PJ, Lang CM, Zagon IS.

(8) http://www.ncbi.nlm.nih.gov/pubmed/9066724
Cancer Lett. 1997 Jan 30;112*(2)*:167-75. Opioid growth factor *(*OGF*)* inhibits human pancreatic cancer transplanted into nude mice.Zagon IS, Hytrek SD, Smith JP, McLaughlin PJ.

(9) http://www.ncbi.nlm.nih.gov/pubmed/6867737
Science. 1983 Aug 12;221*(4611)*:671-3. Naltrexone modulates tumor response in mice with neuroblastoma.Zagon IS, McLaughlin PJ.

(10) http://www.ncbi.nlm.nih.gov/pubmed/6300232
Matthew, PM, Froelich CJ, Sibbitt WL, Jr., Bankhurst AD, Enhancement of natural cytotoxicity by beta-endorphin, J Immunol 130, pp.1658-1662, Apr 1983.

(11) http://www.ncbi.nlm.nih.gov/pubmed/6867737
Zagon IS, McLaughlin PJ, Naltrexone modulates tumor response in mice with neuroblastoma, Science 221, pp.671-3, Aug 12, 1983.

(12) http://www.ncbi.nlm.nih.gov/pubmed/6867737
Hytrek SD, McLaughlin PJ, Lang CM, Zagon IS, Inhibition of human colon cancer by intermittent opioid receptor blockade with naltrexone, Cancer Lett 101*(2)*, pp. 159-64, Mar 29, 1996.

(13) http://www.ncbi.nlm.nih.gov/pubmed/8853403
Zagon IS, Hytrek SD, Lang CM, Smith JP, McGarrity TJ, Wu Y, McLaughlin PJ, Opioid growth factor *(*[Met5]enkephalin*)* prevents the incidence and retards the growth of human colon cancer, Am J Physiol 271*(*3 Pt 2*)*, pp.R780-R786, Sep 1996

(16) http://www.ncbi.nlm.nih.gov/pubmed/6087062
Zagon IS, McLaughlin PJ, Duration of opiate receptor blockade determines tumorigenic response in mice with neuroblastoma: a role for endogenous opioid systems in cancer, Life Sci 35, pp. 409-416, 1984.

(17) http://www.ncbi.nlm.nih.gov/pubmed/6087062
Zagon IS, McLaughlin PJ, Opioid antagonist modulation of murine neuroblastoma: A profile of cell proliferation and opioid peptides and receptors, Brain Res 480, pp. 16-28, 1989.

(18) http://commons.wikimedia.org/wiki/ImageDuane_Hanson_Drug_Addict_Louisiana_1975.jpg
Duane Hanson's sculpture "Drug Addict" from 1974 *(*together with an unidentified museum guest*)*. Picture taken at an exhibition at the Louisiana Museum of Modern Art, Denmark. Source Own work Date Spring 1975 Public domain.

(19) http://en.wikipedia.org/wiki/Naloxone
Wikipedia: "Naloxone is a drug used to counter the effects of opioid overdose, for example heroin or morphine overdose."

(20) http://en.wikipedia.org/wiki/Naltrexone
wikipedia:"Naltrexone is an opioid receptor antagonist used primarily in the management of alcohol dependence and opioid dependence.."

(22) http://www.thecompounder.com/index.php
The Compounder Pharmacy 340 Marshall Ave Unit 100 ~ Aurora, IL 60506-2956
Phone: 630-859-0333 Fax: 630-859-0114

(23) http://wcbstv.com/topstories/lo.dose.naltrexone.2.732830.html
Drug Addiction Medication May Treat Other Diseases Dr. Max Gomez NEW YORK *(*CBS*)* May 2008.

(24) http://www.skipspharmacy.com/sppress/?cat=8
Skip's Pharmacy LDN PAGE 21000 Boca Rio Rd Suite A-29 Boca Raton, Florida 33433
561-218-0111 800-553-7429 Fax: 561-218-8873

Chapter 32

Chapter Debbie Depressed Case Report

A Young Woman with Depression and PMS Gets Off SSRI Drugs, and Reclaims Her Life, a Case Report

Thirty Two old Debbie came into my office along with her Dad, complaining of severe PMS, painful periods with irregular cycles for which birth control pills had been tried and discontinued because of side effects.

Debbie is so depressed that she spends much of her time alone in her room. She is on two different antidepressants, Zoloft 200 mg/day and Wellbutrin 300 mg/day prescribed by her psychiatrist. She has been unable to sleep for many years without Ambien, a prescription sleep medication touted on television ads. Her Fast Food Diet from McDonald's, Wendy's and Taco Bell, and lack of exercise has left her overweight. She takes no nutritional supplements. Her physical exam shows dilated pupils, dry skin, and brittle thin nails. Her reflexes, although hyperactive, are delayed *(*230 msec*)*.

Laboratory Studies

Debbie's labs showed a low Vitamin B-12 level of 304 *(*normal above 400*)*, and an extremely low Vitamin D level of 14 *(*deficiency is below 20*)*. Her thyroid labs were low with a TSH of 4.0 *(*normal less than 2.5*)*, and a free T3 of 270 *(*normal 230-420*)*.*(17)* Debbie's luteal phase progesterone level was low, as well.

Deciding to Get OFF the SSRI's

I explained to Debbie, that her insomnia, dilated pupils and hyperactive reflexes were due to the SSRI antidepressant drugs which are over-stimulating her nervous system. When I suggested that she taper off the SSRI drugs, she and her dad breathed a sigh of relief, and said "that was the main reason they came to see me, to get off the drugs."

I suggested that Debbie and her Dad go back to her psychiatrist and ask the doctor to work with them in getting off the drugs by providing a tapering schedule.

The Psychiatrist Drags His Feet

Later, I learned that her psychiatrist was in general agreement, yet was dragging his feet and refused to provide the tapering schedule for Debbie to get off the SSRI drugs. After waiting a few weeks realizing we were just wasting time, I finally went ahead and called into her pharmacy the authorization to reduce her SSRI dosage in half every week until the dosage was small enough to stop altogether. Tapering is required because the SSRI drugs are chemically addictive and can produce withdrawal effects.

5-HTP for Sleep, acts as an Antidepressant

For sleep during the SSRI tapering period, I recommended 5-HTP capsules which increases serotonin naturally with no side effects.*(20)* She was encouraged to stop the prescription sleep drugs *(*Ambien*)*.

I explained to Debbie that low Vitamin B-12, low Vitamin D and low thyroid function could all be possible causes of depression.

John R Lee MD, Pioneered Use of Progesterone

Natural Progesterone for PMS

The PMS and painful periods were treated with natural progesterone capsules, 50 mg twice a day for the last two weeks of her cycle *(*days 14-28*)*. The night-time progesterone had the added benefit of helping her sleep.

Debbie was started on natural thyroid half grain daily, high quality multivitamin, B12, vitamin D, and iodine supplementation, stopped the fast food, and began going out more for daily activities.

A month later, Debbie had tapered down to Zoloft 50 mg per day and Wellbutrin 100 mg per day. She says, "I am feeling good in general. I have a lot of energy. I am out of my room more. I am basically in a good mood, and sleeping about 4 hours a night."

Two more weeks later, Debbie was off the SSRI drugs and off the sleeping pills.

A Dramatic Improvement

Another 6 weeks later, Dad calls in and says , "Debbie is doing so much better. She has more energy and is sleeping well. The difference is between Night and Day."

That same day, Debbie calls in and says, "I feel a lot better. My energy is pretty good. I am back to work at my mother-in-law's business at the sales counter. I am sleeping good at night 6½ to 7 hours. My mood is stable, pretty much happy. More normal than before. I'm not snappy, and not in my room as much. I am getting out and doing stuff."

Regarding her last menstrual cycle, Debbie remarked "This time, no cramps, no PMS, no mood swings. The progesterone capsules are definitely helping, I have never had a period without pain before. It was awesome to have no pain. Now, I can do normal stuff. Before, when I had my menstrual period, I would be in bed for 7 days because of the pain."

Adverse Side Effects of SSRI drugs

My previous chapter discussed adverse side effects of SSRI antidepressants, namely akathesia, a form of agitation which drives people to commit suicide, sexual dysfunction *(*impotence*)*, tremor, involuntary body and facial movements, tardive dyskinesia, and hyperactive reflexes indicating a hyperactive nervous system. The SSRI induced loss of sexual function may be irreversible even after discontinuation of the drug.*(1)*

In many studies, SSRI efficacy was no better than placebo raising questions about SSRI efficacy. It is astonishing that today, SSRI antidepressants are the standard mainstream medical treatment for PMS *(*Pre-Menstrual Syndrome*)*. In addition, BCP's, birth control pills are frequently given as treatment for PMS, irregular periods, or any female complaint for that matter *(*relating to cycles*)*. Natural, bioidentical Progesterone is a far better and more effective alternative for PMS. *Broda Barnes* found irregular cycles frequently responded to natural thyroid in spite of "normal" thyroid labs.

SSRI drugs for PMS - The Wrong Way, A Practice Which Should Be Abandoned

SSRI antidepressants may have some justifiable uses as a temporary treatment in the severely depressed. However, the widespread usage of SSRI antidepressants for PMS and Menopause should be abandoned.

Women on SSRI antidepressants for PMS, or menopausal symptoms should be encouraged to taper off the SSRI drugs *(*under a physician's supervision*)*. The correct diagnostic workup includes hormone levels, thyroid panel, vitamin D and B12 levels. Treatment with natural bio-identical progesterone, natural thyroid and vitamin supplementation is more effective with fewer side effects than the current mainstream use of SSRI antidepressants or BCP's *(*birth control pills*)*.

A Successful Outcome

The case of Debbie Depressed illustrates a successful outcome treating depression and PMS with progesterone, natural thyroid, vitamins D and B12, and by modifying diet and lifestyle. It is very gratifying to see Debbie make such a dramatic recovery after discontinuing the SSRI drugs.

References for Causes of Depression:

Low vitamin B12 levels are associated with depression. *(2)(3)(4)(5)*

Low Vitamin D levels are associated with depression.*(6)(7)(8)(9)*

Low thyroid function is also associated with depression.*(10)(11)(12)*

Lastly, **bioidentical progesterone** has been widely used as an effective treatment for PMS *(*Pre-Menstrual Syndrome*)*. *(13) (14) (18)(19)*

References

(1) http://jeffreydach.com/2007/05/14/paxil-prozac-and-ssri-induced-suicide-by-jeffrey-dach-md.aspx
Adverse side effects of SSRI drugs, Paxil, Prozac and SSRI Induced Suicide by Jeffrey Dach MD

Low B12 and Depression

(2) http://www.biomedcentral.com/1471-244X/3/17
High vitamin B12 level and good treatment outcome may be associated in major depressive disorder Jukka Hintikka , Tommi Tolmunen , Antti Tanskanen and Heimo Viinamäki Department of Psychiatry, Kuopio University Hospital, Kuopio, Finland BMC Psychiatry 2003, 3:17 December 2003

(3) http://ajp.psychiatryonline.org/cgi/content/abstract/157/5/715
Vitamin B12 Deficiency and Depression in Physically Disabled Older Women: Epidemiologic Evidence From the Women's Health and Aging Study Brenda W.J.H. Penninx, Ph.D., Jack M. Guralnik, M.D., Ph.D., Luigi Ferrucci, M.D., Ph.D., Linda P. Fried, M.D., Ph.D., Robert H. Allen, M.D., and Sally P. Stabler, M.D. Am J Psychiatry 157:715-721, May 2000

(4) http://jop.sagepub.com/cgi/content/abstract/19/1/59
Treatment of depression: time to consider folic acid and vitamin B12, Journal of Psychopharmacology, Vol. 19, No. 1, 59-65 *(*2005*)*. Alec Coppen

(5) http://ajp.psychiatryonline.org/cgi/content/abstract/159/12/2099
Vitamin B12, Folate, and Homocysteine in Depression: The Rotterdam Study, Am J Psychiatry 159:2099-2101, December 2002. Henning Tiemeier, M.D., et al. "Hyperhomocysteinemia, vitamin B12 deficiency, and to a lesser extent, folate deficiency were all related to depressive disorders."

Low Vitamin D and Depression

(6) http://www.oasisadvancedwellness.com/learning/depression-vitamin-d.html
Major Depression and Vitamin D, By John J. Cannell, MD, The Vitamin D Council.

(7) http://www.ncbi.nlm.nih.gov/pubmed/10888476
Vitamin D vs broad spectrum phototherapy in the treatment of seasonal affective disorder. J Nutr Health Aging. 1999;3(1):5-7. Gloth FM 3rd, Alam W, Hollis B. Seasonal Affective Disorder (SAD) is prevalent when vitamin D stores are typically low. Improvement in 25-OH D was significantly associated with improvement in depression scale scores.

(8) http://www.corepsychblog.com/2007/02/depression_and__1.html
Depression and Vitamin D Deficiency: Overlooked Vitamin D Deficiency and Depression: Undetected is Untreated, Dr Charles Parker Blog.

(9) http://www.corepsychblog.com/files/Depression.D3.pdf
MAJOR DEPRESSION AND VITAMIN D The Vitamin D, John J. Cannell, MD March 20, 2004 The Vitamin D Council

Low Thyroid and Depression

(10) http://www.stopthethyroidmadness.com/thyroid-depression-mental-health/inspiring-stories/
Inspiring Stories on Depression that Went Away (and other mental health issues) These are actual stories from real patients whose depression went away using desiccated thyroid on the Stop the Thyroid Madness Blog.

(11) http://www.pubmedcentral.nih.gov/articlerender.fcgi?tool=pmcentrez&artid=149799
Should thyroid replacement therapy be considered for patients with treatment-refractory depression? J Psychiatry Neurosci. 2002 January; 27(1): 80. by Russell T. Joffe

(12) http://www.pubmedcentral.nih.gov/articlerender.fcgi?tool=pmcentrez&artid=1635797
Is the thyroid still important in major depression? Russell T. Joffe, J Psychiatry Neurosci. 2006 November; 31(6): 367–368.

Progesterone for PMS:

(13) http://www.pmstreatmentclinic.com/index.html
The PMS Treatment Clinic- the nation's leading PMS Clinic was established in 1982 and began treatment of Premenstrual Syndrome with natural progesterone therapy

according to the method of PMS world authority Katharina Dalton M.D. of London, England.

(14) *http://www.natural-progesterone-advisory-network.com/PDFs/dalton.pdf*
Interview with Katharina Dalton, MD Progesterone and Related Topics, Dr. Dalton successfully treated PMS, pre-eclampsia, eclampsia and post-partum depression with natural progesterone.

Thyroid for Irregular Menstrual Cycles

(15) *http://www.amazon.com/review/RVRC3UKH8XQ22/ref=cm_cr_rdp_perm*
Hypothyroidism the Unsuspected Illness, by Broda Barnes MD, An observation by Dr. Barnes is that low thyroid is associated with menstrual irregularties, miscarriages and infertility. Barnes treated thousands of young women with thyroid which restored cycle regularity and fertility. In his day, the medical system resorted to the drastic measure of hysterectomy for uncontrolled menstrual bleeding. Although today's use of birth control pills to regulate the cycles is admittedly a far better alternative, Barnes found that the simple administration of desiccated thyroid served quite well. Again, Barnes noted that blood testing was usually normal in these cases which respond to thyroid medication.

What is the Normal TSH Level?

(16) *http://www.aace.com/public/awareness/tam/2003/explanation.php*
American Association of Clinical Endocrinologists, Until recently, physicians accepted the normal TSH range of 0.5 to 5.0 mIU/L. The National Academy of Clinical Biochemistry (NACB guidelines believes that a sustained TSH level above 2.5 mIU/L might not be normal.

(17) *http://thyroid.about.com/od/gettestedanddiagnosed/a/garbertsh.htm*
The TSH Normal Range: Why is There Still Controversy? Insights from One of the Nation's Leading Endocrinologists, Dr. Jeffrey Garber said in practice, he doesn't hesitate to treat a patient who is in the 2.5 to 5.5 TSH range In late 2002, the National Academy of Clinical Biochemistry (NACB issued new guidelines for TSH of 0.4 and 2.5. January 2003, the American Association of Clinical Endocrinologists (AACE), issued their TSH range of 0.3 to 3.0. (Normal range for free T3 is 230-420).

Progesterone for PMS

(18) *http://www.johnleemd.com/*
John R Lee MD web site, pioneered use of natural progesterone.

(19) *http://www.johnleemd.com/store/drphil_anderson.html*
Dr. Phil Interviews Holly Anderson on Treating PMS with Natural Progesterone

5-HTP for Depression

(20) http://www.thorne.com/altmedrev/.fulltext/5/1/64.pdf

5-HTP, Use of Neurotransmitter Precursors for Treatment of Depression by Stephen Meyers, MS. *(* Altern Med Rev 2000;5*(*1*)*:64-71.*)*In a 1988 open study of 25 patients, the therapeutic efficacy of 5-HTP was found to be equal to traditional antidepressants.

(21) http://medicine.plosjournals.org/archive/1549-1676/5/2/pdf/10.1371_journal.pmed.0050045-L.pdf

Initial Severity and Antidepressant Benefits: A Meta-Analysis of Data Submitted to the Food and Drug Administration Irving Kirsch, Brett J. Deacon, Tania B. Huedo-Medina, Alan Scoboria, Thomas J. Moore, Blair T. Johnson. Compared with placebo, the new-generation antidepressants **do not** produce clinically significant improvements in depression in patients who initially have moderate or even very severe depression, but show significant effects only in the most severely depressed patients.

Vitamin D

(22) http://ajgponline.org/cgi/content/abstract/14/12/1032

Vitamin D Deficiency Is Associated With Low Mood and Worse Cognitive Performance in Older Adults. Consuelo H. Wilkins et al. Am J Geriatr Psychiatry 14:1032-1040, Dec 2006

Chapter 34

All About Celiac Disease and Gluten

Fifty three year old Sally McCann came to my office with menopausal symptoms of hot flashes and night sweats. Sally has trouble sleeping, chronic fatigue, and patchy hair loss. For the past nine years, she has taken anti-anxiety medication *(*Buspar*)* for daily anxiety attacks, and Ambien for sleep. Sally is from West Ireland, and has typical features with red hair, green eyes and a fair complexion. She mentions GI symptoms of "irritable bowel", i.e. bloating, gas, alternating constipation and diarrhea. She mentions neurological symptoms of tingling and numbness in her hands and feet. Sally has been to many doctors over the years and has tried many different treatments, and so far nothing has helped her.

Examination

Upon examination Sally had a small bald spot on her scalp, loss of outer third of the eyebrows, and brittle cracking nails.

Laboratory Findings

Sally's lab studies showed a microcytic anemia. Her blood cells were smaller and fewer than normal. This usually indicates Iron deficiency anemia. Her serum Iron, however was not too low because she has been taking Iron supplements. Sally informs me that her blood count has always been low and she has been taking Iron supplements for years. Sally's blood test also showed Hashimoto's thyroiditis with elevated thyroglobulin and peroxidase antibody levels.

Sally's blood test also showed Celiac Disease; *(*IgA TTG and EMA*)* were both positive indicating that Sally has intolerance of wheat gluten, also called celiac disease. I explained that many of her symptoms of peripheral neuropathy *(*tingling sensations*)*, hair loss, anemia, and anxiety are caused by her inability to tolerate wheat gluten in her diet, and all of her symptoms should resolve on a gluten free diet.

Sally was also started on bioidentical hormones for her menopausal symptoms, and natural thyroid for her low thyroid Hashimoto's Disease. Of course, she would need a further consultation with a gastroenterologist, and other family members should have genetic screening.

Treatment Program

The major treatment for Celiac Disease is a Gluten Free Diet.

Sally's Salivary Cortisol test showed a reversed pattern with low cortisol in the morning and high cortisol at night, explaining her morning fatigue and inability to sleep. The treatment for this is a nutritional supplement called Seriphos, *(*phosphorylated serine*)* which resets the biological cortisol clock and the pattern returns to normal in about 6 weeks.

To address adrenal fatigue, an adrenal vitamin program was also started which includes Vitamin C, B5, biotin, and adrenal herbs such as ashwaganda and licorice.

For sleep, Sally was started on melatonin and 5-HTP which replaces the Ambien. And to increase morning energy, Sally was started on D-ribose, L-Carnitine and Co-enzyme Q-10.

For the peripheral neuropathy, Sally is given B12, R-Alpha Lipoic Acid and thiamine.

A Successful Outcome

Six weeks after starting a Gluten free diet, Sally says she is much better. The neuropathy symptoms of tingling and numbness in the hands and feet have improved, she has more energy, sleeping better, and her hot flashes and night sweats are gone. The hair loss is better as well. In short she is a happy camper.

Symptoms of Celiac Disease

Celiac Disease is commonly associated with Hashimoto's Thyroid Disease, Adrenal disorders, Osteoporosis, Alopecia areata, chronic abdominal pain, Skin disorder called Dermatiformis Herpetica, Vitamin K and B12 deficiency, Iron deficiency Anemia, Peripheral Neuropathy, and other neurological disorders. It tends to run in families and has a genetic component.

Symptoms of celiac disease may include one or more of the following:

- gas
- recurring abdominal bloating and pain
- chronic diarrhea
- constipation
- pale, foul-smelling, or fatty stool
- weight loss/weight gain
- fatigue
- unexplained anemia (a low count of red blood cells causing fatigue)
- bone or joint pain
- osteoporosis, osteopenia
- behavioral changes
- tingling numbness in the legs (from nerve damage)
- muscle cramps
- seizures
- missed menstrual periods (often because of excessive weight loss)
- infertility, recurrent miscarriage
- delayed growth
- failure to thrive in infants
- pale sores inside the mouth, called aphthous ulcers
- tooth discoloration or loss of enamel
- itchy skin rash called dermatitis herpetiformis

TTG Blood Testing

A word of caution on blood testing for antibodies for gluten sensitivity and Celiac disease. We were disappointed to find that all tests were negative on a large group of high risk patients indicating the lack of utility of these tests *(*TTG and Endomyseal antibodies from Quest and LabCorp*)*. On the other hand, we have had two positive results using the Enterolab Stool test kit ordered over the internet. *(*enterolab.com, Dr. Kenneth Fine*)* We no longer routinely do the TTG antibody test, and instead recommend the enterolab test kit. An added advantage of the enterolab kit is that genetic typing is included.

References:

Review Articles on Celiac Disease

http://findarticles.com/p/articles/mi_m0ISW/is_2002_Dec/ai_94538644/pg_2
Gluten intolerance: a paradigm of an epidemic. Townsend Letter for Doctors and Patients, Dec, 2002 by Stacy Astor Shaul

http://www.aafp.org/afp/980301ap/pruessn.html

Detecting Celiac Disease in Your Patients. HAROLD T. PRUESSNER, M.D., University of Texas Medical School at Houston Am Fam Physician Mar 1998. excellent revw in American Academy of Family Physicians.

http://www.ajcn.org/cgi/content/full/69/3/354

American Journal of Clinical Nutrition, Vol. 69, No. 3, 354-365, March 1999
Review Article The widening spectrum of celiac disease1,2 Joseph A Murray

http://www.aafp.org/afp/20021215/2259.html

Gluten-Sensitive Enteropathy (Celiac Disease): More Common Than You Think
DAVID A. NELSEN, JR., M.D., M.S., University of Arkansas for Medical Sciences, Little Rock, Arkansas 1: Am Fam Physician. 2002 Dec 15;66(12):2259-66 Excellent review clinical

http://www.gastrojournal.org/article/PIIS0016508501701618/fulltext

Volume 120, Issue 6, Pages 1522-1525 (May 2001)

American Gastroenterological Association medical position statement: Celiac sprue. Official recommendations of the American Gastroenterological Association (AGA) on Celiac Sprue.

http://consensus.nih.gov/2004/2004CeliacDisease118main.htm

1: NIH Consens State Sci Statements. 2004 Jun 28-30;21(1):1-23.
NIH Consensus Development Conference on Celiac Disease.

Symptoms and Prevalence of Celiac Disease

http://digestive.niddk.nih.gov/ddiseases/pubs/celiac/

NIH. How common is celiac disease?

http://www.ncbi.nlm.nih.gov/pubmed/16772832

Eur J Gastroenterol Hepatol. 2006 Jul;18(7):747-54.
Health-related quality of life in adult coeliac disease in Germany: results of a national survey.

http://www.celiacdisease.net/assets/pdf/CDCFactSheetsAntibodyScreening3.pdf

University of Chicago CeliacDisease Center 773.702.7593 *www.CeliacDisease.net.*

Incidence of Celiac Disease, Epidemiology

http://www.eurojgh.com/pt/re/ejgh/abstract.00042737-200305000-00003.htm

High prevalence of coeliac disease in apparently healthy Iranian blood donors. European Journal of Gastroenterology & Hepatology. 15(5):475-478, May 2003. Shahbazkhani et al.

http://www.celiachealth.org/pdf/epidem.pdf
Slide show of Celiac Disease epidemiology

http://www.doctorgluten.com/cms/index.php?option=com_mamblog&task=show&action=view&id=232&Itemid=377
Doctor Gluten. For a fact, about 1% (one in a hundred) of the population has celiac disease.

Pattern of Presentation of Celiac Disease

http://adc.bmj.com/cgi/content/abstract/91/12/969
The changing clinical presentation of coeliac disease M Ravikumara, D P Tuthill, H R Jenkins Department of Paediatric Gastroenterology, University Hospital of Wales, Cardiff, UK

http://www.nutritionj.com/content/5/1/24
Patterns of clinical presentation of adult coeliac disease in a rural setting. Sián Jones Charles D'Souza et al. Nutrition Journal 2006,5:24

Celiac Disease Gluten Free Diets

http://www.healthsystem.virginia.edu/internet/digestive-health/nutritionarticles/dennisarticleapril.pdf
Going Gluten-Free: A Primer for Clinicians PRACTICAL GASTROENTEROLOGY, 2004
One Mom's Experence with Celiac Disease

http://sortacrunchy.typepad.com/sortacrunchy/2008/02/qa-whats-the-de.html
Sorta Crunchy One moms experience with Son having celiac disease, gluten free diet.

News about Gluten Free Restaurants

http://biz.yahoo.com/prnews/080227/law057.html?.v=101
Gluten-Free Restaurant Recommendations Double in Less Than 3 Months. Wednesday February 27, Glutenfreeonthego.com Answers Exploding Demand from Celiacs / Coeliacs, Gluten-Free Guests & Food Allergic Customers

http://www.vaildaily.com/article/20080226/AE/685641038
The challenge of cooking gluten-free, David Hagedorn, L.A. Times-Washington Post News Service Vail CO, Colorado February 26, 2008

Celiac.com Web Site *http://www.celiac.com/ Celiac Com Gluten Free Diets etc.*

http://www.celiac.com/articles/21521/1/How-Early-Can-Celiac-Disease-Be-Diagnosed/Page1.html
How Early Can Celiac Disease Be Diagnosed? Rodney Ford

http://www.doctorgluten.com/cms/ Rodney Ford Web Site Celiac Disease
http://www.doctorgluten.com/cms/index.php?option=com_content&task=view&id=1 11&Itemid=162

Rodney Ford. To diagnose coeliac disease

Alopecia Areata

http://www.ncbi.nlm.nih.gov/pubmed/7557104

Gastroenterology. 1995 Oct;109*(4)*:1333-7. Links
Celiac disease and **alopecia areata**: report of a new association.
Corazza GR, Andreani ML, Venturo N, Bernardi M, Tosti A, Gasbarrini G.

Celiac Disease and Osteoporosis

http://archinte.ama-assn.org/cgi/content/full/165/4/393

Increased Prevalence of Celiac Disease and Need for Routine Screening Among Patients With Osteoporosis

Cardiomyopathy and Celiac Disease

http://www.ncbi.nlm.nih.gov/pubmed/15887437

Mayo Clin Proc. 2005 May;80*(5)*:674-6. Cardiomyopathy associated with celiac disease. Goel NK, McBane RD, Kamath PS.Department of Internal Medicine, Mayo Clinic College of Medicine, Rochester, Minn 55905, USA.

Myopathy and Celiac Disease

http://www.ncbi.nlm.nih.gov/pubmed/16967485

Muscle Nerve. 2007 Jan;35*(1)*:49-54,
Celiac disease and antibodies associated with celiac disease in patients with inflammatory myopathy. Selva-O'Callaghan A, Casellas F, de Torres I, Palou E, Grau-Junyent JM, Vilardell-Tarrés M.

Sarcoidosis and Celiac Disease

http://www.sciencedirect.com/science?_ob=ArticleURL&_udi=B6T1B-49KJMHH-2M0&_user=10&_rdoc=1&_fmt=&_orig=search&_sort=d&view=c&_acct=C000050221&_version=1&_urlVersion=0&_userid=10&md5=6e0ae5fae10b9ea418047ed3ccca7bba

SARCOIDOSIS AND COELIAC DISEASE: AN ASSOCIATION? Science Volume 324, Issue 8393, 7 July 1984, Pages 13-15. J. G. Douglas, R. F. A. Logan1, J. Gillon, I. W. B. Grant and G. K.

http://www.ncbi.nlm.nih.gov/pubmed/17934825

Sarcoidosis in Patients with Celiac Disease. Dig Dis Sci. 2007 Oct 13. Hwang E, McBride R, Neugut AI, Green PH.

Screening and Detection, Lab Testing for Celiac Disease

http://www.Enterolab.com
Dr. Kenneth Fine Enterolab

http://www.inovadx.com/Posters/GLIADIN%20PEPTIDE%20POSTER%202005.pdf
http://www.celiac.com/articles/57/1/Interpretation-of-Celiac-Disease-Blood-Test-Results/Page1.html
INOVA Diagnostics, Inc., Interpretation of Celiac Disease Blood Test Results.

http://cas2.questdiagnostics.com/scripts/webdos.wls?MGWLPN=QDCIAP22&wlapp=DOS&SearchString=celiac &auto=false&tmsearch=Search&tmradio=alias&SITE=9&SearchString2
Quest Lab test Panel for Celiac Disease.

http://www.blackwell-synergy.com/doi/full/10.1046/j.1365-2796.2001.00891.x
Screening for adult coeliac disease – which serological marker(s) to use? J Intern Med 2001; 250: 241–248.

http://www.blackwell-synergy.com/doi/full/10.1046/j.1365-2796.2001.00793.x
Identification of a new coeliac disease subgroup: antiendomysial and anti-transglutaminase antibodies of IgG class in the absence of selective IgA deficiency. J Intern Med 2001; 249: 181–188. Picarelli A et al.

http://www.blackwell-synergy.com/doi/abs/10.1111/j.1572-0241.2001.03754.x
Radioimmunoassay to detect antitransglutaminase autoantibodies is the most sensitive and specific screening method for celiac disease.

http://www.ncbi.nlm.nih.gov/pubmed/17355413
Detection of Celiac disease in primary care: a multicenter case-finding study in North America. Am J Gastroenterol. 2007 Jul;102(7):1454-60. Catassi C et al.

Neuropathy and Neurological Disorders and Celiac Disease

http://www.sciencedirect.com/science?_ob=ArticleURL&_udi=B6WFX-4FVC7DW-R&_user=10&_rdoc=1&_fmt=&_orig=search&_sort=d&view=c&_acct=C000050221&_version=1&_urlVersion=0&_userid=10&md5=c85f5245bad24700b3b13794e13cf125
Neurologic presentation of celiac disease. Khalafalla O. Bushara, Neurology Department, Minneapolis VA Medical Center and University of Minnesota, Minneapolis, Minnesota Gastroenterology Volume 128, Issue 4, Supplement 1, April 2005, Pages S92-S97

http://pediatrics.aappublications.org/cgi/content/full/113/6/1672
PEDIATRICS Vol. 113 No. 6 June 2004, pp. 1672-1676. Range of Neurologic Disorders in Patients With Celiac Disease Nathanel Zelnik, MD, Avi Pacht, MD, Raid Obeid, MD and Aaron Lerner, MD

http://archneur.ama-assn.org/cgi/content/full/62/10/1574
Small-Fiber Neuropathy/Neuronopathy Associated With Celiac Disease Skin Biopsy Findings. Thomas H. Brannagan III, MD et al. Arch Neurol. 2005;62:1574-1578. All patients had asymmetric numbness and paresthesias.

http://jnnp.bmj.com/cgi/content/abstract/76/7/1028
Journal of Neurology Neurosurgery and Psychiatry 2005;76:1028-1030 Gluten sensitivity and neuromyelitis optica: two case reports S Jacob1, M Zarei1, A Kenton2, H Allroggen2

Multiple Sclerosis and Gluten

http://www.ncbi.nlm.nih.gov/pubmed/15355487
Acta Neurol Scand. 2004 Oct;110(4):239-41. IgA antibodies against gliadin and gluten in multiple sclerosis. Reichelt KL, Jensen D. Institute of Pediatric Research, University of Oslo, Oslo, Norway.

http://www.ncbi.nlm.nih.gov/pubmed/17537569
Clin Neurol Neurosurg. 2007 Oct;109(8):651-3. Epub 2007 May 29. Multiple sclerosis and gluten sensitivity.Borhani Haghighi A, Ansari N, Mokhtari M, Geramizadeh B, Lankarani KB.

http://www.direct-ms.org/pdf/NutritionMS/Gluten%20sensitivity%20and%20MS%20 Wills.pdf
Multiple sclerosis and occult gluten sensitivity. NEUROLOGY 2004;62:2326–2327 Connie D.S.N.A. Pengiran Tengah, MRCP; Robert J. Lock, MPhil; D. Joseph Unsworth, PhD; and Adrian J. Wills, MD

http://www.celiac.com/articles/124/1/Multiple-Sclerosis-and-Celiac-Disease/Page1.html
Multiple Sclerosis and Celiac Disease

Wikipedia

http://en.wikipedia.org/wiki/Celiac_sprue
coeliac disease.

Genetic Basis for Celiac HLA DQ2

http://en.wikipedia.org/wiki/Celiac_Disease#_note-pmid17785484
In the United Kingdom (NICE) recommends screening for coeliac disease in patients with newly diagnosed 1) chronic fatigue syndrome 2) irritable bowel syndrome 3) autoimmune thyroid disease. Hashimotos 4) type 1 diabetes,5) unexplained iron-deficiency anemia 6) lupus

http://www.ncbi.nlm.nih.gov/pubmed/8851726
Tissue Antigens. 1996 Feb;47*(2)*:127-33. HLA-DR, DQ genotypes of celiac disease patients and healthy subjects from the West of Ireland.Michalski JP, McCombs CC, Arai T, Elston RC, Cao T, McCarthy CF, Stevens FM.

http://www.nicholsinstitute.com/Transplant/HLA%20TM%20D.pdf
Nichols DNA Test for Celiac 17135X HLA Typing for Celiac Disease 86817
Assess risk of celiac disease in symptomatic*(*HLA-DQ2 and -DQ8*)* patients and in family members of patients with celiac disease

http://en.wikipedia.org/wiki/CELIAC1
HLA-DQB1

http://www.aetna.com/cpb/medical/data/500_599/0561.html
Aetna considers testing of anti-gliadin, anti-reticulin, IgA anti-human tissue transglutimase *(*TTG*)*, and IgA anti-endomysial antibodies *(*EMA*)* medically necessary for any of the following indications:

On Line Genetic Testing for Celiac Disease

https://www.enterolab.com/Home.htm
Enterolab celiac disease testing. Dr Kenneth Fine.

http://www.prometheus-labs.com/
Prometheus celiac disease testing

http://www.timesonline.co.uk/tol/news/uk/science/article3463550.ece
Online genetic testing for 20 diseases From The Times March 1, 2008.

http://www.decodeme.com/
Decodeme. For only $985, we scan over one million variants in your genome

https://www.23andme.com/
23 and me online genetic testing.

Adrenal Insufficiency, Adrenal Fatigue

http://www.ncbi.nlm.nih.gov/pubmed/17595243
J Clin Endocrinol Metab. 2007 Sep;92*(9)*:3595-8. Epub 2007 Jun 26. Risk of primary adrenal insufficiency in patients with celiac disease. .Elfström P, Montgomery SM, Kämpe O, Ekbom A, Ludvigsson JF.

Neurological Disease and Celiac Disease, polyneuropathy

http://www.ncbi.nlm.nih.gov/pubmed/17509100
A population-based study of coeliac disease, neurodegenerative and neuroinflammatory diseases. Aliment Pharmacol Ther. 2007 Jun 1;25(11):1317-27. Ludvigsson JF, Olsson T, Ekbom A, Montgomery SM.

http://www.ncbi.nlm.nih.gov/pubmed/17688758
A case-control study of presentations in general practice before diagnosis of coeliac disease. Br J Gen Pract. 2007 Aug;57(541):636-42.

Celiac and Hashimoto's, B12, K

http://www.clinmedres.org/cgi/content/full/5/3/184
Clin Med Res. 2007 Oct;5(3):184-92. Celiac disease and autoimmune thyroid disease. Ch'ng CL, Jones MK, Kingham JG. Department of Gastroenterology, Singleton Hospital, Swansea, United Kingdom.

http://www.ncbi.nlm.nih.gov/pubmed/17461476
World J Gastroenterol. 2007 Mar 21;13(11):1715-22.
Coeliac disease in Dutch patients with Hashimoto's thyroiditis and vice versa. Hadithi M, de Boer H, Meijer JW, Willekens F, Kerckhaert JA, Heijmans R, Peña AS, Stehouwer CD, Mulder CJ.

http://edrv.endojournals.org/cgi/content/full/23/4/464
Endocr Rev. 2002 Aug;23(4):464-83. Endocrinological disorders and celiac disease. Collin P, Kaukinen K, Välimäki M, Salmi J. Department of Medicine, Tampere University Hospital and University of Tampere, 33014 Tampere, Finland.

http://www.blackwell-synergy.com/doi/abs/10.1111/j.1572-0241.2001.03616.x
The American Journal of Gastroenterology Vol. 96 Issue 3 Page 745 March 2001
Vitamin B12 deficiency in untreated celiac disease Anna Dahele M.R.C.P. (UK), Subrata Ghosh M.D., (Edin)

http://en.wikipedia.org/wiki/Gluten-free_diet
Vitamin K-deficiency, A small proportion (10%) have abnormal coagulation due to deficiency of vitamin K, and are slightly at risk for abnormal bleeding.

Video on Celiac Disease

http://thenewsroom.com/details/1872868
Video from Mayo Clinic on Celiac Disease, Gluten Free Diet

Chapter 35

Fosamax, Actonel, Osteoporosis and Toulouse Lautrec

Osteoporotic Compression Fractures

While working as a radiologist for 25 years, a large part of my day was spent reading X-rays of osteoporotic compression fractures of the spine. These commonly found fractures typically involve the mid thoracic spine causing loss of height and curvature of the spine, and considerable pain.

Vertebroplasty for Compression Fracture

Working in the hospital over the years, I saw many procedures come and go. A procedure called vertebroplasty, still in vogue, is used for treatment of compression fractures. This involves injecting glue into the collapsed vertebral body under x ray control.*(1)* Although the procedure may seem somewhat barbaric, it does provide pain relief and restores height to the collapsed vertebral body. The vertebroplasty procedure was invented in 1984 by the French and introduced into the US by Mary Jensen MD. The procedure is not for the light hearted because, during the actual acrylic glue injection, the acrylic cement may flow into the epidural venous plexus leading to venous thrombosis or pulmonary embolus.*(2)* The more refined Kyphoplasty version involves inflation of a balloon to expand the collapsed vertebral body just prior to injection of cement into the cavity. These procedures are quite useful at providing pain relief.

Prevention Makes More Sense

On the surface, it might appear callous for the medical system to wait years until thousands of women develop severe osteoporosis with compression fractures, and then intervene with glue injections. Perhaps some form of prevention would make more sense. The usual preventive recommendation to take calcium tablets apparently was not effective for these women presenting with osteoporotic compression fractures. Perhaps the best preventive plan can be found in Russell Jaffe's article, Acid-Alkaline Balance and its Effect on Bone Health.*(3)* Russell Jaffe MD is a charming and humorous fellow who informed our small group of docs at his medical seminar that in the old days he ran a lab at the NIH, and was actually offered the job of Assistant Surgeon General, but he declined the offer after trying it for a day. He is also the founder of a supplement company called Perque.*(15)*

Excess Acid in the American Diet Causes Osteoporosis

According to Dr. Jaffe's article, excess acid production from the American diet causes the chronic calcium loss leading to osteoporosis.*(3)* The calcium is pulled away from the bones, and used up as a buffering agent for the acids which can then be excreted in the urine. The solution is to alkalinize the diet, and with the help of alkaline food charts, and pH test strips along with the usual calcium and vitamin supplements, osteoporosis can be arrested and gradually reversed in a process which may take years. I would add that a bio-identical hormone program is also useful for preventing and reversing osteoporosis.

Bisphosphonate Drugs and Toulouse Lautrec

For the impatient ones who wish to see a prompt increase in bone density, the FDA approved the bisphosphonate drug Fosamax *(*alondronate*)* which was first introduced in 1995. Merck made 3.2 Billion on 22 million Fosamax prescriptions in 2006. A major drug study, *(FIT)* the Fracture Intervention Trial, showed lower fracture rates in the drug group.*(4)* And it is true that the bisphosphonate drugs will reward the user with a prompt increase in bone density. The main question remains however, how strong is the bone with the increased density? This is an important question because we know from studies of Toulouse Lautrec that his increased bone density was not stronger, in fact his bones were much weaker leading to spontaneous fracture and jaw necrosis. This is explained below.

Genetic Bone Disease

What could fosamax *(*alondronate*)* have in common with Toulouse Lautrec, the famous French Impressionist artist? One day, Toulouse Lautrec's name came up in conversation, and we puzzled over the cause of Lautrec's short stature. After looking up the question on the internet, we discovered that Toulouse Lautrec's parents were first cousins giving Toulouse the autosomal recessive genetic disease, pycnodysostosis, which means dense bones. I had seen X-Rays of this bone disease in text books while studying for the radiology board exams, but I have never seen it in actual practice.

Dr. Gelb found Toulouse Lautrec's dense bone disease was caused by a genetic defect in cathepsin K, a protease enzyme of the osteoclast cells responsible for removing and remodeling bone.*(5)(6)* Osteoclast cells are bone cells involved in resorption and remodeling of bone. In this genetic disease, the abnormal bone is very dense on xray, yet looking under the microscope, one sees profound deterioration in trabecular architecture and lamellar arrangement. This is presumably the reason for spontaneous fracture and jaw necrosis which occurs in Lautrec's genetic bone disease, and also occurs as an adverse side effect of the bisphosphonate drugs.*(7)*

This osteoclast dysfunction and resulting bone fragility explains why Toulouse had spontaneous fractures of both mid femurs at the age of 12 and 14. The mid-femur fractures never healed properly. The non-healing mid femur fractures caused

Toulouse Lautrec to have short stature, attaining a final height of only four and a half feet.*(8)*

Bisphosphonate Mechanism of Action

Bisphosphonate drugs *(*fosamax and actonel*)* are taken up by osteoclasts, causing disruption of osteoclast activity. The osteoclasts are bone cells involved in bone resorption and remodeling. This loss of the osteoclast activity inhibits bone resorption and bone remodeling, tasks otherwise performed by the osteoclasts.*(9)* Thus, the bisphosphonate drugs produce a chemical disruption of osteoclast activity same as the genetic disease of Toulouse Lautrec. The bisphosphonate drugs also produce the same adverse side effects, namely jaw necrosis and spontaneous fracture.

Questions About Long Term Safety

The conventional medical test for bone density is the DEXA bone scan. And, indeed DEXA bone scanning does confirm that bisphoshonate drug treatment increases bone density, and studies such as the FIT *(*Fracture Intervention Trial*)* report drug treatments reduce fracture rates in severly osteoporotic women over the short term. However, Susan Ott, MD raises questions about the long term safety of bisphosphonates.*(10)* Although the bisphosphonate drugs appear to have short term benefits, Dr. Susan Ott speculates that over the long term, after 5 years of use, the drugs cause severe suppression of bone formation, and negative effects such as microdamage and brittleness.

Reports of Spontaneous Fractures

Jennifer P. Schneider, MD, PhD reports a 59-year old previously healthy woman on long-term alendronate.*(11)* While on a subway train in New York City one morning, the train jolted, and the woman shifted all her weight to one leg, felt a bone snap, and fell to the floor, suffering a spontaneous mid -femur fracture. In the months following, it became clear that the fracture was not uniting. Schneider speculates that increased bone density from the bisphosphonate drug does not necessarily equate with good bone quality. By decreasing osteoclast activity and bone resorption, and therefore bone formation as well, microdamage, and brittle bone may result in fractures.*(11)*

Odvina reports on a series of 9 patients who suffered spontanous fracture while on fosamax *(*alendonate*)*. Five of the nine cases were spontaneous mid femur fractures.*(12)* Two had bilateral mid femur fractures just like those sustained by Toulouse Lautrec. Six of the fractures showed delayed or absent fracture healing. Analysis of the cancellous bone showed markedly suppressed bone formation, and Odvina raised the possibility that severe suppression of bone turnover could develop during long-term fosamax *(*alendronate*)* therapy, resulting in increased susceptibility and delayed healing of fractures.

Dimitrakopoulos report on 11 patients presenting with necrosis of the jaw, claiming this to be a new complication of bisphosphonate therapy administration, i.e. osteonecrosis of jaws.*(13)* He advised clinicians to reconsider the merits of the rampant use of bisphosphonates. Osteonecrosis of the jaw is also common to pycnodysostosis. The bisphosphonate drugs create the same adverse effects of spontaneous mid femur fracture, and failure of bone healing and jaw necrosis which tormented Toulouse Lautrec.

In spite of these adverse effects of bisphosphonates, there are four more drugs in clinical trials specifically designed to inhibit cathepsin K, the enzyme defect in Lautrec's genetic bone disease.*(14)* FDA approval for use in osteoporosis treatment is expected. Excuse me here, but perhaps this thinking needs re-evaluation. In essence, these drugs are creating a population of women with Toulouse Lautrec's bone disease.

Ironically, women who sustain fractures while on Fosamax are told by their docs that the fractures are due to the underlying osteoporosis, not the drug. For a recent example that I know of, a 60 year old female sustained a fractured elbow after minor trauma at home in the kitchen. She claims that, if not for the biphosphate drug, her fracture would have been much worse. When patients continue to fracture while on the bisphosphonate drugs, the medical system tends to blame it on the underlying osteoporosis, not the drug. Sound familiar?

Conclusion:

The obvious conclusion is that this entire class of bisphosphonate drugs should be banned, and I predict that they will be banned within the next few years.

References

(1) http://www.ajronline.org/cgi/reprint/182/2/319.pdf
Treatment of Chronic Symptomatic Vertebral Compression Fractures with Percutaneous Vertebroplasty, Daniel B. Brown et al. AJR 2004;182:319–322.

(2) http://www.emedicine.com/RADIO/topic871.htm
Vertebroplasty and Kyphoplasty, Percutaneous. Jeffrey P Kochan, MD

(3) http://www.betterbones.com/research/articles/bjaffe.PDF
Acid-Alkaline Balance and Its Effect on Bone Health Susan E. Brown, Ph.D., CCN, and Russell Jaffe, MD, Ph.D., CCN International Journal of Integrative Medicine Vol. 2, No. 6 – Nov/Dec 2000

(4) *http://www.ncbi.nlm.nih.gov/pubmed/8950879*
Randomised trial of effect of alendronate on risk of fracture in women with existing vertebral fractures. Fracture Intervention Trial Research Group. Black DM and Cummings SR et al. Lancet. 1996 Dec 7;348(9041):1535-41

(5) *http://www.pubmedcentral.nih.gov/articlerender.fcgi?tool=pubmed&pubmedid=9529353*
Paternal uniparental disomy for chromosome 1 revealed by molecular analysis of a patient with pycnodysostosis. B D Gelb et al. Am J Hum Genet. 1998 April; 62(4): 848–854.

(6) *http://www.ncbi.nlm.nih.gov/entrez/dispomim.cgi?id=265800*
OMIMTM - Online Mendelian Inheritance in Man TM #265800 GeneTests, PYCNODYSOSTOSIS A number sign (#) is used with this entry because pycnodysostosis can be caused by mutation in the cathepsin K gene (CTSK; 601105).

(7) *http://jcem.endojournals.org/cgi/content/full/89/4/1538*
Decreased Bone Turnover and Deterioration of Bone Structure in Two Cases of Pycnodysostosis. Nadja Fratzl-Zelman et al. The Journal of Clinical Endocrinology & Metabolism Vol. 89, No. 4 1538-1547

(8) *http://www.ejbjs.org/cgi/reprint/60/8/1128*
Pycnodysostosis. A case report. J Bone Joint Surg Am Taylor et al. 60 (8): 1128.

(9) *http://lib.bioinfo.pl/pmid:16831938*
Bisphosphonates: from bench to bedside. R Graham G Russell. Ann N Y Acad Sci. 2006 Apr; 1068 :367-401 16831938

(10) *http://jcem.endojournals.org/cgi/content/full/90/3/1897*
Long-Term Safety of Bisphosphonates, Susan M. Ott MD. The Journal of Clinical Endocrinology & Metabolism Vol. 90, No. 3 1897-1899

(11) *http://geriatrics.modernmedicine.com/geriatrics/data/articlestandard/geriatrics/022006/283268/article.pdf*
Should bisphosphonates be continued indefinitely? Case Report Jennifer P. Schneider, MD, PhD Jan 2006 Volume 61, Number 1 Geriatrics.

(12) *http://jcem.endojournals.org/cgi/content/full/90/3/1294*
Severely Suppressed Bone Turnover: A Potential Complication of Alendronate Therapy Clarita V. Odvina et al. The Journal of Clinical Endocrinology & Metabolism Vol. 90, No. 3 1294-1301

(13) *http://www.ncbi.nlm.nih.gov/pubmed/16687238?dopt=AbstractPlus*
Bisphosphonate-induced avascular osteonecrosis of the jaws: a clinical report of 11 cases.

Dimitrakopoulos I, Magopoulos C, Karakasis D. Int J Oral Maxillofac Surg. 2006 Jul;35*(7)*:588-93. Epub 2006 May 9.

(14) http://www.nature.com/nrd/journal/v5/n9/full/nrd2092.html
Nature Reviews Drug Discovery 5, 785-799 *(*September 2006*)* Targeting proteases: successes, failures and future prospects. Boris Turk. Cathepsin K and osteoporosis. Cathepsin K is a lysosomal cysteine cathepsin predominantly located in osteoclasts and is the major enzyme involved in bone resorption. The first evidence for this role came from a genetic study on pycnodysostosis, a rare genetic disorder associated with severe defects in bone growth, which revealed that an inactivating mutation in the gene encoding cathepsin K is a causative factor.

(15) http://www.perque.com/
Russell Jaffe MD Perque Supplements

(16) http://jeffreydach.com/2008/03/09/bisphosphonates-for-osteoporosis-a-closer-look-at-the-data-by-jeffrey-dach-md.aspx
Bisphosphonates for Osteoporosis, A Closer Look at the Data by Jeffrey Dach MD

Chapter 36

Bisphosphonates for Osteoporosis, A Closer Look at the Data

While sitting in my office, 51 year old Jane Smith told me her story. She had seen a TV commercial which showed the actress, Sally Field, suggesting to everyone to have their bones checked for osteoporosis. This prompted a doctor's visit and a DEXA bone scan which showed a T score of minus 2.3. Even though Janet did not have osteoporosis, and has never had an osteoporotic fracture, she was neverthless prescribed a bisphosphonate drug to "prevent" osteoporosis. The most commonly used drugs in this class Fosamax, Boniva, and Actonel which are all bisphosphonates. Jane has no risk factors, doesn't smoke or drink, avoids soda pop and caffeine, exercises regularly, eats organic food and takes a handful of vitamins each day. Jane informs me that she did an internet search and found out that Fosamax and Actonel cause necrosis of the jaw, and bone pain. She wanted to know if there was a more natural way to increase bone density without drugs. The following information was shared with Jane.

Bisphosphonates?

This chapter will take a closer look at the data and current recommendations for bisphosphonate drugs for osteoporosis. We will weigh the possible benefits versus the adverse side effects of the bisphosphonate drugs. The main goal of bisphosphonate drug treatment for osteoporosis is the prevention of hip and vertebral fractures, and the major diagnostic tool is the DEXA bone density scan which is reported as the T-score.

What is Difference Between Primary Prevention and Secondary Prevention?

The **Primary** prevention group is defined as those women who have T scores greater than -2.5 and do **not** have osteoporotic fractures. The more severe Osteporosis is defined as a T-score less than -2.5 , and the less severe Osteopenia has a T score of greater than -2.5. The **Secondary** prevention group is defined as those women who already have fractures from osteoporosis and T scores less than -2.5.

The current NICE *(*National Institute for Clinical Excellence*)* guidelines recommend the bisphosphonate drugs for Secondary prevention of osteoporotic fracture in women who already have osteoporosis *(*T-score less than -2.5*)*, and have a history of osteoporotic fracture. *(21)*

Bisphosphonates Not Recommended for Primary Prevention

For primary prevention of osteoporotic fracture in women with osteopenia, *(*T-score greater than -2.5*)*, the use of bisphosphonates is NOT recommended because the Fracture Intervention Trial *(*FIT*)* data shows **increased** fracture rate with bisphosphonates.*(15)* This is discussed in detail below.

Failure of Treatment

What if the osteoporotic woman continues to fracture while on bisphosphonate drugs? This is called failure of treatment and there are no current guidelines for this scenario.*(22)*. Susan Ott MD, however, would then recommend a trial of intermittent PTH.*(30)*

FDA Issues Alert About Severe Bone Pain from Bisphosphonates

On Jan 7 2008, the FDA issued an alert highlighting "the possibility of severe and sometimes incapacitating bone, joint, and/or muscle *(*musculoskeletal*)* pain in patients taking bisphosphonates. " which may be overlooked, delaying diagnosis, prolonging pain requiring pain medications.*(1)* Could this pain be caused by microdamage and cracks in the bones?*(2)*

Adverse Side Effects Posted on Message Message Boards

For those interested in adverse effects, there are Message Boards on the web posting thousands of messages from patients with adverse side effects from Fosamax and Actonel.*(3)(3A)*

The Adverse Side Effect of Bis- Fossy Jaw *(*4*)*

A number of reports have found similarities between bisphosphonate induced avascular necrosis of the jaw and a 19th century occupational disease in workers in match factories from inhalation of white phosphorus. Not only did these workers have necrosis of the jaw, they also had systemic weakness of all other bones.

> "There is evidence that occupational exposure to white phosphorus affects bones other than those in the jaw; this implies a systemic effect for inhaled white phosphorus. Two middle-aged men occupationally exposed to white phosphorus for 20-30 years had a history of breaking their femurs in accidents not normally expected to result in breakage of bones *(*Dearden 1899*)*."*(10)(5)-(*11*)*

Avascular Necrosis of the Jaw

Some argue that the adverse side effect of jaw necrosis is seen exclusively in cancer patients receiving intravenous bisphosphonates, rather than in those who take the oral form of the medication. However, there are also cases reported in the medical literature of jaw necrosis after dental procedures in patients taking the oral bisphosphonate tablets. For this reason, bisphosphonates are under litigation for jaw necrosis as discussed in the chapter, Protect Your Family from Bad Drugs.*(41)* The issue raised here is: Why is jaw necrosis happening at all? To me, this raises the serious concern about the whole class of bisphosphonate drugs which seriously disturbs the underlying physiology of bone formation.

Toulouse Lautrec's Disease

My previous chapter, *Fosamax, Actonel, Osteoporosis and Toulouse Lautrec*, discussed reports of spontaneous fractures in patients on bisphosphonates and the similarity with pycnodysostosis, a genetic disease of the osteoclast bone cells.*(24)* These are unusual non-healing fractures of the mid femur indicating weak bone matrix. Toulouse Lautrec suffered this exact type of femur fracture bilaterally at a young age.

Avascular Necrosis of the Femoral Head from Bisphosphonates

Another new report is the revelation of a tripled incidence of avascular necrosis of the femoral head in women taking Fosamax. *(13)* Again, the issue is why should this adverse event be increased at all? To me it suggested deranged or abnormal bone physiology as a result of drug treatment.

P and G Hiding Data, Again?

According to a correspondence letter by Paul C. Royce, M.D., Ph.D. *(31)*, Proctor and Gamble, the maker of the bisphosphonate Actonel, omitted data in a large clinical trial that they sponsored whose lead author was McClung. The McClung data included 9,331 elderly women with low bone density. P&G announced that their bisphosphonate risedronate *(*Actonel*)* increased bone mineral density by one per cent *(*1%*)*. However, when they conducted their follow-up phase of the trial, the information about the outcome of 3,324 women *(*slightly over a third of the trial subjects*)*, was not made available. This data was omitted from publication and peer review in the final article.*(32)* The whistle blower, Aubrey Blumson has previously documented extensive scientific misconduct by this same company, Proctor and Gamble, the soap company that makes Actonel. *(17)*

Dr. Cummings did not hide the data in his 1998 JAMA FIT article.

Why Does Fracture Rate Go Up WIth Fosamax in Osteopenia?

Although Fosamax and Actonel reduces fracture rates modestly *(*1-2% absolute*)* in elderly women with severe osteoporosis and compression fractures, why does fosamax **increase** fracture rates in women with osteopenia *(*T greater than -2.5*)*? Fosamax is supposed to make bones stronger, not weaker. Dr. Cummings' original FIT JAMA article in 1998 did not explain why hip fracture rates went up 84% for fosamax in women with osteopenia (a less severe than osteoporosis with T score greater than -2.5)

John Abramson MD Says in his book, Overdosed America*(25)*:

> "In a study published in JAMA in 1998, for example, women with an average age of 68 and a T score of - 2.5 or less who took Fosamax for four years were **56 percent less likely to suffer a hip fracture** than women in the control group. This sounds like very good news for women with osteoporosis, but how many hip fractures were really prevented? With no drug therapy at all, women with osteoporosis had a 99.5 percent chance of making it through each year without a hip fracture -- pretty good odds. With drug therapy, their odds improved to 99.8 percent. In other words, **taking the drugs decreased their risk of hip fracture from 0.5 percent per year to 0.2 percent per year**. This tiny decrease in absolute risk translates into the study's reported 56 percent reduction in relative risk. The bottom line is that 81 women with osteoporosis have to take Fosamax for 4.2 years, at a cost of more than $300,000, to prevent one hip fracture. (This benefit does not include a reduction of less serious fractures, including wrist and vertebral fractures. Most vertebral fractures cause no symptoms.)
>
> What about using these drugs to prevent osteoporosis? The study of Fosamax published in JAMA in 1998 (mentioned earlier) also included women with osteopenia. Did Fosamax reduce their risk of fracture? The results show that the risk of hip fractures **actually went up 84 percent with Fosamax treatment.*** The risk of **wrist fractures increased by about 50 percent.***(25)*"

Here is the Cummings FIT publication in JAMA:

Effect of Alendronate on Risk of Fracture in Women With Low Bone Density but Without Vertebral Fractures Results From the Fracture Intervention Trial. Steven R. Cummings, MD et al. JAMA. 1998;280:2077-2082. *(15)*

HIP Fractures Reduced for 56% for Osteoporosis, But Increased 84% in Osteopenia

> "Alendronate (Fosamax) **reduced the risk of hip fractures by 56%** among women with a femoral neck T score of -2.5 or less: 18 (2.2%) in the placebo group vs 8 (1.0%) in the alendronate group (RH, 0.44; 95% CI, 0.18-0.97; placebo-treatment difference, 1.2%; NNT, 81). There was **no reduction** in risk among those whose femoral neck T scores

were more than -2.5: **6** *(0.4%)* in the placebo group vs **11** *(0.8%)* in the alendronate group *(RH,* **1.84**; 95% CI, 0.70-5.36*)."*

Fosamax Treatment Increases Wrist Fractures by 53% for T score above -2.5

"The effect of alendronate on the risk of wrist fractures also varied by baseline femoral neck BMD. There was no significant reduction among women with a T score of -2.5 or less: 38 *(4.7%)* in the placebo and 34 *(4.2%)* in the alendronate group *(*RH, 0.88; 95% CI, 0.55-1.40*)*.

Similarly, we observed no reduction in risk among women with T scores of -2.0 to -2.5: 20 *(2.8%)* in the placebo group vs 27 *(3.7%)* in the alendronate group *(*RH, 1.33; 95% CI, 0.75-2.4*)*. Among those whose femoral neck T scores were more than -2.0, more fractures occurred in the treatment group *(*n = 22, 3.3%*)* than in the placebo group *(*n = 12, 1.7%; RH, 1.9; 95% CI, 1.0-4.0; placebo-treatment difference, 1.6%*)*. For T score greater than -2.5 *(*49 fxs alendronate vs 32 fxs placebo*)* = RH 1.53". *(15)(16)*

The Osteopenia Group Has No Benefit from the Drug

The FIT data is very clear. For the Osteopenia group, wrist fractures are clearly increased by Fosamax treatment, and there is an increase in hip fractures in the osteopenia group. Why should there be increased fractures in any group? This revelation indicates a serious problem which has been ignored, and suggests there is something seriously wrong with the bone physiology of bisphosphonate drug treatment.

Spontaneous Mid Femur Fractures on Bisphosphonates

Reports by Odvina*(28)* of spontaneous femur fractures and similarities with Pycnodysostosis, Toulous Lautrec's rare genetic bone disease, raises even more questions about the bisphosphonate class of drugs. The report by Odvina of spontaneous mid femur fractures has been duplicated by Goh with his 2007 report of subtrochanteric femur fractures with minimal trauma in women on long term fosamax.*(29)* A third report of spontaneous fractures in menopausal women on fosamax was reported in the New England Journal March 20, 2008 by Dr. Joseph M Lane.*(42)* How many menopausal women on bisphosphonates must suffer spontaneous mid femur fracture before we declare enough is enough and ban this entire class of drugs?

Why is Sally Field Misleading Millions of Women with TV Ads?

Does Sally Field know that her paid television ads for Boniva are targeting women with Osteopenia? If Sally knew the above information about bisphosphonates, would Sally Field again stand up, and tell women that Boniva, like all bisphosphonates, **INCREASES** fracture rates for hip and wrist in women with Osteopenia *(*a less severe form of Osteoporosis with T score greater than -2.5*)*. Perhaps Sally would like to explain this to John Dingle's House Committee which has been investigating celebrity drug endorsement ads.*(37)*

Questions for Sally Field

For example, does Sally really have Osteoporosis with a T score less than -2.5? Or, does Sally have the less severe Osteopenia with a T score of greater than -2.5. Why is Sally taking a bisphosphonate even though she has never had an osteoporotic fracture? Is Sally taking the Boniva drug for prevention? Why is Sally Field misleading millions of women *(*with osteopenia*)* into taking a drug for prevention of osteoporosis when this will clearly harm them by causing increased fracture rate in their group? This is another good example of why all Direct-to-Consumer Ads, including Sally's for bisphosphonates, should be banned. *(33)(34)(35)(36)* Contact John Dingle's Committee at the below address, and send a letter of concern about the Boniva television ads which target millions of women with osteopenia.*(37)* Mr. Dingle's committee has been investigating celebrity drug ads, such as the Jarvik Lipitor ads, and the Vytorin ads. Perhaps the Boniva ads are next.

Send your letter to: the Honorable John Dingle, Dean of the House of Representatives,
Chairman of the Committee on Energy and Commerce
2328 Rayburn House Office Building
Washington, DC 20515, *(*202*)* 225-4071

Also, a convenient web site is available to contact your representative and send an email or letter of concern. *(38) https://forms.house.gov/wyr/welcome.shtml*

Disease Mongering or Prevention?

A January 2008 BMJ report by Pablo Alonso-Coello makes the case that the drug industry's bisphosphonate marketing program is actually a form of disease mongering designed to convince osteopenic women to take bisphosphonates even though there is no evidence of benefit for this group.*(18)* In order to obtain informed consent, all women offered these drugs must be informed about potential risks and benefits, and then be allowed to make their own decision. I have found that most women with osteopenia who are made aware of this information will decline the bisphosphonates class of drugs, and instead use a natural program to build strong bones.

Aubrey Blumsohn says:

> "These are good drugs when used appropriately. However, I'm not sure that the risks and benefits *(*and possibility of unknown risk*)* have

> been appropriately weighed so as to allow correct, cost effective and safe targeting of therapy. We know nothing about the long term (30 year) benefits or risks of bisphosphonates."*(17)*

Dr. Blumsohn was the lead researcher in an Actonel study in Sheffield England. The data was blinded, and the paper published by ghost writers hired by P and G without Blumsohn seeing the actual unblinded data. When Blumsohn objected, he was fired from his job at the university.*(40)*

Susan Ott, MD at the University of Washington says:

> "Many physicians do not even consider the possibility that **bisphosphonates could have some adverse effects on the bone**. The interesting results described in the paper by Odvina et al. along with reports from animal studies and biopsy data from clinical trials, should heighten awareness of the actions of these drugs. The profound suppression of bone formation could have negative effects that occur after long-term accumulation in the skeleton. There is no good surrogate for the passage of time, and **it will be at least a decade before we have any data about whether the potential negative effects would ever predominate over the known positive effects**. Until then, bisphosphonates should be used carefully. **Men and women with established osteoporosis have a high risk of fragility fractures within the 5 yr after diagnosis, and in these cases the proven benefits outweigh the theoretical long-term risks**. These benefits, however, are proven only for the first 5 yr. **I believe the current evidence suggests that bisphosphonates should be stopped after 5 yr.** Those patients who remain at a high risk of fractures or who have had fractures despite bisphosphonate therapy could be considered for treatment with **intermittent PTH**." *(30)*

Preventing the Fall is May be More Important Than the Osteoporosis Drug

My grandmother lived to be 100 with severe osteoporosis, many spinal compression fractures and rib deformities, yet she never had a hip fracture because she never sustained a fall. A recent BMJ article has called for a more logical approach, shifting away from osteoporosis drugs to instead, preventing the falls that produce the deadly hip fractures.*(23)*

Reverse Osteoporosis Naturally Without Drugs

Perhaps the most important concept to reverse osteoporosis is acid base balance which is described in this *article*, Acid-Alkaline Balance and Its Effect on Bone Health by Susan E. Brown, Ph.D., CCN, and Russell Jaffe, MD, Ph.D., CCN, International Journal of Integrative Medicine, Vol. 2, No. 6 Nov/Dec 2000.*(39)* For more information on natural ways to improve bones with diet, lifestyle modifications and supplements to reverse osteoporosis, see my web page on reversing osteoporosis. *(24)*

Conclusion: The bisphosphonates class of drugs actually make the bones weaker, not stronger, and have associated adverse side effects. This entire class of drugs should be banned.

References

(1) http://www.fda.gov/cder/drug/InfoSheets/HCP/bisphosphonatesHCP.htm
FDA: Alert , Information for Healthcare Professionals. Bisphosphonates (marketed as Actonel, Actonel+Ca, Aredia, Boniva, Didronel, Fosamax, Fosamax+D, Reclast, Skelid, and Zometa)

(2) http://www.medicine.indiana.edu/news_releases/viewRelease.php4?art=552
September 15, 2006 Skeletal Microdamage Stable After First Year, Study Shows.

(3) http://www.askapatient.com/viewrating.asp?drug=20560&name=FOSAMAX
Message Board adverse side effects of Fosamax (600 messages)

(3A) http://www.askapatient.com/viewratings.asp?drug=20835&name=ACTONEL&sort =age
Message Board with 530 messages about adverse effects of Actonel.

(4) http://scholar.google.com/scholar?hl=en&lr=&q=phossy+jaw&btnG=Search
Fossy Jaw list of articles

(5) http://www.nzma.org.nz/journal/119-1246/2341/
Journal of the New Zealand Medical Association, 01-December-2006, Vol 119 No 1246
Jaw osteonecrosis associated with bisphosphonates. Jodie Battley et al.

(6) http://www.annals.org/cgi/reprint/144/10/753.pdf
Systematic Review: Bisphosphonates and Osteonecrosis of the Jaws
Sook-Bin Woo, DMD; John W. Hellstein, DDS, MS; and John R. Kalmar, DMD, PhD

(7) http://www.annals.org/cgi/eletters/144/10/753
Bisphosphonates can cause hypocalcemia and vitamin D deficiency.
(8) Berthold HK, Diel IJ, Gouni-Berthold I. Phossy jaw revisited -- do bisphosphonates cause "bisphossy jaws"? Drug Safety. 2004;27:92

(9) http://en.wikipedia.org/wiki/Phossy_jaw
Wikipedia Phossy Jaw

(10) *http://www.atsdr.cdc.gov/toxprofiles/tp103-c2.pdf*
There is evidence that occupational exposure to white phosphorus affects bones other than those in the jaw; this implies a systemic effect for inhaled white phosphorus.

(11) *http://www.mja.com.au/public/issues/183_03_010805/letters_010805_fm-2.html*
Letters, Bisphosphonates and osteonecrosis: analogy to phossy jaw MJA 2005; 183 *(3)*: 163-164

(12) *http://www.mja.com.au/public/issues/182_08_180405/pur10144_fm.html*
ADRAC Report Bisphosphonates and osteonecrosis of the jaw Patrick M Purcell and Ian W Boyd MJA 2005; 182 *(8)*: 417-418

(13) *http://www.jrheum.com/abstracts/abstracts08/13/0120.html*
Use of Oral Bisphosphonates and the Risk of Aseptic Osteonecrosis: A Nested Case-Control Study Oct 2007 Mahyar Etminan et al. A**n association was observed between oral bisphosphonate use and aseptic osteonecrosis.**

(14) *http://content.nejm.org/cgi/content/full/344/5/333*
McClung MR, Geusens P, Miller PD, Zippel H, Bensen WG, Roux C, Adami S, Fogelman I, Diamond T, Eastell R, Meunier PJ, Reginster JY. Effect of risedronate on the risk of hip fracture in elderly women. Hip Intervention Program Study Group. New England Journal of Medicine Feb 1, 2001; 344: 333 - 340. full text of article

(15) *http://jama.ama-assn.org/cgi/content/full/280/24/2077*
Effect of Alendronate on Risk of Fracture in Women With Low Bone Density but Without Vertebral Fractures Results From the Fracture Intervention Trial. Steven R. Cummings et al. JAMA. 1998;280:2077-2082.

(16) *http://jama.ama-assn.org/cgi/content/full/280/24/2119*
Bone Mass, Bone Fragility, and the Decision to Treat Robert P. Heaney, MD JAMA. 1998;280:2119-2120.

(17) *http://scientific-misconduct.blogspot.com/2008/01/bisphosphonate-induced-pain-in.html*
Bisphosphonate induced pain in osteoporosis - statistical analysis discovered, Aubrey Blumson

(18) *http://www.bmj.com/cgi/content/full/336/7636/126*
BMJ 2008;336:126-129 (19 January), doi:10.1136/bmj.39435.656250.AD **Drugs for pre-osteoporosis: prevention or disease mongering**? Pablo Alonso-Coello, family practitioner, Alberto López García-Franco, family practitioner, Gordon Guyatt, professor, Ray Moynihan, conjoint lecturer

(19) *http://jeffreydach.com/2007/05/14/fosamax-actonel-osteoporosis-and-toulouse-lautrec-by-jeffrey-dach-md.aspx*
Fosamax, Actonel, Osteoporosis and Toulouse Lautrec by Jeffrey Dach M.D.

(20) *http://www.keele.ac.uk/schools/pharm/MTRAC/ProductInfo/verdicts/R/Risedronate%20osteo.pdf*
MTRAC information on Actonel

(21) *http://www.nice.org.uk/nicemedia/pdf/TA087guidance.pdf*
NICE guidance recommends bisphosphonates be used as secondary prevention for postmenopausal women who present with osteoporotic fragility fracture

(22) *http://www.ccjm.org/PDFFILES/Carey11_05.pdf*
What is a 'failure' of bisphosphonate therapy for osteoporosis? JOHN J. CAREY, MD Department of Rheumatic and Immunologic Diseases, The Cleveland Clinic Foundation

(22) *http://www.bmj.com/cgi/content/full/324/7342/886*
BMJ 2002;324:886-891 *(* 13 April *)* Education and debate,

Selling sickness: the pharmaceutical industry and disease mongering

(23) *http://www.bmj.com/cgi/content/full/336/7636/124* BMJ 2008;336:124-126 *(*19 January*)*
Shifting the focus in fracture prevention from osteoporosis to falls. Teppo L N Järvinen et al. Falling, not osteoporosis, is the strongest single risk factor for fractures in elderly people. Bone mineral density is a poor predictor of an individual's fracture risk. Drug treatment is expensive and will not prevent most fractures in elderly people.

(24) *http://www.drdach.com/wst_page6.html*
Osteoporosis web page on jeffrey dach md Web site

(25) *http://overdosedamerica.com/excerpts.php?id=2*
Exerpt from OverDosed America by John Abramson MD

(26) *http://www.medicalconsumers.org/pages/OSTEOPOROSISHowEffectiveisPrevention.html*
Bisphosphonates will modestly reduce the hip and spinal fracture rate, but the published evidence for this benefit is primarily confined to elderly women with low bone mineral density and at least one other major risk, such as a previous spinal fracture.

(27) *http://www.gilliansanson.com/index.htm*
The Myth of Osteoporosis by Gillian Sanson MCD Century Publications, 2003.

(28) *http://jcem.endojournals.org/cgi/content/full/90/3/1294*
The Journal of Clinical Endocrinology & Metabolism Vol. 90, No. 3 1294-1301, 2005 Severely Suppressed Bone Turnover: A Potential Complication of Alendronate Therapy. Clarita V. Odvina et al.

(29) *http://www.jbjs.org.uk/cgi/content/abstract/89-B/3/349*
Journal of Bone and Joint Surgery - British Volume, Vol 89-B, Issue 3, 349-353. 2007 Subtrochanteric insufficiency fractures in patients on alendronate therapy, A CAUTION. S.-K. Goh et al.

(30) *http://jcem.endojournals.org/cgi/content/full/90/3/1897*
The Journal of Clinical Endocrinology & Metabolism Vol. 90, No. 3 1897-1899 2005 by The Endocrine Society, Long-Term Safety of Bisphosphonates, Susan M. Ott University of Washington Seattle, Washington

(31) *http://content.nejm.org/cgi/content/extract/344/22/1720*
Royce PC, Goodman RL, Schott AM, Dargent-Molina P, Meunier PJ, McClung M New Engl J Med May 31, 2001; 344: 1720 Letter to Editor.

(32) *http://content.nejm.org/cgi/content/full/344/5/333*
McClung MR, Geusens P, Miller PD, Zippel H, Bensen WG, Roux C, Adami S, Fogelman I, Diamond T, Eastell R, Meunier PJ, Reginster JY. Effect of risedronate on the risk of hip fracture in elderly women. Hip Intervention Program Study Group. New England Journal of Medicine Feb 1, 2001; 344: 333 - 340.

(33) *http://gotbones.healthdiaries.com/sally-field-boniva-and-media-ethics.html*
Sally Field, Boniva, and Media Ethics

(34) *http://www.bonehealth.com/default.aspx*
Sally Field Blog on Osteoporosis and Boniva

(35) *http://video.msn.com/dw.aspx/?mkt=en-us&from=truveo&vid=9bb72f61-a267-428c-9e0c-ac60e281f646&wa=wsignin1.0*
video, Sally Field plugs here website for boniva

(36) *http://www.boniva.com/default.aspx*
Boniva Web Site

(37) *http://www.house.gov/dingell/*
The Honorable John Dingle, Dean of the House of Representatives, Chairman of the Committee on Energy and Commerce. 2328 Rayburn House Office Building. Washington, DC 20515 *(202)* 225-4071

(38) *https://forms.house.gov/wyr/welcome.shtml*
Use this link to Contact Your representative.

(39) *http://www.betterbones.com/research/articles/bjaffe.PDF*
Acid-Alkaline Balance and Its Effect on Bone Health by Susan E. Brown, Ph.D., CCN, and Russell Jaffe, MD, Ph.D., CCN, International Journal of Integrative Medicine, Vol. 2, No. 6 Nov/Dec 2000

(40) *http://www.slate.com/id/2133061/*
Rent-a-Researcher Did a British university sell out to Procter & Gamble? By Jennifer Washburn Dec. 22, 2005

(41) *http://jeffreydach.com/2007/08/26/protect-your-family-from-bad-drugs-by-jeffrey-dach-md.aspx*
Protect Your Family from Bad Drugs, Drugs in Litigation by Jeffrey Dach MD

(42) *http://content.nejm.org/cgi/content/full/358/12/1304*
NEJMVolume358:1304-1306 March20,2008 Number12AtypicalFracturesoftheFemoral Diaphysis in Postmenopausal Women Taking Alendronate Brett A. Lenart, B.S. Dean G. Lorich, M.D. Joseph M. Lane, M.D. Weill Cornell Medical College New York, NY 10021

All references hyperlinked at
www.naturalmedicine101.com

www.ingramcontent.com/pod-product-compliance
Lightning Source LLC
Chambersburg PA
CBHW081105170526
45165CB00008B/2334